STEM CELLS AND REGENERATIVE MEDICINE

MAGNETIC RESONANCE IMAGING OF STEM CELL APPLICATIONS

STEM CELLS AND REGENERATIVE MEDICINE

Additional books in this series can be found on Nova's website
under the Series tab.

Additional e-books in this series can be found on Nova's website
under the e-book tab.

STEM CELLS AND REGENERATIVE MEDICINE

MAGNETIC RESONANCE IMAGING OF STEM CELL APPLICATIONS

XIAOMING YANG, M.D., PH.D.
EDITOR

New York

Library of Congress Cataloging-in-Publication Data

ISBN: 978-1-63463-910-1

Library of Congress Control Number: 2014959998

Published by Nova Science Publishers, Inc. † New York

To Hongxiu, Kristiina & Karoliina
and
My mentors in China, Finland & USA

Contents

Foreword ix

Preface xi

Contributing Authors xiii

SECTION I. OVERVIEW 1

Chapter 1 Stem Cells: The Basic Concept 3
Hongxiu Ji and Kristiina O. Yang

Chapter 2 Magnetic Resonance Imaging of Stem Cells: The Principles 19
Rohan Dharmakumar, Avinash Kali and Debiao Li

Chapter 3 Direct Magnetic Labeling of Stem Cells 45
Bensheng Qiu, Thomas Matula, Norman Beauchamp Jr. and Xiaoming Yang

Chapter 4 Indirect Magnetic Labeling of Stem Cells 57
Anna V. Naumova and Charles E. Murry

Chapter 5 Strategies for Delivery of Stem Cells 81
Sandeep Vaidya and Manjiri Dighe

SECTION II. APPLICATIONS 87

Chapter 6 Magnetic Resonance Imaging of Stem Cell Application in Neurology 89
Antje Arnold, Miroslaw Janowski and Piotr Walczak

Chapter 7 Magnetic Resonance Imaging of Stem Cell Application in Liver 105
Weitao Ye, Changhong Liang and Bin Zhou

Chapter 8 Magnetic Resonance Imaging of Stem Cell Application in Oncology 117
Mariangela Sottili, Chiara Gerini and Monica Mangoni

Chapter 9 Magnetic Resonance Imaging of Stem Cell Application in Heart 137
Morteza Mahmoudi and Phillip C. Yang

Chapter 10	Creation of Animal Models for Magnetic Resonance Imaging of Stem cell Application in Vasculatures *Feng Zhang, Yaoping Shi and Xiaoming Yang*	**159**
Chapter 11	Magnetic Resonance Imaging of Stem Cell Application in Vasculatures *Yanfeng Meng and Xiaoming Yang*	**177**
Chapter 12	Magnetic Resonance Imaging in Clinical Application of Stem Cells: Current Status *Wayne L. Monsky*	**187**
Index		**199**

Foreword

Stem cells have the potential to usher in a new era of modern medicine, one where damaged organs are regenerated and the root causes of currently intractable diseases are treated. Diseases as disparate as heart failure, stroke, spinal cord injury, retinal blindness, diabetes mellitus, Parkinson disease and osteoarthritis share a defining feature: they result from a deficiency in a critical cell population. Over the last two decades there have been breathtaking advances in stem cell science, including the derivation of human embryonic stem cells, cloning of entire mammals, reprogramming adult cells into induced pluripotent stem cells (iPSCs), the ability to direct the differentiation of stem cells into previously unattainable human cell populations, and most recently, the use of stem cells to model genetic diseases and to identify new drugs. With such rapid progress in the basic science of stem cells, medical breakthroughs seem tantalizingly close.

Despite the promise, translating stem cell science into new diagnostics or therapeutics has proven quite a challenge. We have learned, for example, that many cell populations do not work through the direct "bricks and mortar" approach that we initially imagined. Rather than incorporating as new building blocks of tissue, many cell types like bone marrow derivatives live only a few days or weeks and act by secreting factors that control the host response to injury. Other cell types, such as cardiomyocytes, dopaminergic neurons or pancreatic beta-cells, do function directly to build new tissue, but these raise a different set of challenges. For example, delivering cells to the target tissue is tremendously inefficient. Few cells have innate homing abilities, and after intravenous delivery they are first filtered by the lungs and subsequently cleared by the liver and spleen. Direct injection is some better, but even here most leak from the injection site, and most of those that are retained die due to ischemia, inflammation and other transplant-related stresses. The hardy survivors need to grow a blood supply and functionally integrate with their host tissue, while overcoming the host tissue's natural response of isolating them by scar tissue. Despite these challenges, there are exciting examples of tissue regeneration and restoration of function in animal models, and there are a small but growing number of successes in clinical trials.

Biomedical imaging is an essential component of regenerative medicine. Indeed, most of the lessons described above were learned via imaging technologies. For example, imaging allows us to perform longitudinal monitoring of stem cell transplants, watching their biodistribution and population dynamics like death, proliferation and differentiation. Imaging also permits important physiological data to be obtained, e.g., myocardial infarct size, chamber dimensions and mechanical function of the damaged heart. Imaging can thereby guide therapy optimization and can serve as surrogate clinical endpoints for studies not statistically powered for hard outcome measurements like death and rehospitalization.

A critically important, and perhaps under-recognized, point is that imaging helps understand the mechanistic underpinnings of stem cell therapies. By correlating the fate of the transplanted cells with the physiological outcome, we can understand why therapies don't work (e.g., the cells do not home to the tissue) or how they do work (e.g., since many cells don't persist long term, any benefits must work through paracrine pathways). Only by understanding the mechanism of benefit can one hope to rationally improve a therapy, and in my opinion, all those who would use stem cells as therapies need to incorporate imaging into their programs.

Magnetic resonance imaging offers spatial resolution unparalleled amongst the various imaging modalities. Its lack of toxicity makes it well suited for longitudinal monitoring of stem cell therapies, and there are increasing numbers of direct chemical labels and indirect genetic labels that give MRI contrast to transplanted cells. This book summarizes recent advances in the application of MRI to stem cell therapeutics. It will be a good primer for those in the field looking to enhance their knowledge of the field's fundamentals such as stem cells, MRI principles and strategies for cell labeling. It also delves into applications such as cardiac repair, liver regeneration, cancer, vascular biology and clinical trials. In addition to outlining the benefits, these chapters deal with many of imaging's current limitations. We hope that, in pointing out both current successes and shortcomings, imaging researchers will be motivated to improve this key technology and use it to make new stem cell therapeutics a clinical reality.

Charles E. Murry, MD, PhD
Arra and Eva Woods Professor of Pathology, Bioengineering and Medicine/Cardiology
Director, Center for Cardiovascular Biology
Co-Director, Institute for Stem Cell and Regenerative Medicine
University of Washington
Seattle, Washington, US

Preface

Stem cell-based regenerative therapy has become a fronter in modern medicine. For the success of both basic research and clinical application of stem cell technology, it is essential to have noninvasive methods to monitor the delivery of transplanted stem cells, track migration/homing of stem cells to the targets, and assess survival and function of the transplanted stem cells at the targets. Magnetic resonance imaging (MRI) represents a promising technology fitting in this necessity.

So far, scientists from various disciplines around the world have done outstanding works in developing different MR techniques for in vivo imaging of stem cells, so-called cellular MRI. With its primary advantages of high spatial resolution (at cellular level) and excellent contrast between abnormal and healthy tissues with no risk of ionizing radiation injury, cellular MRI is becoming an important modality for in vivo imaging of stem cell applications in repair of damaged or diseased tissues and organs. The core of cellular MRI technology includes (i) direct (chemical) or indirect (genetic) labeling of stem cells with different MRI-visible agents; (ii) improving the capability of using cellular MRI to track the transplanted MR-labeled stem cells; and (iii) precisely assessing the survival and functions of these transplanted stem cells after their migrating/homing to the targets.

As continuous refinements of techniques take place with intensification on their subsequent clinical translation, MRI of stem cell-based regenerative medicine will have significant impact on improving global health care in the near future. The aim of writing this book is to facilitate such translation of advanced cellular MRI techniques from laboratory benches to pre-clinical animal studies, and, ultimately, to clinical practice. The authors are from several continents around the world, with their expertise in the fields of stem cell science, biomedical engineering, medicine, pathology, medical imaging, and interventional radiology. We hope this book will provoke common interests, brainstorming and cooperation among professionals in both stem cell science and medical imaging, and bring regenerative medicine one step closer to benefitting the patients.

Xiaoming Yang, MD, PhD
Professor of Radiology
Attending Physician of Interventional Radiology
Director, Image-Guided Bio-Molecular Interventions Research
Department of Radiology
University of Washington School of Medicine
Seattle, USA

Contributing Authors

Antje Arnold, MS
Russell H. Morgan Department of Radiology
& Radiological Science
Division of Magnetic Resonance Research and Institute for Cell Engineering
The Johns Hopkins University School of Medicine
Baltimore, Maryland, US

Norman J. Beauchamp Jr., MD, MHS
Professor and Chairman
Department of Radiology
Professor of Industrial & Systems Engineering
University of Washington School of Medicine
Seattle, Washington, US

Rohan Dharmakumar, PhD
Associate Professor
Department of Medicine
University of California at Los Angles
Associate Director
Biomedical Imaging Research Institute
Cedars-Sinai Medical Center
Los Angles, California, US

Manjiri Dighe, MD
Associate Professor
Director, Body Imaging
Director, Ultrasound Imaging
Department of Radiology
University of Washington School of Medicine
Seattle, Washington, US

Chiara Gerini, MS
Radiotherapy Unit
Department of Experimental & Clinical Biomedical Sciences
University of Florence
Firenze, Italy

Miroslaw Janowski, MD, PhD
Assistant Professor
Russell H. Morgan Department of Radiology
& Radiological Science
Division of Magnetic Resonance Research and Institute for Cell Engineering
The Johns Hopkins University School of Medicine
Baltimore, Maryland, US

Hongxiu Ji, MD, PhD
Attending Physician of Pathology
Department of Pathology
Overlake Hospital
Belleview, Washington, US
Adjunct Assistant Professor
Department of Radiology
University of Washington School of Medicine
Seattle, Washington, US

Avinash Kali, MS
Scientist
Department of Bioengineering
University of California at Los Angles
Los Angles, California, US

Debiao Li, PhD
Professor
Department of Medicine and Bioengineering
University of California at Los Angles
Director
Biomedical Imaging Research Institute
Cedars-Sinai Medical Center
Los Angles, California, US

Changhong Liang, MD
Professor and Chairman
Department of Radiology
Guangdong General Hospital
Guangzhou, Guangdong, China

Morteza Mahmoudi, PhD
Division of Cardiovascular Medicine
Department of Medicine
Stanford University School of Medicine
Stanford, California, US

Monica Mangoni, MD, PhD
Radiotherapy Unit
Department of Experimental & Clinical Biomedical Sciences
University of Florence
Firenze, Italy

Thomas J. Matula, PhD
Director, Center for Industrial and Medical Ultrasound
Applied Physics Laboratory
Director, Center of Ultrasound-Based Molecular Imaging and Therapy
Affiliate Associate Professor of Electrical Engineering and Bioengineering
University of Washington,
Seattle, Washington, US

Yanfeng Meng, MD, PhD
Instructor
Image-Guided Bio-Molecular Intervention Research
Department of Radiology
Institute for Stem Cell and Regenerative Medicine
University of Washington School of Medicine
Seattle, Washington, US
Attending physician and Vice Chairman
Department of Radiology
Taiyuan Central Hospital
Taiyuan, Shanxi, China

Wayne Monsky, MD, PhD
Associate Professor
Director, Harborview Medical Center, Interventional Radiology
Department of Radiology, Section of Interventional Radiology
University of Washington Medical Center
Seattle, Washington, US

Charles E. Murry, MD, PhD
Arra and Eva Woods Professor of Pathology,
Bioengineering and Medicine/Cardiology
Director, Center for Cardiovascular Biology
Co-Director, Institute for Stem Cell and Regenerative Medicine
University of Washington
Seattle, Washington, US

Anna V. Naumova, PhD
Assistant Professor
Department of Radiology
Center for Cardiovascular Biology
Institute for Stem Cell and Regenerative Medicine
University of Washington
Seattle, Washington, US

Bensheng Qiu, PhD
Image-Guided Biomolecular Intervention Research
Department of Radiology
University of Washington School of Medicine
Seattle, Washington, US

Yaoping Shi, MD, PhD
Image-Guided Bio-Molecular Intervention Research
Department of Radiology
University of Washington School of Medicine
Seattle, Washington, US
Department of Radiology
Sir Run Run Shaw Hospital
Zhejiang University School of Medicine
Hangzhou, Zhejiang, China

Mariangela Sottili, PhD
Radiotherapy Unit
Department of Experimental & Clinical Biomedical Sciences
University of Florence
Firenze, Italy

Sandeep Vaidya, MD
Associate Professor
Division of Interventional Radiology
Department of Radiology
University of Washington School of Medicine
Seattle, Washington, US

Piotr Walczak, MD, PhD
Associate Professor
Russell H. Morgan Department of Radiology
& Radiological Science
Division of Magnetic Resonance Research and Institute
for Cell Engineering
The Johns Hopkins University School of Medicine
Baltimore, Maryland, US

Kristiina O. Yang, BS
University of Pennsylvania
Philadelphia, Pennsylvania, US

Phillip C. Yang, MD
Associated Professor
Director, Laboratory for Cellular and Molecular Imaging of Cardiovascular Stem Cells
Director, Cardiothoracic MRI Program
Division of Cardiovascular Medicine
Department of Medicine
Stanford University School of Medicine
Stanford, California, US

Xiaoming Yang, MD, PhD
Professor of Radiology
Attending Physician of Interventional Radiology
Director, Image-Guided Bio-Molecular Intervention Research
Department of Radiology
University of Washington School of Medicine
Seattle, Washington, US

Weitao Ye, MD
Radiologist
Department of Radiology
Guangdong General Hospital
Guangzhou, Guangdong, China

Feng Zhang, MD, PhD
Research Assistant Professor
Image-Guided Bio-Molecular Intervention Research
Department of Radiology
University of Washington School of Medicine
Seattle, Washington, US

Bin Zhou, MD
Associate Professor
Department of Radiology
Third Affiliated Hospital
Sun Yat-sen University
Guangzhou, Guangdong, China

SECTION I. OVERVIEW

In: Magnetic Resonance Imaging of Stem Cell Applications ISBN: 978-1-63463-910-1
Editor: Xiaoming Yang

Chapter 1

Stem Cells: The Basic Concept

Hongxiu Ji* and Kristiina O. Yang
University of Washington School of Medicine,
Seattle; and Incyte Diagnostics, Bellevue, Washington, US

Abstract

Stem cells are defined as cells capable of unlimited proliferation (self-renewal) and of giving rise to specialized cells (differentiation). Some stem cells are tissue- and organ-specific (multipotent) while others are pluripotent. The latter are derived either from embryonic origin obtained through in vitro fertilization or somatic cell nuclear transfer, or through transcription factor-induced dedifferentiation from adult somatic cells. Stem cells hold great promise in cell and tissue replacement therapy to treat a wide range of diseases and conditions that are beyond the reach of current medical technologies. In addition, the theory of cancer stem cell highlights the complexity of cancer biology and invigorates the exploration of alternative treatment options, in addition to conventional therapy, for better cancer control. This chapter introduces the major types of stem cells and their potential clinical applications.

Keywords: Stem cell, multipotent, pluripotent, cancer

Introduction

The term, stem cell, first appeared in scientific literature in 1868. It was introduced by the eminent German biologist Ernst Haeckel to describe the original unicellular organism from which he presumed all multicellular organisms evolved. Later, he proposed that the fertilized egg also be called a stem cell [1]. In the 1960s, James Till and Ernest McCulloch provided definitive evidence of the existence of hematopoietic stem cells in the bone marrow [2].

* Corresponding author: Hongxiu Ji, MD, PhD, (hji@incdx.com).

These are primitive and undifferentiated cells, but capable of self-renewal and differentiation to all types of mature blood cells. Over time, the concept of stem cell has expanded to include cells along the germline lineage between the fertilized egg and lineage committed cells, the common precursor cells of the hematopoietic system and other organs and tissues, and cancer stem cells [1, 3-6]. Today, stem cells are defined as cells capable of unlimited proliferation (self-renewal) and of giving rise to specialized cells (differentiation).

Stem cells can be found in all living multicellular organisms, including plants, animals and humans. In the human body, stem cells exist in many tissues and organs. They are essential for tissue and organ growth, regeneration, repair, and healing. When stem cells are destroyed or inadequate, proper regeneration of the functional mature cells will either be lost or diminished, so that diseases and adverse conditions take place. Examples of these are countless, including loss of vision in patients with age-related macular degeneration and hereditary retinitis pigmentosa, heart failure post myocardial infarction, paralysis after traumatic spinal cord injury, and type I diabetes due to the destruction of pancreatic beta cells, to name a few. For such conditions, cell replacement therapy represents the most desirable treatment option, and in some instances, is the only hope for regaining proper cell and tissue function. If successful, stem cell replacement therapy will not only improve the everyday lives of millions of patients, but also relieve enormous burdens from their caregivers, and society as a whole. Therefore, stem cells represent the greatest hope in combatting conditions that have no cure by conventional treatment. And this hope is not unrealistic. In fact, since the first successful attempt by Dr. E. Donnall Thomas on identical twins in 1958, bone marrow transplantation of hematopoietic stem cells has helped hundreds of thousands of patients surviving leukemia, lymphoma and multiple myeloma [7].

One crucial factor for a successful stem cell replacement therapy is the sufficient availability of such cells for transplantation. This has been achieved with hematopoietic stem cells that are harvested through bone marrow aspiration or more recently, peripheral blood apheresis following stem cell mobilization. Another successful approach for obtaining a sufficient number of hematopoietic stem cells is harvesting them from umbilical cord blood at delivery, which has become a routine clinical practice in recent years [8]. On the other hand, isolating adequate number of stem cells from other tissues remains a significant challenge. This is because stem cells in solid organs are scarce, approximately 1 in 1,000 to 3,000 cells. Once harvested, they could be difficult to propagate in vitro or could lose the ability of self-renewal.

Multipotent Stem Cells

The stem cells mentioned above share a common quality; they can be found in many tissues or organs in the human body, but are limited to cell lineages present in the organs from which they are derived. Examples of those cells include bronchial epithelial reserve cells giving rise to bronchial epithelial lining cells and mucous-secreting gland cells, skin and hair follicle stem cells responsible for skin regeneration and hair growth, as well as, intestinal stem cells in the crypts to replenish epithelial cells lining the intestinal mucosa. In addition, there are neural stem cells in the brain, enamel stem cells in the teeth, and cardiac stem cells in the heart. All these stem cells belong to the category of multipotent stem cells. They have been called “reserve cells”, “progenitor cells”, “tissue stem cells”, “adult stem cells” and “somatic stem cells”.

Most adult stem cells can only give rise to mature cells naturally residing in the specific tissue or organ. But by manipulating in vitro culture conditions, scientists have been able to generate more diverse mature cells from the somatic stem cells [9]. For example, mesenchymal stem cells of mesodermal lineage, found in bone marrow and other tissues, can differentiate towards cells of both mesodermal lineage including endothelial cells, fibroblasts, adipocytes, and ectodermal lineage, such as cardiomyocytes and hepatocytes (Figure 1.1).

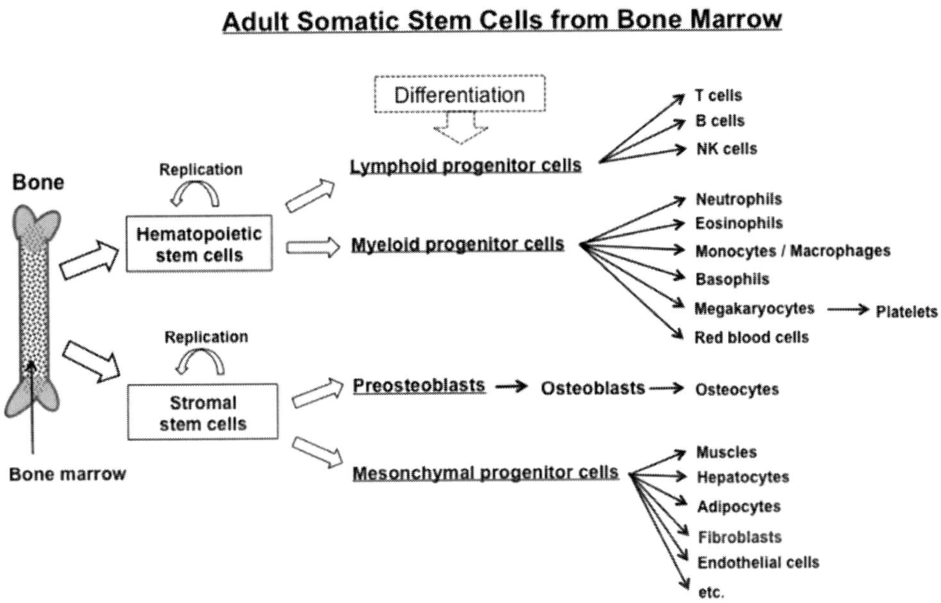

Figure 1.1. Bone marrow hematopoietic and mesenchymal stem cells with potential for differentiation to a variety of mature cells.

Hematopoietic Stem Cells (HSCs)

HSCs are the most famous multipotent stem cells. They are immature cells found in bone marrow, peripheral blood and umbilical cord blood. They express stem cell surface markers including CD34, CD90, CD38 and CD133 and can replicate and differentiate towards all types of blood cells (Figure 1.1). They are used for bone marrow transplantation, to replenish bone marrow cells and blood cells in patients with a severe lack of functional blood cells or with hematologic malignancies after ablative therapy. The transplantation can be allogeneic with donor cells after appropriate HLA matching followed by immune suppressive therapy, or autologous using patient’s own bone marrow cells. The common procedure is to aspirate an appropriate amount of bone marrow from healthy donors or patients. The cells are processed and enriched in vitro. After infused into patient’s bloodstream, the bone marrow cells are expected to migrate to the bone marrow microenvironment and to restore the patient’s ability to produce an adequate number of functional blood cells. This process has recently been replaced by apheresis procedure when the peripheral blood is pumped out of and back to a donor's circulation and the hematologic stem cells are harvested and later infused to the patient [10].

Recently, hematopoietic stem cell transplantation has been expanded to treat many other disease conditions, especially in patients with immune-mediated diseases (IMDs) that are refractory to conventional therapy. This is based on the notion that the transplant of HSCs can reset the immune system by increasing the proportion of naïve and immunotolerant lymphocytes. Autologous HSC transplantation for IMDs is similar to that for hematological malignancies. HSCs are harvested from the patient via peripheral blood apheresis and then purified by selecting CD34 positive stem cells and eliminating lymphocytes using monoclonal antibodies anti-CD52, CD3, CD19 and CD20. The patient is pre-conditioned to eliminate self-reactive T cells, such as receiving cyclophosphamide and anti-thymocyte immunoglobulin. This step achieves the goal of lymph ablation without irreversible destruction of the hematopoietic cells in the bone marrow. On the other hand, allogeneic systemic transplant, i.e., replacement of patient's immune system with donor immune system, can correct genetic predisposition or defects of the patient by conforming a new immune system that of the donor. Currently allogeneic HSC transplantation for IMDs carries high mortality and complications [11].

Mesenchymal Stem/Progenitor Cells (MSCs)

A more recent example of potentially useful multipotent cells is mesenchymal stem cells [12, 13]. They are rare, non-hematopoietic cells natively present throughout a variety of postnatal tissues, most famously in bone marrow, where they typically participate in perivascular stem cell niches and play key supportive and trophic roles [14]. The cells are able not only to differentiate into cardiomyocytes, neurons and other cells, but also to form supporting cells to reestablish favorable microenvironment for other crucial cells to grow (Figure 1.1).

In addition to autologous transplantation, MSCs can be applied for exogenous stem cell delivery. There is evidence both from in vitro experiments and animal studies that MSCs can safely augment cardiac repair post-myocardial infarction through pleiotropic mechanisms. So far, the results on clinical efficacy in patients with myocardial infarction remain controversial. It is observed that the therapy provides some improvement of left ventricular ejection fraction, reduced infarct size and reduced left ventricular end systolic and end diastolic volume, but improvement in overall survival is yet to be demonstrated [15-17]. In addition, bone marrow MSCs, through either systemic or local administration, have demonstrated immunomodulation and tropic action in treating IMDs [18, 19]. Since this type of treatment does not alter the genetic factors for IMDs, the diseases might reappear after exposure to triggering antigens. But the treatment may serve as interim between more definitive treatment or as an attempt to change the natural course of disease. Furthermore, MSCs are being tested in multiple ongoing clinical trials for a variety of diseases and conditions, although favorable results are yet to be observed or confirmed.

Other Multipotent Stem Cells

Other multipotent stem cells include neural stem cells, adipose stem cells, dental enamel stem cells, cardiac stem cells, bone and cartilage stem cells, intestinal stem cells, and skin stem cells. It has been reported that autologous somatic stem cells can deliver treatment directly to the central nervous system [20]. Another successful instance of using tissue-specific stem/progenitor cells in a clinical setting is skin grafts for burn victims. Skin cells harvested from a healthy area can be cultured and enriched in vitro, and can then be implanted in areas that have been burnt. The cells will grow, re-epithelize the skin, and heal the wound. This is particularly efficient, because the cells are autologous with no risk of immune rejection. Further, Limbal stem cell treatment is shown to be successful in corneal regeneration in patients with burn and corneal limbal cell deficiency [21].

Pluripotent Stem Cells

Although useful, multipotent somatic stem cells have a narrow therapeutic range. An ideal stem cell for cell replacement therapy should be capable of in vitro replication to produce an unlimited number of identical cells, and of differentiating to any cell type in the human body. This demand can only be fulfilled with pluripotent/totipotent stem cells. Currently, there are three types of stem cells that fulfill the requirements of pluripotent stem cells (Figure 1.2).

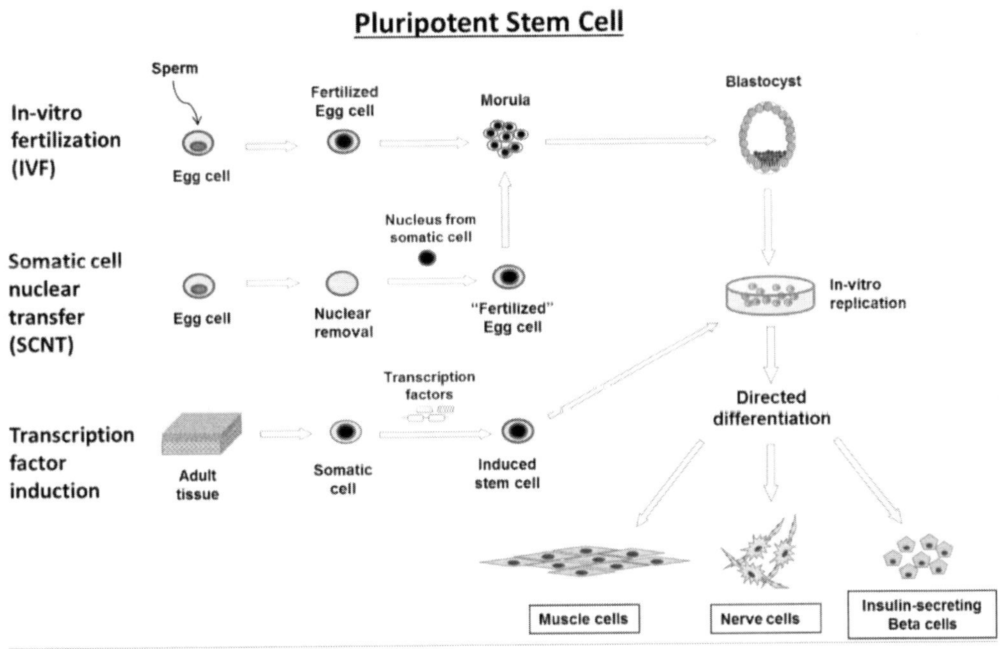

Figure 1.2. Three approaches in obtaining pluripotent stem cells.

Human Embryonic Stem Cells

It is well known that the inner cell mass of an early embryo contains the ultimate pluripotent stem cells that are primitive and capable of differentiating to all cell types needed to form the human body, namely, the ectoderm (skin, brain, etc.), endoderm (stomach, intestine, etc.) and mesoderm (skeletal muscle, heart, bone, cartilage, etc.). The inner cell mass is formed approximately 8-10 days post-conception, as one part of the blastocyst. The other part of the blastocyst is a layer of cells that form the shell of the blastocyst, which will become the fetal membranes and placenta, functioning to protect and nourish the growing fetus after implantation into the gestational endometrium. In 1998, a group of developmental biologists led by James Thomson at the University of Wisconsin published their initial success in isolating and cultivating human embryonic stem cells from inner cell masses of blastocyst-stage embryos that are discarded from in vitro fertilization [3]. The researchers were able to document that the cells: (1) are immature by cytomorphology; (2) express markers of undifferentiated cells; (3) proliferate unlimitedly in Petri dish; (4) endure freeze and thaw process for cell cryopreservation; (5) form immature teratomas containing endoderm, ectoderm and mesoderm elements; and (6) are able to differentiate to desired cell types under specific culture environment in vitro. Gearhart et al. produced similar cells from human primordial germ cells, which were isolated from the gonadal ridge and mesenteries of 5-9 week post-fertilization human embryos obtained as a result of therapeutic termination of pregnancy [4]. Since then, many embryonic stem cell lines have been established.

The discovery of embryonic stem cells was discouraged for religious and ethical concerns [22]. Harvesting stem cells from an early embryo would require the destruction of the embryo, which is unacceptable to groups who believe that life begins at the moment of fertilization, albeit the embryos being used for research so far having been obtained from excess embryos from in vitro fertilization procedures. The concern is that without setting a strict boundary for what is ethical and allowable, and what is not, a slippery slope will emerge. The controversy over embryonic stem cells has also been subject to public policy-making. In 2001, President George W. Bush banned federal funding for research related to embryonic stem cells, although this decision was overturned by President Barack Obama in 2009.

In addition to ethical concerns, embryonic stem cells pose two other significant hurdles. The first is its tumorigenicity. As demonstrated both by Thomson and Gearhart, when injected to severe combined immunodeficiency (SCID) mice, the undifferentiated stem cells form immature teratomas in all cases [3, 4]. Therefore strict and complete in vitro differentiation is a mandatory step to complete before introduction to the human body, ensuring that the cells are matured to a specific cell type, such as pancreatic Beta cells [23]. This crucial step may be easily defined, but difficult to accomplish in practice. In any given cell culture condition, a minority of cells may remain immature, and theoretically, a single undifferentiated cell could pose potential risk of forming teratomas after transplantation.

The second hurdle of embryonic stem cells is that they are foreign cells to the recipient. The host will recognize the cells as invaders, and immune rejection will take place. Therefore, the recipient will need life-long immune suppression in order to tolerate the transplanted cells, which is an issue since immunosuppression is not without its own cost or health consequences. The patient may be more susceptible to infections, malignancy, and may be forced to bear enormous economic burdens.

So far, clinical applications of human embryonic stem cells have been limited. Studies have been undertaken in Europe with patients requiring retina treatment showing significant improvement. The first FDA-approved clinical trial on human embryonic stem cells was initiated in California by company named Geron [24]. This trial intended to test whether stem cells can help nerves regrow in cases of traumatic spinal cord injury. It is done by surgically implanting embryonic stem cells into the damaged site, and coaxing the cells to become myelinated glial cells, which could insulate and protect nerve fibers. The first patient was treated in 2010. Due to financial reasons, however, the trial was halted, but has been recently restarted. No final results have been reported thus far. Recently, Advanced Cell Technologies led by Dr. Robert Lanza, has published their human studies using embryonic stem cells in treating macular degeneration and multiple sclerosis [25, 26].

Somatic Cell Nuclear Transfer (SCNT)

The second method for producing pluripotent stem cells is somatic cell nuclear transfer (SCNT), a cloning technique that introduces an adult cell nucleus into an empty oocyte, from which the oocyte nuclear material is removed. Given the suitable nutritional environment of the oocyte, the newly formed cell can develop into an embryo, and pluripotent stem cells can then be harvested from its inner cell mass (Figure 1.2). This method has proven to be very successful in animal models [27], and was used to produce the famous Dolly sheep [28]. Although there are less ethical concerns compared to embryonic stem cells obtained from in vitro fertilization, SCNT also possesses the problems of allogeneic rejection and immature teratoma formation. In addition, obtaining fresh oocytes from reproductive age women is not an easy task and is ethically questionable. Lastly, SCNT as a procedure is technically challenging. Only recently has there been success with human adult cell SCNT - stem cells were generated via using dermal fibroblasts from adult human cells [29]. This, however, does support SCNT as a strategy for regenerative medicine.

Induced Pluripotent Stem Cells (iPS Cells)

Giving the potentials and limitations of embryonic stem cells, it became important to develop methods of obtaining pluripotent stem cells without paying the price of destroying early embryos [30]. At Kyoto University in 2006-2007, Dr. Shinya Yamanaka's team published their results in obtaining pluripotent stem cells from cultured animal and human fibroblasts [5, 31]. They introduced a retrovirus carrying four genes (Oct3/4, Sox2, Klf4 and c-Myc) to human fibroblasts in a cell culture. Through viral expression of transcription factors, the fibroblasts acquired the quality of undifferentiated stem cells, those capable of self-renewal and differentiation to various mature cells (Figure 1.2). They were named "induced pluripotent stem cells (iPS cells)". The beauty of iPS cells is multifold [32]. First, they come from patient's own somatic cells and can be any cells in the body, such as fat cells, skin cells, bone cells, etc. There is no risk of immune rejection after implantation back to the patient's body. Second, the cells are easy to produce - only four genes need to be introduced. Third, they have all the features of undifferentiated cells for the potential to develop into any cells in the body. Fourth, they can be mass produced and repeatedly introduced to the patient.

In addition to cell replacement therapy, iPS cells can be used for a variety of other applications, such as establishing new disease models for many slow-developing human diseases, and for drug discovery and toxicity studies. Lastly, these cells are not ethically dubious and have not been shown to form tumors [33].

However, iPS cells do offer some cause for concern. First, iPS cells are prone to epigenetic and transcriptional aberrations. Second, as in the case of culturing embryonic stem cells, iPS cells often require a layer of feeder cells. The purification of stem cells from contaminated feeder cells before injecting human body can be a daunting task. Recently, however, a feeder-free system was developed [34]. Third, like embryonic stem cells, iPS cells also need to be differentiated to specific functional mature cells before being introduced into human body. Fourth, iPS cells are adult somatic cells, which can be short lived depending on the natural lifespan of the parental cell before reprograming. Fifth, the initial reprogramming of iPS cells is completed utilizing a retrovirus carrying oncogenes, including c-myc. Both the retained virus and oncogene may potentially cause genetic mutations of the cell through viral integration, and can produce cancer [35]. This problem can be alleviated with transient viral infections, such as through non-integrating adenoviruses [36] and non–viral or non-transgene (chemical) approaches [37]. Finally, with current technology, iPS cells require a long production cycle composed of multiple steps, including initial cell culture, transfection of genes, stem cell selection, growth to adequate number of viable cells, modifying culture condition for specific cell differentiation, injection to patient, homing to specific body site, adapting to local environment, and establishing desired function. All of these steps would take months to complete. Therefore, iPS cells are not useful in emergencies or acute situations, such as traumatic spinal cord injury and myocardial infarction, when the need of replacement would be immediate. To reduce the length of production, researchers have been developing a system to bank iPS cells for future use. According to a recent estimation, enough human leukocyte antigen (HLA)-matched iPS cells can be banked from selected HLA donors to satisfy the needs in 90% of Japanese population with minimal immune rejection. However, other researchers in Europe are skeptical about this approach [38].

In addition to producing iPS cells in a Petri dish, theoretically, reprograming (trans-differentiation) of adult somatic cells could be accomplished in vivo. For example, fibroblasts in scar tissue of myocardial infarction may be reprogramed in situ to behave like iPS cells and then be directed to differentiate into cardiomyocytes. This would eliminate many in vitro steps of cell reprograming and ensure accurate localization of stem cells to the site of injury.

The first clinical trial using iPS cells has recently been initiated in Japan for patients with macular degeneration [39]. According to the study protocol, skin cells will be harvested from each patient, and will be cultured and reprogramed to become iPS cells. Then, the cells will be directed to mature into pigmented retina cells, which will be locally injected underneath the retina for re-epithelization [40].

When the three types of pluripotent stem cells were compared side-by-side, it appears that iPS cells differed and retained a residual DNA methylation pattern typical of parental somatic cells, whereas similar methylation transcritome profiles were observed in both embryonic stem cells and stem cells obtained by somatic cell nuclear transfer [41].

Taken together, embryonic stem cells have brought great hope for cell replacement therapy. The new discovery of iPS cells could benefit a large number of patients. This pluripotent stem cell approach is particularly useful for diseases that have no cure, but are a result of a simple defect in one type of cell, such as retinitis pigmentosa, ALS, Alzheimer's disease, Parkinson's disease, type I diabetes, etc. The pluripotent stem cells can also be modified to produce tissues and organs for transplantation. The potential is limitless as long as the current huddles can be overcome.

Table 1.1 illustrates the similarities and differences between multipotent and pluripotent stem cells. Extensive bench and animal research has brought us a wealth of knowledge and skills in stem cell biology and technology, although beneficial clinical applications remain limited. However, this will likely start to change in the very near future, given the vast number of clinical trials currently underway. According to recent data from the National Institutes of Health, there are over 4,500 clinical trials using multipotent stem cells, and over 100 clinical trials using pluripotent stem cells, being undertaken (https://clinicaltrials.gov).

Table 1.1. Comparison between multipotent stem cells and pluripotent stem cells

Stem cell type	Multipotent	Pluripotent
Source	Many tissues and organs in the body	IVF, SCNT, induced PS cells
Availability	Harvested/isolated from organs/tissues	Through in vitro replication
Abundance	Scarce, 1 in 1,000 to 3,000 cells	Unlimited
In vitro culture	difficult	Relatively easy
Differentiation potential	Limited, to specific cells in the residing tissue and organ	Unlimited, to all types of cells in the body
Cell preparation	Direct implantation after harvesting and enrichment	Differentiation to mature cells before implantation
Ethical concerns	No	Yes if embryonic Probable if SCNT No if iPS cells
Tumorigenecity	No	Yes, teratomas
Immune rejection	Yes if allogeneic No if autologous	Yes if embryonic No if SCNT & induced from autologous cells
Scope of clinical application	Limited	Unlimited
Clinical indications	Cell and tissue regeneration	Cell replacement therapy
Examples of diseases can be treated with stem cells	Leukemia, lymphoma, immune mediated diseases, myocardial infarction, heart failure, wound repair, etc.	Type I diabetes, retinitis pigmentosa, macular degeneration, traumatic spinal cord injury, Parkinson's disease, myocardial infarction, etc.

Cancer Stem Cells

The concept of stem cells would not be complete without mentioning cancer stem cells. In 1994, John Dick proposed that cancer, too, might originate from particular stem cells [6]. Since then, studies have provided evidence of cancer stem cells in many solid and hematopoietic tumors. It is now generally accepted that cancer develops through a clonal process originating from genetic alterations, such as gene mutation, of a single pre-existing tissue stem/progenitor cell. Another recent hypothesis is that cancer stem cells may also be derived from mature tissue cells through dedifferentiation (Figure 1.3) [42]. This so-called "plasticity" phenomenon has been observed in otherwise mature mucin-secreting glandular cells that acquire stem cell characteristics and behave like stem cells when the stem cell layer of the bronchial mucosa is removed [43]. This may reflect adaptive mechanisms for self-preservation of epithelia to repair injuries, but could also contribute to human cancer development if the repertoires go awry. Other researchers have also observed requisition of stem cell properties in committed and/or differentiated cells [44].

Cancer stem cells possess the same characteristics of other stem cells, being able to replicate and differentiate to more mature cells. They also produce uncontrolled growth with the ability of migrating to other body sites and secreting factors to destroy normal structures. In vivo clonal analysis has revealed that cancer stem cells are capable of geometric expansion, but with limited potential for terminal differentiation [45]. When dormant, the cells are hard to eradicate by conventional methods of treatment, such as chemotherapy and radiation. Instead, cancer stem cells enter the cell cycle years later, and can reinitiate a tumor mass as a recurrent tumor, or can contribute to metastatic tumor [46]. It is also generally believed that cancer stem cells are scarce in number. Currently, there is no in vivo imaging method or biomarker test that is sensitive enough to detect residual cancer stem cells after ablative treatment.

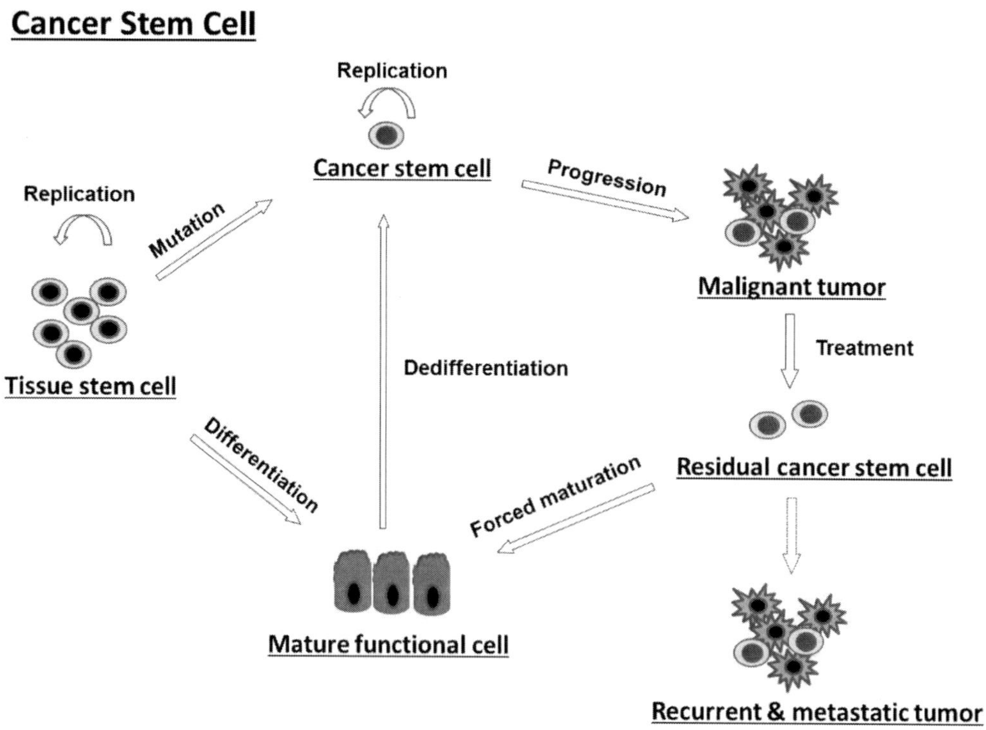

Figure 1.3. The theory and dynamics of cancer stem cells.

Giving the described challenges, instead of taking desperate measures to locate and destroy cancer stem cells, scientists are looking for alternative ways to lead cancer stem cells to maturation. Matured cancer cells can function as normal cells, such as white blood cells, or lose the ability to invade adjacent tissue or migrate to other organs. They may become more susceptible to conventional cancer therapy. This is based on recent evidence that cancer stem cells, although driven by aberrant expression of proteins that are caused by gene mutations, retain normal gene functions. Suppressing abnormal gene function will restore original programming to normal gene function. The successful stories are in Notch pathway for solid tumors, including ovarian cancer, pancreatic cancer and breast cancer. Recent studies have shown that the Notch gene, when mutated, prevents cells from reaching maturation. On the other hand, when the mutated gene is suppressed, the cells are prompted to mature and more closely resemble normal tissue cells. Pre-clinical data has demonstrated that when the mutated Notch gene pathway is blocked, stable disease can be achieved [47].

Another example is acute myeloid leukemia and glioblastoma. These tumors have notable mutations in the genes that produce the enzymes IDH-1/2. Normally, these enzymes help to break down nutrients and generate energy for cells. When mutated, it creates a molecule called 2-hydroxyglotarate, 2-HG, which appears to switch off certain genes in the nucleus. As a result, the cells remain primitive and grow uncontrollably [48]. As it turns out, however, cells containing mutated IDH-1/2 also still contain the healthy enzyme. Once the abnormal enzyme is neutralized, the healthy ones put the cells back on track, coaxing them into maturation into functional blood cells. Recent studies have shown that an IDH-1 inhibitor, ML309, can bind to the enzyme and prevent it from creating 2-HG, causing the primitive malignant cells to then mature into healthy ones [49]. Another drug capable of reversing maturation blockage in acute myeloid leukemia cells is called all-trans-retinoic acid, or ATRA, a derivative of vitamin A. By attacking a fusion gene protein produced as a result of the chromosome translocation (15:17), ATAR can cause a subset of acute myeloid leukemia to abandon their relentless growth and to mature into white blood cells [50].

These examples represent a paradigm shift in cancer treatment- of maturing cancer cells, in addition to killing them. So far, the effect of inhibitors appears short-lived. However, the benefit could be amplified with in combination with conventional chemotherapy. After maturing, the cancer cells become more susceptible to conventional therapy, which may translate into a significant increase of overall survival and an improved quality of life for many cancer patients.

Conclusion

Stem cells, with their capability for self-renewal and their versatility to differentiate into desired mature functional cells, open an exciting avenue for cell replacement therapy and regenerative medicine. If successful, a long list of currently devastating diseases and conditions could be effectively treated or reversed. The scientific research on stem cells over the last 50+ years has already brought us a wealth of knowledge on stem cell biology, and abundant skills in in vitro manipulation. The next focus is to refine the theories and technologies that will allow stem cell therapy to enter into the mainstream of clinical practice. So far, a variety of animal models and limited human studies have been encouraging. But a large body of work, from bench to bedside, needs to be carried out, especially with human studies to guide implantation and to monitor in vivo survival and function of stem cells. Instead of waiting for final functional assessment, imaging modalities, particularly MR imaging, can be developed to evaluate stem cell therapy in real-time, and to help our understanding of why a stem cell therapy regimen is effective or ineffective. This will answer many pressing questions in stem cell therapy, including the desired quantity and quality of stem cells for transplantation, the route of implantation, the local and systemic environment of the host, the migration of stem cells to the desired body sites, the survival and differentiation of implanted cells in the recipient, and the effect to and the ultimate functional improvement of the recipient.

Stem cell research is a unique field that requires collaboration across many disciplines. Expertise is needed not only in cell and molecular biology, but also in tissue and organ engineering, immunology, cell labeling and in vivo imaging, and clinical diagnosis and treatment. It is also essential to gain support from industries, pharmaceuticals, government and regulatory agencies. Efforts should also be aimed for the standardization of procedures, favorable policymaking, and adequate funding of both research and clinical trials. In addition, a sustainable stem cell therapy procedure will require resources and infrastructure for stem cell banking and logistics in the effective distribution of stem cells.

Theories about cancer stem cells require continued refinement. Advances in our understanding of cancer biology will help us, in addition to fine-tuning the methods utilized to rid cancer cells from the body, to look for other options in cancer control, such as maturing cancer stem cells to normal functional cells or to cells more susceptible to conventional therapy. This will provide the opportunity for cancer patients to gain prolonged overall survival and an improved quality of life while living with cancer.

References

[1] Ramalho-Santos M, Willenbring H. On the origin of the term "stem cell". *Cell Stem Cell* 2007;1(1):35-38.

[2] Becker AJ, Mc CE, Till JE. Cytological demonstration of the clonal nature of spleen colonies derived from transplanted mouse marrow cells. *Nature* 1963;197:452-454.

[3] Thomson JA, Itskovitz-Eldor J, Shapiro SS, Waknitz MA, Swiergiel JJ, Marshall VS, et al. Embryonic stem cell lines derived from human blastocysts. *Science* 1998;282(5391):1145-1147.

[4] Shamblott MJ, Axelman J, Wang S, Bugg EM, Littlefield JW, Donovan PJ, et al. Derivation of pluripotent stem cells from cultured human primordial germ cells. *Proc. Natl. Acad. Sci. USA* 1998;95(23):13726-13731.

[5] Takahashi K, Yamanaka S. Induction of pluripotent stem cells from mouse embryonic and adult fibroblast cultures by defined factors. *Cell* 2006;126(4):663-676.

[6] Lapidot T, Sirard C, Vormoor J, Murdoch B, Hoang T, Caceres-Cortes J, et al. A cell initiating human acute myeloid leukaemia after transplantation into SCID mice. *Nature* 1994;367(6464):645-648.

[7] Appelbaum FR. Retrospective. E. Donnall Thomas (1920-2012). *Science* 2012;338(6111):1163.

[8] Butler MG, Menitove JE. Umbilical cord blood banking: an update. *J. Assist. Reprod. Genet* 2011;28(8):669-676.
[9] Clarke DL, Johansson CB, Wilbertz J, Veress B, Nilsson E, Karlstrom H, et al. Generalized potential of adult neural stem cells. *Science* 2000;288(5471):1660-1663.
[10] Bensinger W, DiPersio JF, McCarty JM. Improving stem cell mobilization strategies: future directions. *Bone Marrow Transplant* 2009;43(3):181-195.
[11] Sykes M, Nikolic B. Treatment of severe autoimmune disease by stem-cell transplantation. *Nature* 2005;435(7042):620-627.
[12] Sutton MT, Bonfield TL. Stem cells: innovations in clinical applications. *Stem Cells Int.* 2014;2014:516278.
[13] Hoch AI, Leach JK. Concise review: optimizing expansion of bone marrow mesenchymal stem/stromal cells for clinical applications. *Stem Cells Transl. Med.* 2014;3(5):643-652.
[14] Cordeiro-Spinetti E, de Mello W, Trindade LS, Taub DD, Taichman RS, Balduino A. Human bone marrow mesenchymal progenitors: perspectives on an optimized in vitro manipulation. *Front Cell Dev. Biol.* 2014;2:7.
[15] Clifford DM, Fisher SA, Brunskill SJ, Doree C, Mathur A, Watt S, et al. Stem cell treatment for acute myocardial infarction. *Cochrane Database Syst. Rev.* 2012;2:CD006536.
[16] Traverse JH, Henry TD, Pepine CJ, Willerson JT, Ellis SG. One-year follow-up of intracoronary stem cell delivery on left ventricular function following ST-elevation myocardial infarction. *JAMA* 2014;311(3):301-302.
[17] Psaltis PJ, Spoon DB, Wong DT. Utility of mesenchymal stromal cells for myocardial infarction. Transitioning from bench to bedside. *Minerva Cardioangiol* 2013;61(6):639-663.
[18] Collins E, Gilkeson G. Hematopoetic and mesenchymal stem cell transplantation in the treatment of refractory systemic lupus erythematosus--where are we now? *Clin. Immunol* 2013;148(3):328-334.
[19] Chinnadurai R, Waller EK, Galipeau J, Nooka AK. From single nucleotide polymorphisms to constant immunosuppression: mesenchymal stem cell therapy for autoimmune diseases. *Biomed. Res. Int.* 2013;2013:929842.
[20] Basel MT, Shrestha TB, Bossmann SH, Troyer DL. Cells as delivery vehicles for cancer therapeutics. *Ther. Deliv.* 2014;5(5):555-567.
[21] Rama P, Matuska S, Paganoni G, Spinelli A, De Luca M, Pellegrini G. Limbal stem-cell therapy and long-term corneal regeneration. *N .Engl. J. Med.* 2010;363(2):147-155.
[22] Sandel MJ. Embryo ethics--the moral logic of stem-cell research. *N. Engl. J. Med.* 2004;351(3):207-209.
[23] Fox IJ, Daley GQ, Goldman SA, Huard J, Kamp TJ, Trucco M. Stem cell therapy. Use of differentiated pluripotent stem cells as replacement therapy for treating disease. *Science* 2014;345(6199):1247391.
[24] Alper J. Geron gets green light for human trial of ES cell-derived product. *Nat. Biotechnol.* 2009;27(3):213-214.
[25] Schwartz SD, Hubschman JP, Heilwell G, Franco-Cardenas V, Pan CK, Ostrick RM, et al. Embryonic stem cell trials for macular degeneration: a preliminary report. *Lancet* 2012;379(9817):713-720.

[26] Wang X, Kimbrel EA, Ijichi K, Paul D, Lazorchak AS, Chu J, et al. Human ESC-derived MSCs outperform bone marrow MSCs in the treatment of an EAE model of multiple sclerosis. *Stem Cell Reports* 2014;3(1):115-130.

[27] Wakayama T, Tabar V, Rodriguez I, Perry AC, Studer L, Mombaerts P. Differentiation of embryonic stem cell lines generated from adult somatic cells by nuclear transfer. *Science* 2001;292(5517):740-743.

[28] Wilmut I, Schnieke AE, McWhir J, Kind AJ, Campbell KH. Viable offspring derived from fetal and adult mammalian cells. *Nature 1*997;385(6619):810-813.

[29] Tachibana M, Amato P, Sparman M, Gutierrez NM, Tippner-Hedges R, Ma H, et al. Human embryonic stem cells derived by somatic cell nuclear transfer. *Cell* 2013;153(6):1228-1238.

[30] Yamanaka S. A fresh look at iPS cells. *Cell* 2009;137(1):13-17.

[31] Takahashi K, Tanabe K, Ohnuki M, Narita M, Ichisaka T, Tomoda K, et al. Induction of pluripotent stem cells from adult human fibroblasts by defined factors. *Cell* 2007;131(5):861-872.

[32] Inoue H, Nagata N, Kurokawa H, Yamanaka S. iPS cells: a game changer for future medicine. *EMBO J.* 2014;33(5):409-417.

[33] Kamao H, Mandai M, Okamoto S, Sakai N, Suga A, Sugita S, et al. Characterization of human induced pluripotent stem cell-derived retinal pigment epithelium cell sheets aiming for clinical application. *Stem Cell Reports* 2014;2(2):205-218.

[34] Nakagawa M, Taniguchi Y, Senda S, Takizawa N, Ichisaka T, Asano K, et al. A novel efficient feeder-free culture system for the derivation of human induced pluripotent stem cells. *Sci Rep* 2014;4:3594.

[35] Yu J, Vodyanik MA, Smuga-Otto K, Antosiewicz-Bourget J, Frane JL, Tian S, et al. Induced pluripotent stem cell lines derived from human somatic cells. *Science* 2007;318(5858):1917-1920.

[36] Stadtfeld M, Nagaya M, Utikal J, Weir G, Hochedlinger K. Induced pluripotent stem cells generated without viral integration. *Science* 2008;322(5903):945-949.

[37] Hou P, Li Y, Zhang X, Liu C, Guan J, Li H, et al. Pluripotent stem cells induced from mouse somatic cells by small-molecule compounds. *Science* 2013;341(6146):651-654.

[38] de Rham C, Villard J. Potential and limitation of HLA-based banking of human pluripotent stem cells for cell therapy. *J. Immunol. Res.* 2014;2014:518135.

[39] Reardon S, Cyranoski D. Japan stem-cell trial stirs envy. *Nature* 2014;513(7518):287-288.

[40] Nakano-Okuno M, Borah BR, Nakano I. Ethics of iPSC-Based Clinical Research for Age-Related Macular Degeneration: Patient-Centered Risk-Benefit Analysis. *Stem Cell Rev* 2014;10(6):743-752.

[41] Ma H, Morey R, O'Neil RC, He Y, Daughtry B, Schultz MD, et al. Abnormalities in human pluripotent cells due to reprogramming mechanisms. *Nature* 2014;511(7508):177-183.

[42] Varga J, De Oliveira T, Greten FR. The architect who never sleeps: tumor-induced plasticity. *FEBS Lett.* 2014;588(15):2422-2427.

[43] Tata PR, Mou H, Pardo-Saganta A, Zhao R, Prabhu M, Law BM, et al. Dedifferentiation of committed epithelial cells into stem cells in vivo. *Nature* 2013;503(7475):218-223.

[44] Blanpain C, Fuchs E. Stem cell plasticity. Plasticity of epithelial stem cells in tissue regeneration. *Science* 2014;344(6189):1242281.

[45] Driessens G, Beck B, Caauwe A, Simons BD, Blanpain C. Defining the mode of tumour growth by clonal analysis. *Nature* 2012;488(7412):527-530.

[46] Chen J, Li Y, Yu TS, McKay RM, Burns DK, Kernie SG, et al. A restricted cell population propagates glioblastoma growth after chemotherapy. *Nature* 2012;488(7412):522-526.

[47] Takebe N, Nguyen D, Yang SX. Targeting notch signaling pathway in cancer: clinical development advances and challenges. *Pharmacol. Ther.* 2014;141(2):140-149.

[48] Rakheja D, Konoplev S, Medeiros LJ, Chen W. IDH mutations in acute myeloid leukemia. *Hum. Pathol.* 2012;43(10):1541-1551.

[49] Davis MI, Gross S, Shen M, Straley KS, Pragani R, Lea WA, et al. Biochemical, cellular, and biophysical characterization of a potent inhibitor of mutant isocitrate dehydrogenase IDH1. *J. Biol. Chem.* 2014;289(20):13717-13725.

[50] Huang ME, Ye YC, Chen SR, Chai JR, Lu JX, Zhoa L, et al. Use of all-trans retinoic acid in the treatment of acute promyelocytic leukemia. *Blood* 1988;72(2):567-572.

In: Magnetic Resonance Imaging of Stem Cell Applications ISBN: 978-1-63463-910-1
Editor: Xiaoming Yang

Chapter 2

Magnetic Resonance Imaging of Stem Cells: The Principles

Rohan Dharmakumar*, Avinash Kali and Debiao Li
Biomedical Imaging Research Institute, Cedars-Sinai Medical Center,
Los Angeles, CA, US

Abstract

This chapter provides an overview of magnetic resonance imaging (MRI) principles for detecting, quantifying and tracking stem cells. We begin with a quick overview of all imaging approaches currently used for imaging cells, and then transition into reviewing the commonly used MRI contrast agents in the field. Next, we review the "negative-contrast" and "positive contrast" imaging approaches used for cellular MRI as well as the main aspects of cell tracking with fluorine-19 (^{19}F). We close with the current challenges facing cellular MRI and provide an outlook of the novel contrast agents and imaging approaches that are in the horizon with the potential to significantly advance the capabilities of cellular MRI technology.

Keywords: MRI, cell tracking, ^{19}F MRI, negative contrast imaging and positive contrast imaging

Introduction

General Overview of Cellular Imaging

Imaging methods are expected to play a central role in regenerative medicine. Currently, various imaging modalities, including nuclear imaging (such as Positron Emission

* Correspondence to: Rohan Dharmakumar, PhD, (rohandkumar@csmc.edu).

Tomography (PET) and Single Photon Emission Computed Tomography (SPECT)), Computed Tomography (CT), and Ultrasound Imaging (US), Magnetic Resonance Imaging (MRI), Optical Imaging methods (such as Fluorescence and Bioluminescence imaging as well as Quantum Dot Imaging), are routinely used to study stem cells in vivo. Typically contrast agents or reporter molecules are used to label the cells for visualization. These contrast agents need to be non-toxic, bio-compatible, highly specific to the targeted cells, not interfere with the proliferation and differentiation capacities of the cells, and sufficiently sensitive to facilitate detection by the corresponding imaging method [1, 2]. Each imaging approach has some key advantages and challenges. The key aspects of the imaging approaches are summarized in Table 2.1.

Table 2.1. Key aspects of standard imaging modalities used for cellular imaging

Imaging Modality	Contrast Media	Sensitivity (mol/L)	Advantages	Challenges
Nuclear Imaging (SPECT and PET)	- In-111 Oxin, - Tc-99m - F18-FDG - Cu-64 (and others)	10^{-9} to 10^{-8}	-high sensitivity -high translational capacity	-low spatial resolution -short half-life of label -ionizing radiation -lack of anatomic details
Optical Imaging (Fluorescence and bioluminescence imaging)	-near infra-red fluorophores, -fluorescent enzymes (e.g., luciferase)	10^{-12} to 10^{-9} (fluorescence); 10-17 to 10-15 (bioluminescence)	-high sensitivity -high spatial resolution -no ionizing radiation	-limited penetration depth -photobleaching of the fluorophores
Ultrasound Imaging	-microbubbles -perfluorocarbons -liposomes -gold nanoparticles	N/A	-low scan time -high sensitivity to the tracer -inexpensive	-low spatial resolution -inaccessibility of many anatomical sites - acoustic shadow -dilution of the contrast label upon cell division -unstable tracers
Computed Tomography (CT)	-iodine-based contrast media -gadolinium-based contrast media -barium sulfate labeled microcapsules	N/A	-high spatial resolution -high temporal resolution - short scan time	-very high concentration of contrast needed to visualize stem cells -dilution of the contrast label upon cell division -ionizing radiation
Magnetic Resonance Imaging (MRI)	- iron oxide - gadolinium chelates - perfluorocarbons	10^{-5} to 10^{-3}	-excellent soft tissue contrast -high spatial resolution -no ionizing radiation -excellent correlation with anatomical details -functional imaging can be done simultaneously with cellular imaging	-low sensitivity -dilution of the contrast label upon cell division hampers long-term studies -contrast behavior not specific

Contrast Agents for Cellular MRI

T_1 Agents

Paramagnetic contrast agents such as gadolinium (Gd) chelates have initially been explored for stem cell labeling. At low concentrations, Gd-chelates generate hyperintense contrast primarily through the T_1 shortening effects [3]. However, they cannot easily pass through cell membranes and require long incubation times and high concentrations to achieve significant labeling [4]. At least 50-500 μmol/L of intracellular concentration is needed to generate sufficient signal intensity [5]. The potential toxicity of Gd-chelates upon dechelation within a cell is yet to be explored. Studies suggest that labeling mesenchymal stem cells with gadolinium fullerenol decreased stem cell proliferation, probably by altering mitochondrial function and increased reactive oxygen species within the cells [6, 7].

T_2 and T_2* Agents

A more widely preferred class of contrast agents generate contrast primarily based on shortening of T_2 and T_2* relaxation times. These include superparamagnetic iron-oxide (SPIO) nanoparticles, ultra-small superparamagnetic iron oxide (USPIO) nanoparticles, and micron-sized iron oxide particles (MPIO). Upon incubation, a variety of cells (particularly macrophages) readily internalize these nano and micro-particles. These particles consist of a magnetite (Fe_3O_4) core encapsulated usually in dextran, polymers such as polystyrene, or other agents that enhance internalization by the cells. They have magnetic moments that are at least 3 orders of magnitude greater than paramagnetic agents and very high R_2 /R_1 relaxivity ratio, where $R_1 = 1/T_1$ and $R_2 = 1/T_2$. They generate contrast by promoting dephasing of proton spins and enhancing T2 relaxation due to susceptibility differences in the surroundings and distortion of local magnetic fields. As a result, hypointense areas are generated in the T_2 and T_2* images by the contrast agent labeled cells. Iron oxide contrast agents are preferable to paramagnetic agents because

a. they generate the largest change in signal per unit of the contrast agent, in particular in T_2* weighted images; intracellular concentration of 1.4 – 4 pg Fe/cell is sufficient for detection in a 100 x 100 x 200 μm^3 voxel [8, 9];
b. they are non-toxic and bio-compatible; the iron is eliminated by cells by using normal biochemical pathways for iron metabolism;
c. they are easily internalized by a variety of cells and they can be easily detected by light and electron microscopy; and
d. the magnetic properties of the particles can be varied by controlling the size of the core and coating.

SPIOs and USPIOs are nanometer-sized particles. As a result, thousands of particles need to be internalized by the cell to render the imaging protocol to be sensitive. This requires robust and highly efficient labeling schemes, which is typically achieved via exogenous labeling of cells. Moreover, cell division can dilute the nanoparticles beyond detectability and hamper long-term studies. Recently, micron-sized iron-oxide particles (MPIOs) have been developed, which have higher relaxivities based on equivalent iron content [10]. The particles range from 0.96 μm to 5.80 μm in diameter and easily achieve iron loading of 100 pgFe/cell [10]. As larger iron oxide particles exert stronger T2* effects, individual particles are detectable at 50-μm resolution. Thus, this approach allows for single particle internalized within the cell to be imaged and removes concerns over cell divisions diluting the labels within the cell (Figure 2.1).

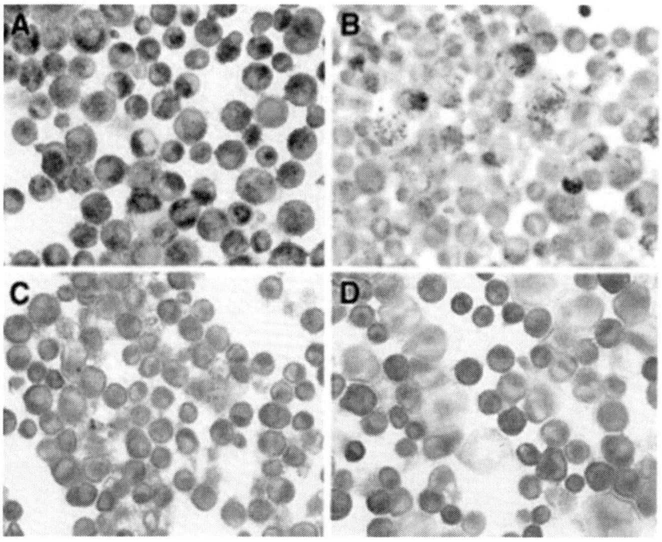

Figure 2.1. Effect of cell division on iron dilution. Microscopy of diaminobenzide-enhanced Prussian blue–stained HeLa cells show the rapid disappearance of stainable iron particles (brown dots) from the fast growing cells. Findings at day 0 (**A**), day 7 (**B**), day 14 (**C**), and day 21 (**D**) after labeling with the ferumoxides/poly L-lysine (PLL) complex are shown. The doubling time of the cells is 2.6 days. By five to eight divisions (i.e., 14–21 days), no detectable iron particles are observed in the cells. The cells are counterstained with nuclear fast red and photographed at a magnification of x20. Reprinted, with permission, from [11].

This also enables direct in-vivo labeling of the cells [12]. MPIOs were successfully used to monitor rejection of allogenic heart transplantation and macrophage infiltration in the rejection sites in rodents at a 4.7T small animal scanner [13]. Single MPIO particles injected into mouse embryos could be detected in-vivo at embryonic day 11.5 [14]. Using wide and confocal fluorescence microscopy techniques and dual-labeling schemes, single hepatocytes loaded with 1.63-μm MPIOs could be detected in-vivo at 7T scanner one month after intra-splenic transplantation [15]. Since comparing identical slices from in-vivo and in-vitro MRI with histological sections is difficult, the following indirect lines of evidence are typically used to confirm single-cell detection with this approach:

- Spacing between the hypointense regions on in-vivo MR images is identical to that observed in the histological sections using a wide field fluorescence microscopy. Dual-labeling schemes and confocal fluorescence microscopy prove that cells observed in the wide field microscopy are the transplanted cells; and

- Sizes and hypointensities of the dark contrast regions in the in-vivo MR images are identical to those of the labeled hepatocytes embedded in an agarose phantom.

A more direct line of evidence for single-cell detection using in-vivo MRI has been provided by Heyn et al. [16].

MPIOs are readily endocytosed by a variety of progenitor and stem cells [17]. Neuronal precursor cells are found to endocytose free MPIOs injected into the lateral ventricles in brain, thereby enabling in-vivo cell labeling [18]. This allows in-vivo labeling and tracking of neural progenitors along the rostral migratory pathway (RMS) to the olfactory bulb (OB). In-vivo cell labeling can be non-specific as the injected MPIOs can be endocytosed by several cell phenotypes apart from the targeted cells. The specific phenotypes labeled by the MPIOs cannot be characterized by MRI in-vivo and histology will still be required [18]. The applicability of MPIOs has been studied using dedicated animal scanners at high magnetic fields. Their applications in clinical settings are yet to be explored.

The physicochemical characteristics and pharmacokinetics of smaller iron oxide agents have been studied [11, 19-21]. These studies have shown that hepatic and splenic macrophages readily phagocytose iron-oxide particles even in the absence of dextran coating. As a result, SPIOs are rapidly cleared from the system. Ultrasmall SPIOs (USPIOs), on the other hand, are not readily recognized by the hepatic and splenic macrophages and hence have a longer half-life in the body.

Application of Iron-based Contrast Agents for Cellular MRI

Numerous studies have demonstrated the ability of these particles to be readily internalized by a variety of cells, particularly macrophages. They have been successfully used to study macrophage infiltration in different disease models: liver metastasis [22, 23], tumor metastases in lymph nodes [24, 25], bone marrow [26], experimental acute encephalomyelitis in rats and mice [27, 28], ischemic brain damage [29], induced arthritis in knees [30], atherosclerotic plaques of hyperlipidemic rabbits [31], ischemic and reperfusion injury in kidneys [32], selective immune-mediated injury to the glomerulus [33], nephrotoxic injury to cortex and medulla of kidney [34], and rejection of allogenic organ transplantation [13, 35, 36].

Labeling of non-phagocytic cells with iron-oxide particles requires modification of the particle surface by transfection agents such as dextran, poly L-lysine [37], protamine sulfate and carboxylated dendrimers [38]. These agents prevent aggregation of particles [39] and nullify the negative charges on them, otherwise repelled by the negatively charged cells. A variety of stem and progenitor cells such as rat neural stem cells, rat oligodendroglial progenitors, mouse muscle progenitors, mouse embryonic stem cells, human mesenchymal stem cells, human neural stem cells, human embryoid body-derived pluripotent stem cells, etc., have been successfully labeled and tracked using these methods [8]. A number of studies have elucidated the applicability of iron oxides for stem cell tracking in various disease models, primarily in central nervous system (CNS) and heart. Some of these are listed below:

- Neural stem cell derived, iron-oxide-labeled oligodendroglial progenitors were transplanted into ventricles, which promoted myelination and functional recovery of dysmyelinated axons in Long Evans Shaker rats (Figure 2.2). These labeled cells were seen as hypointense regions in brain parenchyma in in-vivo MR images at 4.7T. The presence of iron oxide labeled cells in these regions was validated using β-LacZ gene expression by these cells [38].

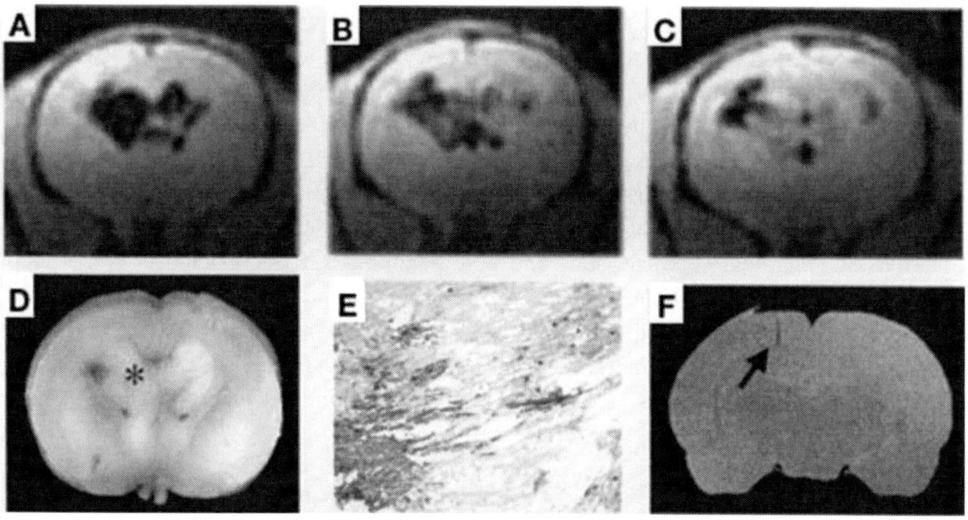

Figure 2.2. In vivo MR tracking of cells in ventricles of rat brain. (**A–C**) Sequential in-vivo MRI (4.7 T, T_2*-weighted multigradient echo consecutive transverse images) obtained from a les rat 42 days after intraventricular transplantation of iron-labeled and LacZ-transfected, neural stem cell-derived oligodendroglial progenitors. (**D**) X-gal staining of the corresponding gross specimen shows a close overlap between the distribution of labeled cells and the MR contrast in the middle image (**B**). (**E**) Immunolabeling shows a close association between LacZ-positive cells and newly formed myelin in this area (**D**, asterisk). (**F**) Control ex vivo MRI of a les rat 32 days following transplantation of unlabeled cells, showing needle track (arrow) without any confounding artifacts. Overall, note the lack of contrast between gray and white matter due to the absence of normal myelin. Reprinted, with permission, from [38].

- Labeled neural precursor cells were injected intravenously into adult experimental autoimmune encephalomyelitis mice. Migration of the cells into inflammatory demyelinating lesions in brain parenchyma was observed using in-vivo MRI at 3T. Quantification of transplanted cells in the focal demyelinating lesions with ex-vivo R_2 * (or $1/T_2$*) relaxometry showed higher R_2 * values in these lesions compared to the normal parenchyma [40].
- Mesenchymal stem cells (MSC) are widely studied because of their therapeutic potential. Hinds et al., have demonstrated that Hematopoietic CD34+ stem cells and MSCs could efficiently uptake MPIOs. MPIO labeling did not affect the proliferative and differentiation capacities of these cells [17].
- Transplanted iron oxide labeled MSCs were tracked in large animal myocardial infarction models using clinical 1.5T scanners [41, 42]. Cells were transplanted through intra-myocardial injections guided by X-ray fluoroscopy. Some authors reported that at least 10^5 transplanted cells could be detected at the injection sites

[41]. Serial cardiac imaging could detect transplanted cells for up to 3 weeks post-injection.

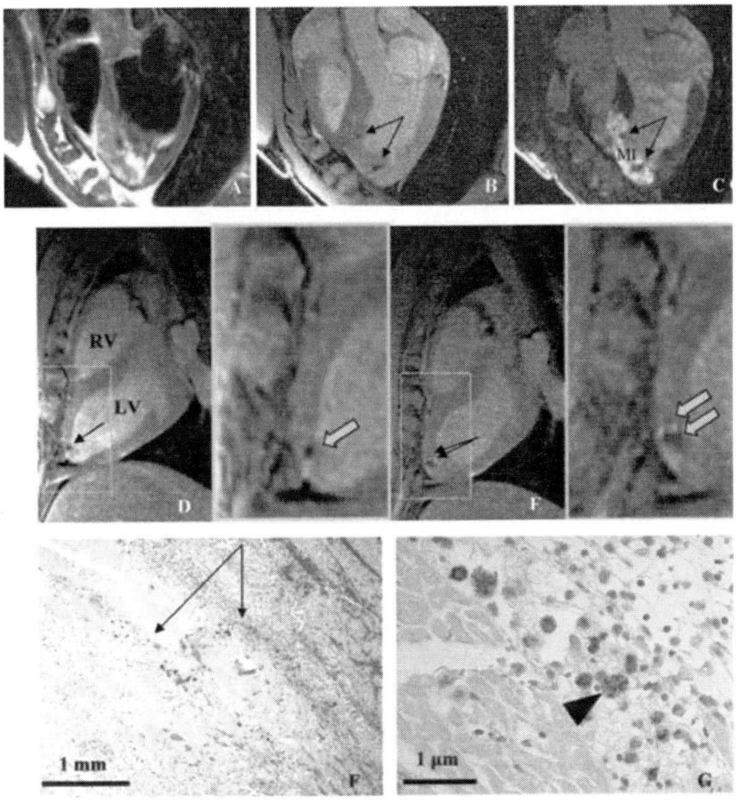

Figure 2.3. MR tracking of iron-labeled stem cell in myocardium. Representative hypointense lesions in fast spin echo (**A**), fast gradient-recalled echo (GRE) (**B**), and late enhancement MRI (**C**) of mesenchymal stem cell (MSC) injection sites (arrows) within 24 hours of injection. MSCs are injected in the myocardial infarct (MI, hyperintense region in **C**). Long-axis MRIs showing hypointense lesions (arrows) caused by MSCs are acquired within 24 hours (**D**) and 1 week (**E**) of injection with inset at right demonstrating expansion of lesion over 1 week. Needle tract (arrow) of MSCs is demonstrated in histological section at 1 week after injection with Prussian Blue staining (**F**) as cells with blue iron inclusions (arrowhead) that are excluded from nucleus (**G**). LV indicates left ventricle; RV, right ventricle. Reprinted, with permission, from [42].

- One study reported that lesions detected within 24 hours post-injection could still be detected after 1 week with an accompanied 15% expansion in the spread of hypointensities and 25% decrease in the contrast (Figure 2.3) [42]. However, 3 weeks post-injection only 26% of the original lesions could be observed, probably owing to the dilution of the label.
- MSCs were also tracked in small animal models such as rats [43]. Other cells such as embryonic ventricular cardiomyocytes were tracked using in-vivo MRI at 7T in ischemic models of mice [44]. MR studies in large animal models, such as dogs and pigs, more appropriately demonstrate the capabilities of the cellular imaging

techniques that may be translated to subsequent human clinical trials [8]. The key aspects supporting this notion are:

a. Closed-chest myocardial infarction models in large animals are minimally invasive and more closely resemble pathophysiology of human myocardial infarction than the small animal models.
b. Interventional imaging techniques used for in-vivo cell transplantation, such as X-ray fluoroscopy, are similar in large animal models and human trials.
c. MR studies with large animals can be performed on clinical 1.5 – 3T MR scanners. The imaging protocols used in these studies can be directly applied to human trials.

Cellular MRI: Negative Contrast Approaches

As discussed earlier, nano- and micron-scale iron-oxide particles are the most widely preferred contrast agents for cellular MRI. SPIO particles have magnetic moments at least 3 orders of magnitude greater than paramagnetic contrast agents and high R_2 /R_1 relaxivity ratio. The particles enhance transverse relaxation of proton spins due to susceptibility differences with the surroundings and strongly distort the local magnetic fields. As a result, they are manifested as blooming hypointensities or dark spots in MR images. The hypointensities become more effective when the particles are internalized by cells or clustered [45] and can be predominantly observed in T_2* MR images. This is because the large magnetic moments of the SPIO particles impose a susceptibility shift between the cells and the surrounding medium, which results in spatially distorted local magnetic fields. Spin diffusion in these filed gradients leads to irreversible loss of phase coherence and enhanced transverse relaxation.

Moreover, the particles have very small effect on T_1 relaxation as compared to the T_1 effects of paramagnetic agents [45]. Studies by Bowen et al. [45] have indicated that the R_2* to R_2 relaxivity ratio dramatically rises upon cellular internalization of these particles. Baseline tissue R_2* relaxation rate of any tissue at any field strength is typically no more than 1 order of magnitude greater than the R_2 values and two orders of magnitude greater than the R_1 values. R_2* values of internalized SPIO particles was found to be 70 times greater than R_2 and 3100 times than R_1 values. This suggests R_2* weighted acquisitions provide greater contrast-to-noise ratio than the R_2 and R_1 acquisitions and hold great potential for SPIO loaded cell quantification. Additionally, R_2* relaxivity is independent of field strength and iron-oxide particle size for both SPIO and USPIO particles [45].

R_2 also demonstrates sensitivity to iron-oxide concentration [45]. However, this sensitivity varies depending on the method chosen to alter iron concentration within a voxel. Iron concentration in a voxel can be varied by either varying the iron mass per cell or the number of cells per voxel. Hence, this method is unsuitable for quantifying SPIO loaded cells. Some authors suggest that R_2' measurements ($R_2' = R_2* - R_2$) is the most sensitive and quantitative parameter for estimating iron oxide concentration [45]. However, R_2' relates to iron concentration only when the iron mass per cell is sufficient to satisfy static-dephasing regime conditions [46], a case when $\Delta\omega\tau_c >>1$, where $\Delta\omega$ is the peak angular frequency shift at the surface of the magnetic perturber and τ_c is the correlation time associated with the mean path length of protons. For a 100 s^{-1} increase in R_2' values, each cell must be loaded with at least 0.07 pg of iron [45]. Most of the commonly used labeling techniques achieve iron concentration of at least 20-pg Fe/cell.

Limits of Detection

R_2* relaxivity is the most sensitive parameter for the estimation of iron concentration in a voxel in the context of negative contrast imaging, and most of the cell quantification MR techniques are based on T_2*-weighted acquisitions. Gradient echo techniques are the most sensitive to the presence of intracellular SPIO. However, they are also sensitive to susceptibility-induced artifacts from macroscopic background field inhomogeneities generated by factors such as air-tissue interface, hemorrhage, blood, endogenous ferritin deposits, and injury caused by the direct injection of stem cells [5]. On the other hand, T_2 approaches are less sensitive to the background inhomogeneities, but also less sensitive to iron labeled cells [5]. Balanced steady-state free precession (SSFP) techniques at high flip angles can provide the sensitivity as high as the gradient echo techniques, and specificity as good as the spin echo techniques [9].

Various groups have attempted to estimate the detection threshold of MRI using T_2 and T_2*-weighted techniques. The detection threshold depends on acquisition parameters, field strength, signal-to-noise ratio and pulse sequence [5]. Apart from that, the number of detectable cells can also depend on the type of cell used, method of labeling and the uptake of iron by these cells [47].

In 1999, Dodd et al. first showed that single SPIO labeled T-lymphocytes could be detected in-vitro in gelatin at 7T. Good correlation was observed between the MR images and corresponding fluorescence microscopy images [48]. In 2000, using HIV-tat peptide bound to SPIO particles, Lewin et al. imaged single hematopoietic and neural progenitor cells ex-vivo in mice bone marrow tissue at 14.1T [49]. In 2002, Majors et al. imaged single MD-100 labeled oocytes in-vitro at 11.7T [50]. Hoehn et al. established an in-vivo detection limit of 500 embryonic stem cells transplanted in rat brain at 7T [51]. In 2003, Jendelova et al. estimated a detection limit of 625 bone marrow stromal cells in-vitro at 4.7T [52]. Kircher et al. demonstrated the ability to image as few as three SPIO labeled cytotoxic lymphocytes in-vivo in mice tumors at 8.5T [53]. Using custom designed gradient and radiofrequency (RF) coils, Foster-Gareau et al. imaged single human monocytic leukemia cells (THP-1) in-vitro in a clinical 1.5T MR scanner [54]. In 2005, Dahnke et al. estimated a detection limit of 28000 cells/voxel and 600 cells/voxel in liver and brain, respectively. The difference in the detection limits can be attributed to the different spatial resolution used for brain and liver [55]. Using a balanced SSFP sequence, some scientists have demonstrated that 1.3-pg Fe/cell is sufficient to detect a single cell at 100μm resolution in a 1.5T clinical MR scanner [9].

Quantification

To date, most of the studies done to quantify the transplanted cells in-vivo have relied on the generation of hypointense regions or negative contrast in T_2 and T_2* MR images containing intracellular SPIO. Attempts have been made to correlate the R_2 and R_2*

relaxation rates to iron concentration, and therefore the number of labeled cells in a given voxel. As mentioned earlier, Bowen et al. have demonstrated the potential of employing R_2 * relaxation rates to estimate iron concentration [45]. They have also suggested that that R_2' is the most sensitive parameter for such quantification.

Early in the clinical development, MR imaging played a major role in the diagnosis of hemochromatosis and subsequent hepatic iron overload [56, 57]. Iron overload in the liver causes a reduction in signal intensity on T_2 -weighted MR images. Using ex-vivo MR of iron-overloaded livers, Stark et al. demonstrated that enhancement of T_2 relaxation rates increased linearly with tissue iron concentration ranging from 250 to 3000μgFe/g of tissue [57]. Bulte et al. demonstrated a linear relationship between R_2 values and tissue iron concentration in marmosets with hepatic hemosiderosis. T_2 relaxation was monoexponential for mild hemosiderosis, while biexponential for moderate to severe hemosiderosis at higher field strengths. Maceration of the moderate to severe hemosiderosis tissue caused the relationship to become monoexponential. This suggested that tissue architecture was important for the observed biexponential relaxation [58].

Rad et al. have demonstrated good linear correlation between the number of labeled cells and R_2 values [47]. However, R_2 values differed for various types but equal number of labeled cells. Moreover, intracellular iron showed lower R_2 values than free iron in all types of cells. The authors have suggested that the detection limit of labeled cells strongly depends on the type of cells, size of cells, and amount of intracellular iron [47]. Bowen et al. suggested that R_2 values were unsuitable for iron quantification, while R_2* was a highly sensitive parameter [45]. Bos et al., demonstrated that the R_2* increase in the liver of a rat model was of the same order as the number of labeled mesenchymal stem cells injected into the portal vein [59]. Politi et al. have demonstrated the selective homing of neural precursor cells in experimental autoimmune encephalomyelitis mice and quantified the number of cells accumulated within the brain lesions [40]. Based on brain phantoms with intra-parenchymal injection of known number of cells to establish the calibration curve, R_2* values and the number of labeled cells in the brain lesions have been estimated. This study showed that the number of cells accumulated in the lesions varied between 33.3 and 164.4 cells per site [40]. However, R_2* based quantification leads to over-estimation of the number of cells due to the background macroscopic magnetic field inhomogeneities. A number of correction techniques have been developed to overcome these background effects, which include:

- Increasing the spatial resolution [60].
- Altering the slice-refocusing gradient – Typically, voxel size is larger along the slice-select direction compared to the in-plane dimensions. Therefore, slice select direction is the most sensitive to background inhomogeneities [55]. If the background gradient is assumed to be constant along the slice select direction in a voxel, the linear phase distribution caused by the gradient can be adjusted by altering the slice refocusing gradient amplitude [61].
- Using a tailored RF pulse – A tailored RF pulse that produces quadratic phase distribution along the slice select direction has also been used to acquire signals simultaneously from regions with homogeneous and inhomogeneous backgrounds [62]. The effect of background inhomogeneities on the signal can then be analyzed

using spectral decomposition [62]. However, this technique causes a reduction in signal strength.

- Employing a B_0 field inhomogeneity correction – Dahnke et al. have employed a B_0 correction technique in which the main field inhomogeneity is obtained from multi-slice T_2* relaxometry data [55]. This is used as an initial value for iterative optimization, and relaxation signal is corrected for each voxel. The corrected T_2* maps showed less sensitivity to background inhomogeneities [55]. Moreover, the correction technique suffers from the fact that redundant data collection and long scan times.

Ultrashort echo time (TE) imaging is suggested to be valuable in estimating the very short T_2* of highly concentrated SPIO labeled cells, where the signal decay is fast [63]. Conventional gradient echo techniques for determining T_2* relaxation rates of the labeled cells are limited by the RF pulses and gradient performance [64]. Based on the long T_2 decay of the intracellular SPIO particles, one study has demonstrated an ultrashort T_2* relaxometry technique, which is based on spin echo images acquired with the readout echo shifted sequentially to increase T_2* weighting [64]. Using this technique, T_2* values as low as 1 ms can be measured. As T_2 decay characteristics of free and intracellular iron are different [65, 66], the method can be used to only obtain T_2* values of labeled cells. The authors reported that the proposed shifted spin echo (SSE) technique could only detect intracellular iron but not free iron, as the T_2 decay of free iron was too fast for the technique [64].

Limitations of Negative Contrast Approaches

Although different correction techniques have been proposed, R_2* based quantification of SPIO loaded cells still suffers from a number of limitations:

- The most predominant limitation of R_2* based methods is the over-estimation due to sensitivity to background field inhomogeneities. The correction techniques proposed assume a linear gradient of background inhomogeneities throughout a given voxel. However, if the gradients are non-linear, the correction methods become corrupted [55]. Redundant data collection and long scan times are also matters of concern.
- The negative contrast generated by the internalized iron extends well outside the boundaries of the cell is another limitation. This 'blooming' artifact leads to over-estimation of iron concentration.
- R_2* based methods suffer from partial volume effects. Ability to detect a signal void depends on the resolution of the image. The negative contrast generated by the intracellular SPIO particles depends on the position of the cell within a voxel. The negative contrast is more ideal for a cell positioned at the center of a voxel than that for a cell positioned at the edge [9].
- Slow flowing venous blood also generates hypointensities [5]. Suppression of the hypointensities can be achieved by administering paramagnetic contrast agent prior to imaging [67], commonly referred as susceptibility matching.

Cellular MRI: Positive Contrast Approaches

Given the inherent drawbacks of the negative contrast techniques, a new class of techniques has been developed to generate positive contrast from SPIO loaded cells. Studies have shown that the hypointense signal surrounding a point magnetic dipole (such as a cell labeled with iron) has a characteristic barbell pattern [68], which emanates from spatially distributed off-resonance frequencies surrounding the perturber. Over the past decade, several different techniques have been proposed, which selectively excite off-resonant protons associated with the iron oxide labeled cells, while suppressing the surrounding of on-resonant protons.

Off-Resonance Projection Imaging with Positive Contrast

Cunningham et al. were one of the first to propose the use of spectrally selective RF pulses that can excite and refocus off-resonant water surrounding the labeled cells while suppressing the on-resonant signal [69]. Therefore, only a thin shell of protons adjacent to the cells offset by particular values from the resonant frequency is excited and become visible as positive contrast in the image [69]. The boundaries of the excited shell vary depending on the excitation pulse profile, center-frequency shift, and the echo time. The authors have reported a detection limit of $5x10^5$ cells at 1.5T in-vitro, and a good correlation between the signal intensity and estimated number of cells. However, this method has a few limitations:

- Susceptibility-shift induced field inhomogeneities can shift background spins into the pass band, which can also be excited. Therefore, care should be taken not to set the off-resonance frequency bandwidth too close to the on-resonant water.
- Since the technique excites only spins that are off resonant by particular values from the on-resonant water, only a small volume surrounding the labeled cell can be excited. Thus, the amount of signal generated is limited.
- To maximize the signal generated, RF bandwidth can be set as wide as possible so that it excites a larger volume of off-resonant spins. However, this would also increase the T_2* decay and limit sensitivity and resolution. Therefore, RF bandwidth needs to be optimized for differently sized groups of cells.
- The technique employs projection imaging making it unsuitable for two-dimensional (2D) slice selection and three-dimensional (3D) spatial encoding [70].
- For slice selection, the gradient needs to be refocused by a negative lobe of half-duration or amplitude. Since the magnetic field gradients cannot be fully refocused by the negative lobe in the presence of iron, this technique is limited to spin echo imaging [70].

Based on the observations of Baklanov et al., [71], Foltz et al. [72] have combined the off-resonance positive contrast technique proposed by Cunningham et al., [69] with simultaneous intravascular injection of paramagnetic contrast agents. Rat fibroblasts labeled with 1-μm iron-oxide particles were intramuscularly injected into the rat hind limbs. They reported an improved signal-to-noise ratio (SNR) of the positive contrast regions at 1.5T following Gd-DTPA administration. The extent of positive contrast was shown to increase with the increase in the number of cells, and Gd-DTPA administration improved the detectability of cells numbering less than 2.5 x 10^5 [72]. The lowest detected number of cells was reported to be 2.5 x 10^4.

White Marker Technique

Seppenwoolde et al. proposed a 'White Marker' technique, in which the rephasing lobe of the slice selection gradient is reduced in strength so that the on-resonant spins are not fully rephased during the echo times [73]. However, in certain spatial regions with local magnetic gradients, the gradient imbalance is totally corrected and the spins are fully refocused and excited at the echo times [73]. While the feasibility of this approach has been demonstrated [73], there are inherent limitations with this technique as well:

- Susceptibility gradients only along the slice selection direction are compensated [5].
- Large gradient imbalances not only suppress on-resonant signal, but also reduce the SNR.
- The technique is still sensitive to any local magnetic gradients since other sources of magnetic gradients (e.g., air-water interface) can also result in background spins to get excited.
- Similar to the method proposed by Cunningham et al., only a small volume of spins surrounding the labeled cell with the correct field gradients is excited. Therefore, the amount of signal generated is limited.
- This method is limited only to the gradient echo techniques [70].

Mani et al., have proposed a derivative of this technique for imaging USPIO labeled cells at 1.5T and 3T [74].

Inversion Recovery with ON-Resonant Water Suppression (IRON)

Stuber et al. developed a technique, in which on-resonant signal is suppressed by saturating on resonant spins with a spectrally selective RF pulse of a limited bandwidth [70]. Off-resonant protons are not excited by this saturation pulse and, therefore, generate positive contrast surrounding the labeled cells [70]. Fat signal is suppressed using a dual inversion pre-pulse. By varying the bandwidth of the saturation pulse, the flip angle can control the size of the positive contrast. Importantly, the technique can be used with both gradient echo and spin echo techniques. The authors reported a linear correlation between volume of positive contrast and number of labeled cells. The technique could detect 1.25 x 10^5 and 2.5 x 10^5 cells at two different injection sites in-vivo [70]. However, the method suffers from B_1 inhomogeneity, and it compensates for B_0 inhomogeneities only along the slice selection direction [5].

Diffusion Mediated Off-Resonance Saturation

Zurkiya and Hu proposed a positive contrast technique using diffusion mediated off-resonance saturation [75]. By selectively applying off-resonance radiation, protons in some shells of the off-resonance region can be saturated, thereby causing signal reduction. Moreover, diffusion of protons into these shells causes an additional small volume of protons near the shells to be saturated. The total volume of saturation depends on the offset frequency, saturation, and the time a proton spends in the shell. The authors have reported increasing off-resonance saturation (ORS) effect with increasing iron concentration in-vitro. However, ORS effect varies linearly with iron at low concentrations. At higher concentrations, the diffusion contribution of adjacent iron particles becomes interdependent, and the relationship becomes non-linear. The authors identified the following limitations of this technique:

- The relationship between image contrast and intracellular iron is complex due to iron particle clustering and restricted diffusion. This renders the technique impractical for in-vivo cell detection and quantification.
- The magnetization transfer effects dominate in-vivo, and, therefore, it is difficult to detect the ORS effects. The authors suggested quantifying magnetization transfer effects prior to labeled cell transplantation.
- Similar to the other positive-contrast techniques, this technique is susceptible to B_0 inhomogeneity and fat.

Post-Processing Techniques for Generating Positive Contrast Images

Various post-processing techniques have also been proposed to derive positive-contrast images from magnetic field maps. Local magnetic gradients induced by the superparamagnetic contrast agent leads to echo shifts in k-space in gradient-echo imaging [76]. Local phase information was obtained through k-space filtering by Posse [77]. By subtracting the complex k-space filtered image from the magnitude-filtered image or by performing 1D Fast Fourier Transform (FFT) along the slice select direction and selecting the appropriate Fourier encoded slice, Reichenbach et al., generated positive contrast images [78]. Bakker et al. generated positive contrast images using a shifted reconstruction window to exploit the echo shifts [79].

Liu et al. proposed a susceptibility gradient mapping (SGM) method to generate a color map of the 3D susceptibility-gradient vector for each voxel by computing echo shifts in all three dimensions [76]. The authors compared the SGM technique with IRON and white marker techniques using SPIO-labeled C6 glioma tumors transplanted in the flanks of nude rats. SGM technique could detect significantly more positive pixels surrounding small and medium tumors compared to IRON and white marker techniques [76]. In large tumors, the number of positive pixels detected by all the methods is similar. Since this is a post-processing technique, it holds the advantage that no dedicated pulse-sequence design and no longer scan time are required.

Off-Resonance Positive Contrast MRI with Steady-State Free Precession (FLAPS)

This approach primarily relies on taking advantage of the flip-angle dependent spectral response profile of the steady-state free precession (SSFP) signals to generate signal enhancement from off-resonant spins, while suppressing the signal from on-resonant spins at relatively low flip angles. A complete theoretical basis for this approach and experimental validation of this approach can be found in [80, 81].

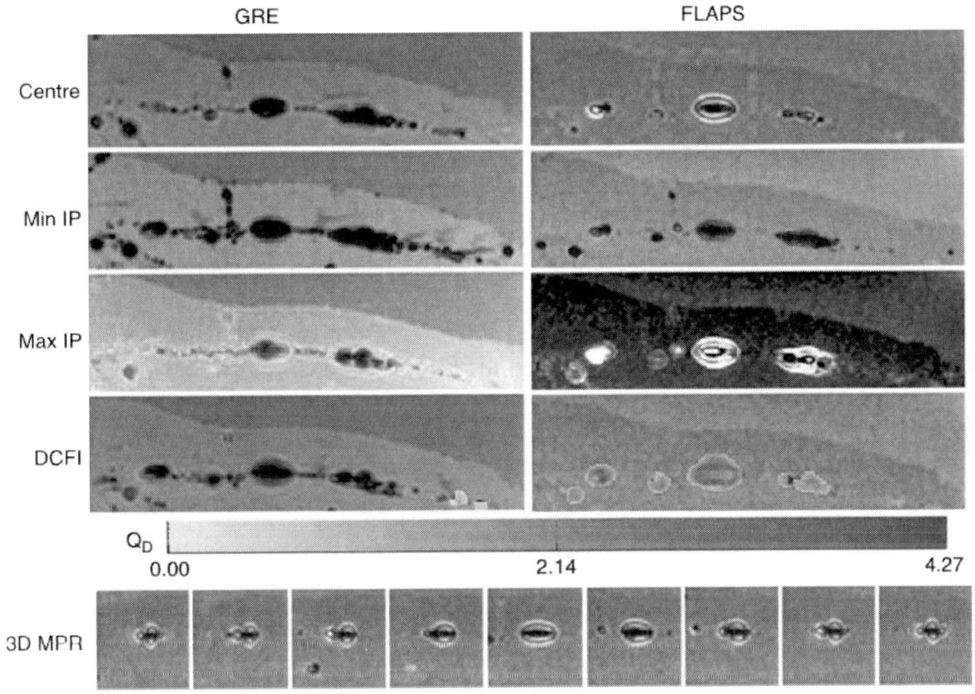

Figure 2.4. Gradient-recalled echo (GRE) and FLAPS images of labeled cells injected into ex vivo skeletal muscle. The results from the three-dimensional GRE and FLAPS acquisitions are shown along the left and right panels, respectively. Panels labeled Centre, Min IP, Max IP, and DCFI show the central slice, thin minimum and maximum intensity projections, and dual-contrast filtered image overlaid on top of the corresponding central GRE and FLAPS slices, respectively. The central slice is an imaging slice from the three-dimensional volume covering a slab thickness of 4.4 mm, with the slice thickness of 0.4 mm. Labeled cells are visualized as dark regions in GRE images, whereas FLAPS images identify them as regions of dark core surrounded bright contours. Min IP shows the dark regions surrounding labeled cells in both GRE and FLAPS images, whereas Max IP through the same slab shows the labeled cells as regions of brightness. DCFI labeled images shows the capacity for preferential identification and visualization of regions containing only labeled cells based on unique image processing filters. The color bar shows the output from DCFI (Q_D). Note that effectively no significant values are generated from the DCFI applied to the central GRE image. Three-dimensional MPR is a multiplanar reformation of the highlighted region (orange box) in the central FLAPS images over the full imaging volume, providing a means for visualizing the labeled cells throughout the imaging volume. Reprinted, with permission, from [82].

Theoretical and experimental studies have shown that the optimal image contrast using FLAPS is uniquely determined by the choice of flip angle and the characteristic flip angle is dependent on T_1/T_2 of the medium. FLAPS approach provides unique benefits:

- FLAPS has been shown to increase the sensitivity for detecting cell by a factor of two over the conventional T2* approach.
- The dual contrast feature of labeled cells within a FLAPS MR image significantly enhances the specificity of detection (Figure 2.4). The presence of low spin density, relaxation changes within the field-of-view, or blooming artifacts, all of which are well-known limitations of GRE imaging, are no longer impediments that decrease the specificity of labeled cells.
- It overcomes several key limitations of standard positive contrast imaging methods, such as the vulnerability to bulk frequency shifts, typically arising from air-tissue interfaces; signal from fat protons; or coil sensitivity variations, all of which appear as hyper-enhancements. Moreover, since a unique and easily identifiable contrast pattern is generated from the labeled cells in FLAPS images, image filters and furthermore detection algorithms that distinctly identify the topologic pattern can be implemented [82]. In addition, other positive contrast methods require fusing an anatomic image with positive contrast image, which has limitations when acquisitions are acquired separately and motion between acquisitions is present. This is not necessary with FLAPS MRI since the desirable contrast and anatomical features are captured within the same image.
- FLAPS MRI is a fast imaging method, a feature that is highly desirable for any imaging approach that can benefit clinical application.
- FLAPS MRI uses low flip angles, compared to standard spin-echo approaches, reducing concerns related to tissue heating in acquisitions that demand ultra-high spatial resolutions, which necessitate multiple averaging. The inability to control or minimize the thermal dose delivered during cell imaging studies may compromise cell function and the overall benefits of imaging studies.

Nonetheless, the optimal contrast-to-noise ratio (CNR) between the labeled cells and the surrounding based on FLAPS diminishes as T_1/T_2 increases, which can limit its use in some applications.

Cell Tracking with ^{19}F MRI

Over the past 5-10 years, fluorine-19 (^{19}F) MRI has attracted significant attention for cell tracking as an alternative to the more commonly utilized proton MRI (^{1}H-MRI) approaches discussed above. The key advantages of ^{19}F compared to ^{1}H-MRI are: (a) long-term cell tracking; (b) the absence of background ^{19}F-MRI signal, which potentially permits accurate detection and quantification of cells; and (c) physiological compatibility, given that perfluorocarbon is a common blood substitute. Importantly, when ^{19}F and standard ^{1}H-MRI are acquired in an interleaved fashion and rapidly fused together, accurate detection of cells of interest (labeled with ^{19}F label) within the anatomy of interest becomes possible (Figure

2.5). However, to generate detectable amount of signal, sufficient ^{19}F must be loaded onto the cell, which is particularly difficult in non-phagocytic cells, such as stem cells. Many different formulations of ^{19}F, such as emulsions, particles, and polymers, have been developed for pre-clinical and clinical use. In general, the in-vivo specificity of ^{19}F is enhanced by (a) functionalization of ^{19}F agents with cell-specific probes; or by (b) the use of "smart" ^{19}F agents that change chemical properties upon interaction with a molecular target. In spite these advances, the binding of the agent to a surface molecule is limited and presents the primary challenge for in vivo ^{19}F-MRI. Moreover, as with iron-based agents, ^{19}F-MRI may not be able to discriminate between live/dead cells or loss of tag by the cells of interest.

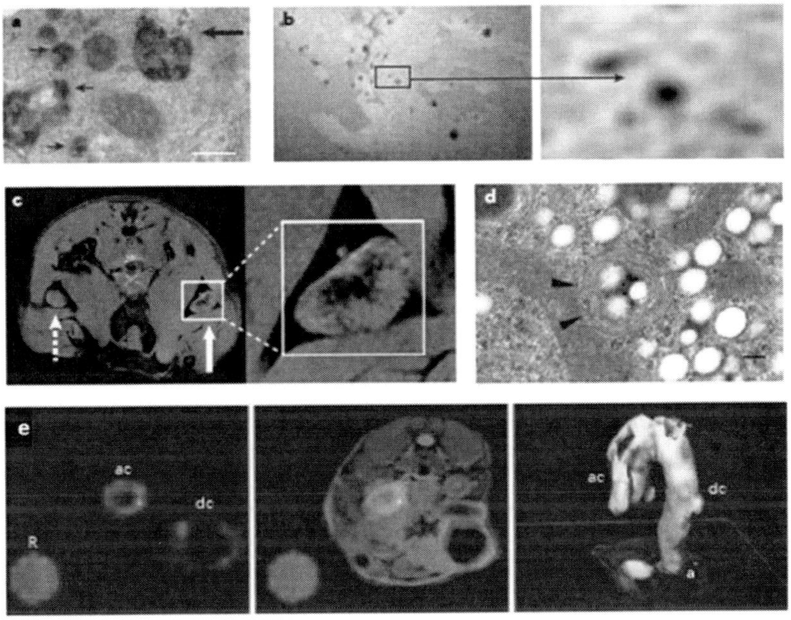

Figure 2.5. Tracking immune cells with MRI using SPIO nanoparticles and perfluorcarbon emulsions. (a) Intracellular labelling of mononuclear cells with magnetoliposomes is shown. The electron micrograph shows SPIO particles in secondary lysosomes (small arrows) and in primary lysosomes that are fusing with endosomes (large arrow). The scale bar represents 200 nm. (b) Imaging of a non-obese diabetic (NOD)–severe combined immunodeficient (SCID) mouse pancreas ex vivo is shown following the adoptive transfer of SPIO-labelled T cells. Image hypointensities represent infiltrating T cells that are observed at 24 hours post transfer. (c) Imaging of in vivo antigen capture and trafficking of dendritic cells (DCs) is shown. Sentinel DCs were labelled in situ by intradermal injection of unlabeled (dashed arrow) or SPIO-labelled (solid arrow) irradiated cancer cells, which function as a vaccine. Following phagocytosis of both SPIO particles and tumor antigens in a process known as magnetovaccination, the hypointense DCs migrate into the medulla of the draining popliteal lymph node, as observed on day 8. (d) An electron micrograph of a perfluorocarbon (PFC)-labeled DC is shown. Numerous bright spots (PFC droplets) are observed inside the cell. Particles appear as smooth spheroids. Arrowheads indicate vesicles. The scale bar represents 200 nm. (e) Inflammatory bowel disease (IBD) in an interleukin-10 (Il10)−/− mouse model was visualized using in situ PFC labelling and ^{19}F MRI in vivo. The ^{19}F image (pseudo-color) is shown on the far left, the composite ^{1}H and ^{19}F image is shown in the middle and a three-dimensional rendering of the in vivo ^{19}F MRI data from the abdomen is shown on the far right. A reference tube that contains PFC emulsion (R) was placed alongside the torso of the mouse. The images through the abdomen show PFC accumulation (indicating inflammation) in the ascending colon (ac) and descending colon (dc), where (a) is the anus. Reprinted, with permission, from [83].

Challenges Facing Cellular MRI

Differentiating Intracellular and Extracellular Iron, Viable and Lysed Cells

Concerns have been raised about the inability of the R_2* based imaging to discriminate between intracellular and extracellular iron. Kuhlpeter et al. have demonstrated that mean R_2 values are greater for free iron than those for the intracellular iron, while the reverse holds true for the R_2* values. Therefore, calculating the difference (R_2') between R_2 and R_2*, intracellular and extracellular iron can be differentiated [65]. However, correction techniques still need to be applied for the correct estimation of R_2 and R_2* values. Concerns have also been raised about the inability to discriminate between viable and lysed cells in-vivo. Henning et al. have demonstrated that the T_2 values markedly decreased upon lysis of the cells and liberation of the iron particles [66]. The authors suggest that this may be due to a more uniform dispersion of the iron particles upon liberation and increased diffusion of water molecules through the microscopic field inhomogeneities. On the other hand, T_2* values remained relatively unaffected upon disruption as the static field inhomogeneity would be less altered upon disruption. Therefore, T_2 weighted spin echo sequences can be employed to discriminate between viable and lysed cells. This limitation is expected to extend to positive contrast imaging approaches as well.

Intracellular Iron Dilution upon Cell Division and Apoptosis

Continuous stem cell proliferation can lead to rapid dilution of the iron oxide particles and loss of signal from the cells. In a study by Walczak et al., significant cell division had led to the rapid dilution of the iron particles between mother and daughter cells towards undetectable levels [84]. In this study, neural stem cells were transplanted into the Shiverer demyelinated mouse brain. There was a strong mismatch between the hypointense MR signal and histological observations 6 days post-transplantation [84]. There was a sharp cut-off in the MR signal rather than a gradual decrease. The authors attribute this observation to rapid asymmetric cell division of neural stem cells. As indicated earlier, MPIOs can be useful in such a case as even single MPIO particle internalized by the cell is sufficient to generate the necessary contrast [12]. Nonetheless, Terrovitis et al. have reported that MRI over-estimates transplanted Ferumoxide labeled stem cells as iron particles from cells undergoing apoptosis can be taken up by macrophages. Histological observations revealed a significant number of iron-loaded macrophages in the injection site as compared to very few transplanted stem cells in a cardiac application [85].

Baklanov et al. have reported that cells delivered to the peri-infarct regions of a one-week old transmural myocardial infarction in pigs can be detected better with a double-contrast mechanism using a combination of paramagnetic and superparamagnetic contrast agents [71]. The authors suggested that the R_2* values of the intracellular iron increases linearly with increasing intravascular concentration of the paramagnetic agent. The concentration of the intravascular paramagnetic agent in turn varies with the micro-architectural differences between normal, infarcted and ischemic myocardium. This can facilitate better detection of the iron labeled cells in-vivo, even upon dilution due to cell division or apoptosis.

Impact of Iron Oxides on Cell Viability, Differentiation, Proliferation and Function

In general, cells labeled with SPIO particles have not shown to affect cell viability or proliferation capacity, although there are exceptions. Kostura and colleagues showed that mesenchymal cells labeled with SPIOs could block cell differentiation along a specific pathway without affecting viability or proliferation [86]. Other studies have shown that human mesenchymal stem cell proliferation can be promoted by SPIOs nanoparticles [87]. Recent studies by Berman et al. have shown that the migratory capacity of neural stem cells is reduced after SPIO labeling [88].

Tissue Hemorrhage

In cases where therapeutic cells are expected to be of great benefit after a traumatic injury, one of the limitations of cellular MRI in tracking the iron-labeled cells is the presence of hemorrhage and its long lasting degradation products, typically in the form of hemosiderin. Hemosiderin has been shown to persist in stroke patients well past a year after an acute injury [89, 90] and at least six months post myocardial infarction [91].

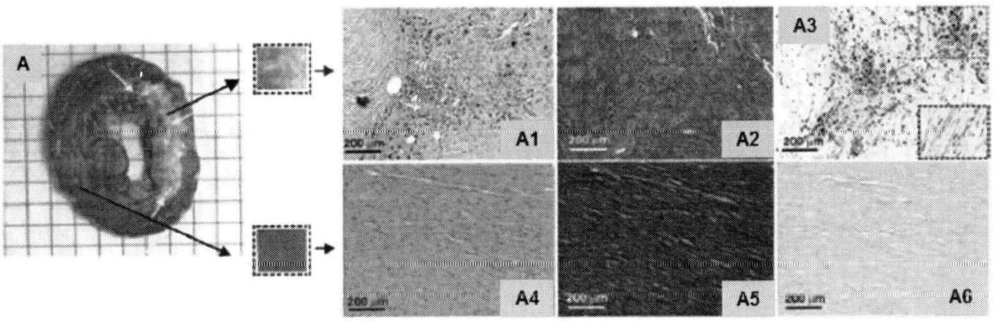

Figure 2.6. Histological validation of chronic iron deposition in hemorrhagic myocardial infarction. (A) Gross histochemical staining (triphenyl tetrazolium chloride [TTC]) of short-axis sections of hearts shows the site of chronic myocardial infarction (pale color, yellow arrows. Histopathology (x 100 magnification) of chronic infarct (A1–A6) and corresponding remote sections shows grossly damaged myocardium (hematoxylin and eosin), dense deposition of collagen (Masson trichrome), and iron (Perls stain; black arrows; inset) in the infarcted section (not observed in remote territories). Insets show detailed views of tissue structures collected from regions indicated by arrows. Note the presence of iron mixed in with viable cells and intact blood vessels (lower inset of A3 obtained from infarct border). Reprinted, with permission, from [91].

While hemorrhage may not always be present at the site of injury, it is often associated with significant tissue damage, a case where therapeutic generation may be of significant value. The MRI signal features of hemosiderin is essentially similar to iron labeled cells as they both impart the same biophysical effects on MR images; hence long-term tracking of labeled cells would need to establish the baseline levels of hemosiderin prior to cell delivery, otherwise, hemosiderin could be mistakenly identified as iron-labeled cells (Figure 2.6). In cases where hemosiderin is present in the damaged tissue, it may also be important to consider the pathogenic features of hemosiderin as it has been shown to facilitate chronic inflammation in the heart [91].

Future of Cellular MRI

Cellular MRI is expected to be an indispensible imaging tool since it is non-invasive, and permits serial imaging to visualize the cells as well as the therapeutic benefit that the cells impart to repair the organ system. Nonetheless, there are a few key areas of investigations that are much needed to further enhance the capabilities of cellular MRI:

- Novel, biologically inert contrast media that can increase the sensitivity of detection without increasing the payload to the cells are still needed. Newer contrast agents [92] that are in the horizon, such as iron-cobalt particles, gadolinium core, and ferrite nano wontons are expected to markedly improve the sensitivity of MRI for detecting cells;
- Regenerative medicine in particular stands to benefit markedly if MRI can be used to successfully track the transplanted cells over multiple cell divisions. Much work is needed in this arena given the current challenges associated with the existing methods to discriminate between endogenous and exogenous iron owing to the presence of tissue hemorrhage, which can mimic labeled cells.
- Accurate quantification of transplanted cells with MRI is also expected to be critical since it will be important to establish the number of cells that are retained following delivery in the overall assessment of therapeutic efficacy of the various cell formulations.
- With the growing availability of multi-modal imaging systems such as hybrid PET/MR scanners, the key advantages of both MRI (soft-tissue contrast) and PET imaging (sensitivity to contrast agents), are expected to be captured together to advance cellular imaging.

References

[1] Zhang SJ, Wu JC. Comparison of imaging techniques for tracking cardiac stem cell therapy. *J. Nucl. Med.* 2007;48(12):1916-1919.

[2] Kraitchman DL, Bulte JW. Imaging of stem cells using MRI. *Basic Res. Cardiol.* 2008;103(2):105-113.

[3] Rogers WJ, Meyer CH, Kramer CM. Technology insight: in vivo cell tracking by use of MRI. *Nat. Clin. Pract. Cardiovasc Med* 2006;3(10):554-562.

[4] Crich SG, Biancone L, Cantaluppi V, Duo D, Esposito G, Russo S, et al., Improved route for the visualization of stem cells labeled with a Gd-/Eu-chelate as dual (MRI and fluorescence) agent. *Magn. Reson. Med.* 2004;51(5):938-944.

[5] Liu W, Frank JA. Detection and quantification of magnetically labeled cells by cellular MRI. *Eur. J. Radiol.* 2009;70(2):258-264.

[6] Anderson SA, Lee KK, Frank JA. Gadolinium-fullerenol as a paramagnetic contrast agent for cellular imaging. *Invest Radiol.* 2006;41(3):332-338.

[7] Brekke C, Morgan SC, Lowe AS, Meade TJ, Price J, Williams SC, et al., The in vitro effects of a bimodal contrast agent on cellular functions and relaxometry. *NMR Biomed.* 2007;20(2):77-89.

[8] Bulte JW, Kraitchman DL. Iron oxide MR contrast agents for molecular and cellular imaging. NMR Biomed 2004;17(7):484-499.

[9] Heyn C, Bowen CV, Rutt BK, Foster PJ. Detection threshold of single SPIO-labeled cells with FIESTA. *Magn. Reson. Med.* 2005;53(2):312-320.

[10] Shapiro EM, Skrtic S, Koretsky AP. Sizing it up: cellular MRI using micron-sized iron oxide particles. *Magn. Reson. Med.* 2005;53(2):329-338.

[11] Arbab AS, Bashaw LA, Miller BR, Jordan EK, Lewis BK, Kalish H, et al., Characterization of biophysical and metabolic properties of cells labeled with superparamagnetic iron oxide nanoparticles and transfection agent for cellular MR imaging. *Radiology* 2003;229(3):838-846.

[12] Shapiro EM, Skrtic S, Koretsky AP. *Long term cellular MR imaging using micron sized iron oxide particles.* in *12th Annual Meeting of ISMRM.* 2004.

[13] Wu YL, Ye Q, Foley LM, Hitchens TK, Sato K, Williams JB, et al., In situ labeling of immune cells with iron oxide particles: an approach to detect organ rejection by cellular MRI. *Proc. Natl. Acad. Sci. USA* 2006;103(6):1852-1857.

[14] Shapiro EM, Skrtic S, Sharer K, Hill JM, Dunbar CE, Koretsky AP. MRI detection of single particles for cellular imaging. *Proc. Natl. Acad. Sci. USA* 2004;101(30):10901-10906.

[15] Shapiro EM, Sharer K, Skrtic S, Koretsky AP. In vivo detection of single cells by MRI. *Magn. Reson. Med.* 2006;55(2):242-249.

[16] Heyn C, Ronald JA, Mackenzie LT, MacDonald IC, Chambers AF, Rutt BK, et al., In vivo magnetic resonance imaging of single cells in mouse brain with optical validation. *Magn. Reson. Med.* 2006;55(1):23-29.

[17] Hinds KA, Hill JM, Shapiro EM, Laukkanen MO, Silva AC, Combs CA, et al., Highly efficient endosomal labeling of progenitor and stem cells with large magnetic particles allows magnetic resonance imaging of single cells. *Blood* 2003;102(3):867-872.

[18] Sumner JP, Shapiro EM, Maric D, Conroy R, Koretsky AP. In vivo labeling of adult neural progenitors for MRI with micron sized particles of iron oxide: quantification of labeled cell phenotype. *Neuroimage* 2009;44(3):671-678.

[19] Jung CW, Jacobs P. Physical and chemical properties of superparamagnetic iron oxide MR contrast agents: ferumoxides, ferumoxtran, ferumoxsil. *Magn. Reson. Imaging* 1995;13(5):661-674.

[20] Wang YX, Hussain SM, Krestin GP. Superparamagnetic iron oxide contrast agents: physicochemical characteristics and applications in MR imaging. *Eur. Radiol.* 2001;11(11):2319-2331.

[21] Islam T, Wolf G. The pharmacokinetics of the lymphotropic nanoparticle MRI contrast agent ferumoxtran-10. *Cancer Biomark* 2009;5(2):69-73.

[22] Stark DD, Weissleder R, Elizondo G, Hahn PF, Saini S, Todd LE, et al., Superparamagnetic iron oxide: clinical application as a contrast agent for MR imaging of the liver. *Radiology* 1988;168(2):297-301.

[23] Weissleder R. Liver MR imaging with iron oxides: toward consensus and clinical practice. *Radiology* 1994;193(3):593-595.
[24] Weissleder R, Heautot JF, Schaffer BK, Nossiff N, Papisov MI, Bogdanov A, Jr., et al., MR lymphography: study of a high-efficiency lymphotrophic agent. *Radiology* 1994;191(1):225-230.
[25] Harisinghani MG, Barentsz J, Hahn PF, Deserno WM, Tabatabaei S, van de Kaa CH, et al., Noninvasive detection of clinically occult lymph-node metastases in prostate cancer. *N. Engl. J. Med.* 2003;348(25):2491-2499.
[26] Seneterre E, Weissleder R, Jaramillo D, Reimer P, Lee AS, Brady TJ, et al., Bone marrow: ultrasmall superparamagnetic iron oxide for MR imaging. *Radiology* 1991;179(2):529-533.
[27] Xu S, Jordan EK, Brocke S, Bulte JW, Quigley L, Tresser N, et al., Study of relapsing remitting experimental allergic encephalomyelitis SJL mouse model using MION-46L enhanced in vivo MRI: early histopathological correlation. *J. Neurosci. Res.* 1998;52(5):549-558.
[28] Rausch M, Hiestand P, Baumann D, Cannet C, Rudin M. MRI-based monitoring of inflammation and tissue damage in acute and chronic relapsing EAE. *Magn. Reson. Med.* 2003;50(2):309-314.
[29] Rausch M, Baumann D, Neubacher U, Rudin M. In-vivo visualization of phagocytotic cells in rat brains after transient ischemia by USPIO. *NMR Biomed.* 2002;15(4):278-283.
[30] Beckmann N, Falk R, Zurbrugg S, Dawson J, Engelhardt P. Macrophage infiltration into the rat knee detected by MRI in a model of antigen-induced arthritis. *Magn. Reson. Med.* 2003;49(6):1047-1055.
[31] Ruehm SG, Corot C, Vogt P, Kolb S, Debatin JF. Magnetic resonance imaging of atherosclerotic plaque with ultrasmall superparamagnetic particles of iron oxide in hyperlipidemic rabbits. *Circulation* 2001;103(3):415-422.
[32] Jo SK, Hu X, Kobayashi H, Lizak M, Miyaji T, Koretsky A, et al., Detection of inflammation following renal ischemia by magnetic resonance imaging. *Kidney Int.* 2003;64(1):43-51.
[33] Hauger O, Delalande C, Trillaud H, Deminiere C, Quesson B, Kahn H, et al., MR imaging of intrarenal macrophage infiltration in an experimental model of nephrotic syndrome. *Magn. Reson. Med.* 1999;41(1):156-162.
[34] Hauger O, Delalande C, Deminiere C, Fouqueray B, Ohayon C, Garcia S, et al., Nephrotoxic nephritis and obstructive nephropathy: evaluation with MR imaging enhanced with ultrasmall superparamagnetic iron oxide-preliminary findings in a rat model. *Radiology* 2000;217(3):819-826.
[35] Kanno S, Wu YJ, Lee PC, Dodd SJ, Williams M, Griffith BP, et al., Macrophage accumulation associated with rat cardiac allograft rejection detected by magnetic resonance imaging with ultrasmall superparamagnetic iron oxide particles. *Circulation* 2001;104(8):934-938.
[36] Zhang Y, Dodd SJ, Hendrich KS, Williams M, Ho C. Magnetic resonance imaging detection of rat renal transplant rejection by monitoring macrophage infiltration. *Kidney Int.* 2000;58(3):1300-1310.
[37] Frank JA, Zywicke H, Jordan EK, Mitchell J, Lewis BK, Miller B, et al., Magnetic intracellular labeling of mammalian cells by combining (FDA-approved)

superparamagnetic iron oxide MR contrast agents and commonly used transfection agents. *Acad. Radiol.* 2002;9 Suppl 2(S484-487.

[38] Bulte JW, Douglas T, Witwer B, Zhang SC, Strable E, Lewis BK, et al., Magnetodendrimers allow endosomal magnetic labeling and in vivo tracking of stem cells. *Nat. Biotechnol.* 2001;19(12):1141-1147.

[39] Sykova E, Jendelova P, Herynek V. MR tracking of stem cells in living recipients. *Methods Mol. Biol.* 2009;549(197-215.

[40] Politi LS, Bacigaluppi M, Brambilla E, Cadioli M, Falini A, Comi G, et al., Magnetic-resonance-based tracking and quantification of intravenously injected neural stem cell accumulation in the brains of mice with experimental multiple sclerosis. *Stem Cells* 2007;25(10):2583-2592.

[41] Hill JM, Dick AJ, Raman VK, Thompson RB, Yu ZX, Hinds KA, et al., Serial cardiac magnetic resonance imaging of injected mesenchymal stem cells. *Circulation* 2003;108(8):1009-1014.

[42] Kraitchman DL, Heldman AW, Atalar E, Amado LC, Martin BJ, Pittenger MF, et al., In vivo magnetic resonance imaging of mesenchymal stem cells in myocardial infarction. *Circulation* 2003;107(18):2290-2293.

[43] Sorger JM, Despres D, Schimel D, McVeigh ER, Hill JM. *MRI tracking of stem cell homing to myocardial infarction.* in *11th Annual Meeting of the International Society for Magnetic Resonance in Medicine*. 2003. Toronto, ON.

[44] Kustermann E, Roell W, Breitbach M, Wecker S, Wiedermann D, Buehrle C, et al., Stem cell implantation in ischemic mouse heart: a high-resolution magnetic resonance imaging investigation. *NMR Biomed.* 2005;18(6):362-370.

[45] Bowen CV, Zhang X, Saab G, Gareau PJ, Rutt BK. Application of the static dephasing regime theory to superparamagnetic iron-oxide loaded cells. *Magn. Reson. Med.* 2002;48(1):52-61.

[46] Yablonskiy DA, Haacke EM. Theory of NMR signal behavior in magnetically inhomogeneous tissues: the static dephasing regime. *Magn. Reson. Med.* 1994;32(6):749-763.

[47] Rad AM, Arbab AS, Iskander AS, Jiang Q, Soltanian-Zadeh H. Quantification of superparamagnetic iron oxide (SPIO)-labeled cells using MRI. *J. Magn. Reson. Imaging* 2007;26(2):366-374.

[48] Dodd SJ, Williams M, Suhan JP, Williams DS, Koretsky AP, Ho C. Detection of single mammalian cells by high-resolution magnetic resonance imaging. *Biophys. J.* 1999;76(1 Pt 1):103-109.

[49] Lewin M, Carlesso N, Tung CH, Tang XW, Cory D, Scadden DT, et al., Tat peptide-derivatized magnetic nanoparticles allow in vivo tracking and recovery of progenitor cells. *Nat. Biotechnol.* 2000;18(4):410-414.

[50] Majors PD, Ackerman EJ, Wind RA, Douglas T, Bulte JW. *MR microscopy of magnetodendrimer uptake in single cells.* in *10th Annual Meeting of the International Society for Magentic Resonance in Medicine*. 2002. Denver, CO.

[51] Hoehn M, Kustermann E, Blunk J, Wiedermann D, Trapp T, Wecker S, et al., Monitoring of implanted stem cell migration in vivo: a highly resolved in vivo magnetic resonance imaging investigation of experimental stroke in rat. *Proc. Natl. Acad. Sci. USA* 2002;99(25):16267-16272.

[52] Jendelova P, Herynek V, DeCroos J, Glogarova K, Andersson B, Hajek M, et al., Imaging the fate of implanted bone marrow stromal cells labeled with superparamagnetic nanoparticles. *Magn. Reson. Med.* 2003;50(4):767-776.
[53] Kircher MF, Allport JR, Graves EE, Love V, Josephson L, Lichtman AH, et al., In vivo high resolution three-dimensional imaging of antigen-specific cytotoxic T-lymphocyte trafficking to tumors. *Cancer Res.* 2003;63(20):6838-6846.
[54] Foster-Gareau P, Heyn C, Alejski A, Rutt BK. Imaging single mammalian cells with a 1.5 T clinical MRI scanner. *Magn. Reson. Med.* 2003;49(5):968-971.
[55] Dahnke H, Schaeffter T. Limits of detection of SPIO at 3.0 T using T2 relaxometry. *Magn. Reson. Med.* 2005;53(5):1202-1206.
[56] Stark DD. Hepatic iron overload: paramagnetic pathology. *Radiology* 1991;179(2):333-335.
[57] Stark DD, Moseley ME, Bacon BR, Moss AA, Goldberg HI, Bass NM, et al., Magnetic resonance imaging and spectroscopy of hepatic iron overload. *Radiology* 1985;154(1):137-142.
[58] Bulte JW, Miller GF, Vymazal J, Brooks RA, Frank JA. Hepatic hemosiderosis in non-human primates: quantification of liver iron using different field strengths. *Magn. Reson. Med.* 1997;37(4):530-536.
[59] Bos C, Delmas Y, Desmouliere A, Solanilla A, Hauger O, Grosset C, et al., In vivo MR imaging of intravascularly injected magnetically labeled mesenchymal stem cells in rat kidney and liver. *Radiology* 2004;233(3):781-789.
[60] Young IR, Cox IJ, Bryant DJ, Bydder GM. The benefits of increasing spatial resolution as a means of reducing artifacts due to field inhomogeneities. *Magn. Reson. Imaging* 1988;6(5):585-590.
[61] Frahm J, Merboldt KD, Hanicke W. Direct FLASH MR imaging of magnetic field inhomogeneities by gradient compensation. *Magn. Reson. Med.* 1988;6(4):474-480.
[62] Cho ZH, Ro YM. Reduction of susceptibility artifact in gradient-echo imaging. *Magn. Reson. Med.* 1992;23(1):193-200.
[63] Liu W, Dahnke H, Rahmer J, Jordan EK, Frank JA. Ultrashort T2* relaxometry for quantitation of highly concentrated superparamagnetic iron oxide (SPIO) nanoparticle labeled cells. *Magn. Reson. Med.* 2009;61(4):761-766.
[64] Crowe LA, Wang YX, Gatehouse P. *Ex vivo MR imaging of atherosclerotic rabbit aorta labeled with USPIO – enhancement of iron loaded regions in UTE imaging*. in *13th Annual Meeting of the International Society for Magentic Resonance in Medicine*. 2005. Miami, FL.
[65] Kuhlpeter R, Dahnke H, Matuszewski L, Persigehl T, von Wallbrunn A, Allkemper T, et al., R2 and R2* mapping for sensing cell-bound superparamagnetic nanoparticles: in vitro and murine in vivo testing. *Radiology* 2007;245(2):449-457.
[66] Henning TD, Wendland MF, Golovko D, Sutton EJ, Sennino B, Malek F, et al., Relaxation effects of ferucarbotran-labeled mesenchymal stem cells at 1.5T and 3T: discrimination of viable from lysed cells. *Magn. Reson. Med.* 2009;62(2):325-332.
[67] Anderson SA, Glod J, Arbab AS, Noel M, Ashari P, Fine HA, et al., Noninvasive MR imaging of magnetically labeled stem cells to directly identify neovasculature in a glioma model. *Blood* 2005;105(1):420-425.
[68] Kim JK, Kucharczyk W, Henkelman RM. Cavernous hemangiomas: dipolar susceptibility artifacts at MR imaging. *Radiology* 1993;187(3):735-741.

[69] Cunningham CH, Arai T, Yang PC, McConnell MV, Pauly JM, Conolly SM. Positive contrast magnetic resonance imaging of cells labeled with magnetic nanoparticles. *Magn. Reson. Med.* 2005;53(5):999-1005.

[70] Stuber M, Gilson WD, Schar M, Kedziorek DA, Hofmann LV, Shah S, et al., Positive contrast visualization of iron oxide-labeled stem cells using inversion-recovery with ON-resonant water suppression (IRON). *Magn. Reson. Med.* 2007;58(5):1072-1077.

[71] Baklanov DV, Demuinck ED, Thompson CA, Pearlman JD. Novel double contrast MRI technique for intramyocardial detection of percutaneously transplanted autologous cells. *Magn. Reson. Med.* 2004;52(6):1438-1442.

[72] Foltz WD, Cunningham CH, Mutsaers AJ, Conolly SM, Stewart DJ, Dick AJ. Positive-contrast imaging in the rabbit hind-limb of transplanted cells bearing endocytosed superparamagnetic beads. *J. Cardiovasc. Magn. Reson.* 2006;8(6):817-823.

[73] Seppenwoolde JH, Viergever MA, Bakker CJ. Passive tracking exploiting local signal conservation: the white marker phenomenon. *Magn. Reson. Med.* 2003;50(4):784-790.

[74] Mani V, Briley-Saebo KC, Itskovich VV, Samber DD, Fayad ZA. Gradient echo acquisition for superparamagnetic particles with positive contrast (GRASP): sequence characterization in membrane and glass superparamagnetic iron oxide phantoms at 1.5T and 3T. *Magn. Reson. Med.* 2006;55(1):126-135.

[75] Zurkiya O, Hu X. Off-resonance saturation as a means of generating contrast with superparamagnetic nanoparticles. *Magn. Reson. Med.* 2006;56(4):726-732.

[76] Liu W, Dahnke H, Jordan EK, Schaeffter T, Frank JA. In vivo MRI using positive-contrast techniques in detection of cells labeled with superparamagnetic iron oxide nanoparticles. *NMR Biomed.* 2008;21(3):242-250.

[77] Posse S. Direct imaging of magnetic field gradients by group spin-echo selection. *Magn. Reson. Med.* 1992;25(1):12-29.

[78] Reichenbach JR, Venkatesan R, Yablonskiy DA, Thompson MR, Lai S, Haacke EM. Theory and application of static field inhomogeneity effects in gradient-echo imaging. *J. Magn. Reson. Imaging* 1997;7(2):266-279.

[79] Bakker CJ, Seppenwoolde JH, Vincken KL. Dephased MRI. *Magn. Reson. Med.* 2006;55(1):92-97.

[80] Dharmakumar R, Koktzoglou I, Li D. Generating positive contrast from off-resonant spins with steady-state free precession magnetic resonance imaging: theory and proof-of-principle experiments. *Phys. Med. Biol.* 2006;51(17):4201-4215.

[81] Dharmakumar R, Koktzoglou I, Li D. Factors influencing fast low angle positive contrast steady-state free precession (FLAPS) magnetic resonance imaging. *Phys. Med. Biol.* 2007;52(11):3261-3273.

[82] Dharmakumar R, Zhang Z, Koktzoglou I, Tsaftaris SA, Li D. Dual-contrast cellular magnetic resonance imaging. *Mol. Imaging* 2009;8(5):254-263.

[83] Ahrens ET, Bulte JW. Tracking immune cells in vivo using magnetic resonance imaging. *Nat. Rev. Immunol.* 2013;13(10):755-763.

[84] Walczak P, Kedziorek DA, Gilad AA, Barnett BP, Bulte JW. Applicability and limitations of MR tracking of neural stem cells with asymmetric cell division and rapid turnover: the case of the shiverer dysmyelinated mouse brain. *Magn. Reson. Med.* 2007;58(2):261-269.

[85] Terrovitis J, Stuber M, Youssef A, Preece S, Leppo M, Kizana E, et al., Magnetic resonance imaging overestimates ferumoxide-labeled stem cell survival after transplantation in the heart. *Circulation* 2008;117(12):1555-1562.

[86] Kostura L, Kraitchman DL, Mackay AM, Pittenger MF, Bulte JW. Feridex labeling of mesenchymal stem cells inhibits chondrogenesis but not adipogenesis or osteogenesis. *NMR Biomed.* 2004;17(7):513-517.

[87] Huang DM, Hsiao JK, Chen YC, Chien LY, Yao M, Chen YK, et al., The promotion of human mesenchymal stem cell proliferation by superparamagnetic iron oxide nanoparticles. *Biomaterials* 2009;30(22):3645-3651.

[88] Cromer Berman SM, Kshitiz, Wang CJ, Orukari I, Levchenko A, Bulte JW, et al., Cell motility of neural stem cells is reduced after SPIO-labeling, which is mitigated after exocytosis. *Magn. Reson. Med.* 2013;69(1):255-262.

[89] Bradley WG, Jr. MR appearance of hemorrhage in the brain. *Radiology* 1993;189(1):15-26.

[90] Schenck JF, Zimmerman EA. High-field magnetic resonance imaging of brain iron: birth of a biomarker? *NMR Biomed.* 2004;17(7):433-445.

[91] Kali A, Kumar A, Cokic I, Tang RL, Tsaftaris SA, Friedrich MG, et al., Chronic manifestation of postreperfusion intramyocardial hemorrhage as regional iron deposition: a cardiovascular magnetic resonance study with ex vivo validation. *Circ. Cardiovasc. Imaging* 2013;6(2):218-228.

[92] Bouchard LS, Anwar MS, Liu GL, Hann B, Xie ZH, Gray JW, et al., Picomolar sensitivity MRI and photoacoustic imaging of cobalt nanoparticles. *Proc. Natl. Acad. Sci. USA* 2009;106(11):4085-4089.

In: Magnetic Resonance Imaging of Stem Cell Applications ISBN: 978-1-63463-910-1
Editor: Xiaoming Yang

Chapter 3

Direct Magnetic Labeling of Stem Cells*

Bensheng Qiu, Thomas Matula, Norman Beauchamp Jr. and Xiaoming Yang*#
Image-Guided Bio-Molecular Intervention Research,
Department of Radiology, Institute for Stem Cell and Regenerative Medicine,
University of Washington School of Medicine, Seattle, Washington, US

Abstract

Noninvasive MRI is an important tool in guiding stem cell delivery, tracking stem cell migration, and accessing stem cell functions *in vivo*. Recent efforts have focused on the development of efficient, convenient and safe techniques for magnetic labeling of stem cells. In this chapter, we first introduce MRI contrast agents (such as T1, T2, ^{19}F contrast agents) for magnetic cell labeling, and then review direct magnetic cell labeling techniques, including simply incubation, magnetoelectroporation, and magnetosonoporation. With the development of direct magnetic cell labeling techniques, MRI-guided stem cell therapy is becoming a promising tool in regeneration medicine.

Keywords: MR contract agent, stem cell, simple incubation, magnetoelectroporation, magnetosonoporation

Introduction

Stem cells have being explored for regenerative repair of damaged or diseased tissues and organs [1]. Non-invasive *in vivo* imaging of stem cell therapies is essential for the success of

* This work was supported by National Institutes of Health R01EB012467 grant, RSNA RSD 0719 grant, Royalty Research Fund, and Washington State Life Science Discovery Fund.
# Corresponding author: Xiaoming Yang, MD, PhD, (xmyang@uw.edu).

both basic research and clinical applications of stem cell technology. Cellular magnetic resonance imaging (MRI), with its high spatial resolution and excellent tissue contrast, is becoming an important tool in guiding stem cell delivery, tracking stem cell migration/homing, and assessing survival and functions of transplanted stem cells. One of the key steps for *in vivo* MR imaging of stem cells is to pre-label the cells with sufficient MRI contrast agents, so-called direct magnetic cell labeling, and then transplant the pre-labeled cells into the body, which can be followed up by cellular MRI [2, 3]. Recently, tremendous effort has focused on the development of direct magnetic cell labeling techniques to label stem cells with MR contrast agents in an efficient, convenient and safe manner, with specific emphasis on their potential clinical application. In this chapter, we first summarize the currently available MRI contrast agents for cell labeling, and then review recent progress on direct magnetic cell labeling.

MR Contrast Agents for Stem Cell Labeling

Most of the previous works were to label the cells with superparamagnetic iron oxide (SPIO) particles, a T2 magnetodendrimer contrast agent, for MR visualization of stem cells *in vivo*. These SPIO particles include commercially available contrast agents, such as Feridex I.V.® and Combidex® (AMAG Pharmaceuticals Inc., Cambridge, MA). The reason of using these superparamagnetic particles is that T2 contrast agents can induce strong field inhomogeneities and create a significant dephasing of protons, which predominantly reduces the T2 and T2* relaxation times for MR imaging [2, 4]. As a result of creating strong hypointensity, the T2 contrast agents have the major advantage of enabling sensitive detection of even few SPIO-labeled cells. However, the strong hypointensity (or "negative" manifestation) created by SPIO-labeled cells may (i) affect visibility of the target and its surrounding tissues; and (ii) be confused as a normal anatomic signal void and artifacts on T2-weighted MRI.

To overcome these problems, some scientists used T1 MRI contrast agents, such as gadophrin-2 (Schering AG, Berlin, Germany) [5] and motexafin gadolinium (MGd, Pharmacyclics, Inc., Sunnyvale, CA), to label stem cells, which can produce bright or "positive" signal on T1-weighted MRI, enabling visualization of both the target and its background [6]. Among these contrast agents, MGd is composed of aromatic rings and a fluorophore, which can be detected by both MRI and fluorescence microscopy, which allows precise histological confirmation of the transplanted stem cells migrated to or homed at targets [7] (Figure 3.1). Compared with T2 contrast agents, T1 contrast agents have less sensitivity of detecting MR-labeled cells, and could be confused with background and artifacts as well. Because of this, some scientists developed a T1/T2 dual-mode contrast agent, which can display both T1 and T2 signal enhancements simultaneously. In order to avoid the confusion of MR-labeled cell signal with the surrounding tissues, ^{19}F-based perfluorocarbons (PFC) emulsion nanoparticles (nominal size ranging from <100 nm to several hundreds of nanometers) are formulated to label stem cells [8] (Figure 3.2). The formulated PFC nanoparticle comprises a liquid PFC core encapsulated by a lipid monolayer, resulting in a high concentration of ^{19}F atoms. Because the resonance frequency of ^{19}F is different with that of proton, the labeled cells can be specifically detected by ^{19}F-based cellular MRI based on their positive signal with no background of proton. In addition, the biodistribution of cells can be visualized by overlaying ^{19}F image of labeled cells on the ^{1}H anatomical image acquired at the same location, while the local concentration of labeled cells can be determined by quantitative ^{19}F MRI [9-12].

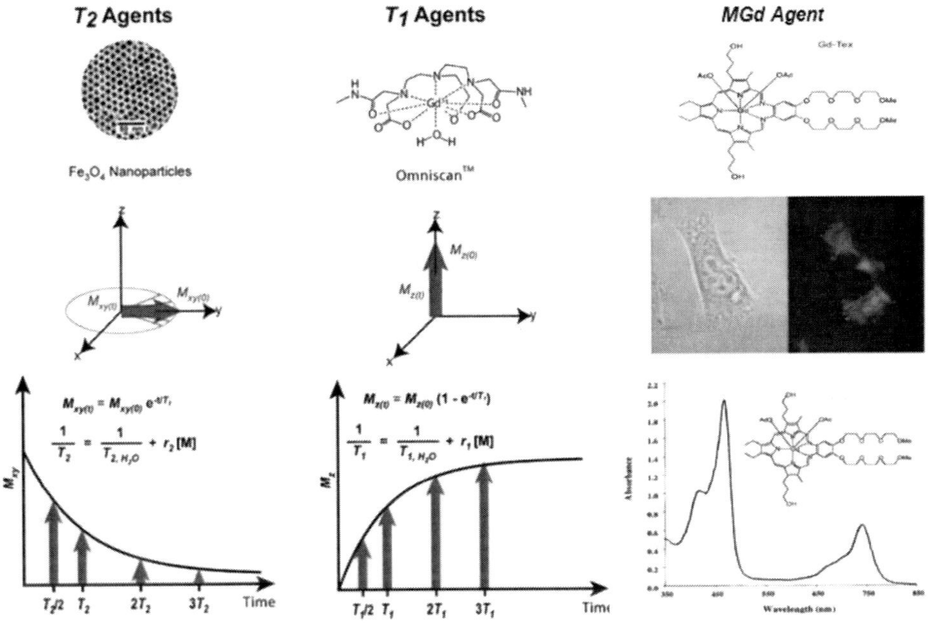

Figure 3.1. Representative chemical structures and compositions for three different types of MRI contrast agents. Left column: transmission electron microscopy (TEM) image of a T2 agent, 9 nm Fe_3O_4 nanoparticles, and T2 relaxation. Middle column: Chemical structure of a T1 agent, Omniscan, and T1 relaxation mechanism. Right column: Chemical structure of MGd and an absorption spectrum of 25 mg/ml MGd in phosphate-buffered saline with 10% Fetal Bovine Serum (FBS). MGd has a large sort band at 473 nm. Due to its extended porphyrin aromatic conjugation system, the texaphyrin macrocycle has a low-energy band occurring at 740 nm. The_signature fluorescence emission band of MGd is centered at 758 nm and used to monitor MGd biolocalization in EMT 6 cells treated for 4 h with 25 mg/ml MGd. Reprinted, with permission, from [14] and [7].

In recent years, a new MR contrast agent based on chemical exchange saturation transfer (CEST) has been reported [13-15]. CEST uses the chemical exchange phenomena between bulk water protons and exchangeable protons with a different chemical shift (d = 4.78 ppm) (Figure 3.2). To create a large chemical shift difference between bound water and bulk water, a Europium (III) DOTA–based paramagnetic metal CEST contrast agent was developed [16]. When bound water protons in pool B are irradiated with a saturation RF pulse, their net magnetization becomes zero, and then saturation transfer from pool B to pool A occurs, causing a decrease in MRI signal of bulk water protons in pool A. In MRI, as given RF pulse is turned ‘‘on’’ and ‘‘off’’ with identical imaging conditions, the CEST contrast is distinguished from the target background. Therefore, if stem cells are labeled with either ^{19}F or CEST contrast agents, it is easy to differentiate MR-labeled stem cells from the target background. However, the MRI scanner needs a multinuclear transceiver or a saturation transfer imaging protocol, while the sensitivity of detecting ^{19}F or CEST-labeled cells is still low.

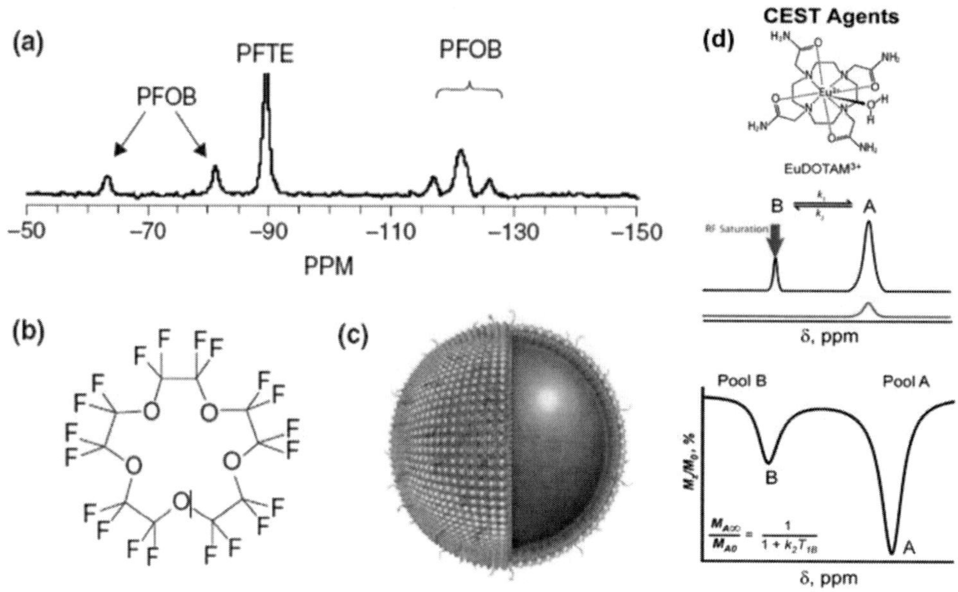

Figure 3.2. (a) Representative ^{19}F spectrum of perfluoropolyether (PFPE) and perfluorooctylbromide (PFOB) nanoparticles, showing the chemical shift of 19F signatures. The single PFPE peak and five discernible PFOB peaks are easily detected and individually resolved. (b) Chemical structure of PFPE shows its 20 ^{19}F atoms. (c) Schematic of a PFPE nanoparticle functionalized with homing ligands in the outer phospholipid monolayer (shown in green). The PFPE nanoparticle provides ^{1}H magnetic resonance (MR) contrast by its surface payload of ~90, 000 Gd3+ (shown in gold) and ^{19}F MR contrast by ~100 M ^{19}F in its core. (d) The chemical structure of EuDOTAM3+, a PARACEST agent. A two-pool exchange model for CEST mechanism and a representative Z-spectrum are illustrated. Reprinted, with permission, from [8] and [14].

Direct Magnetic Cell Labeling Techniques

Simple Incubation

The most commonly used method for direct cell labeling is simple incubation of cells with a selected contrast agent and various transfection reagents, such as polycationic transfection agents, lipofectamine [17], poly-l-lysine (PLL) [3] and protamine sulfate [18]. Since the transfection reagents are positively charged, their coated transfection reagents on the negatively charged MR contrast agents can create positive compounds on the surface, which facilitate the attraction and binding of positively charged contrast agents to the negative cell membranes. Through attraction, disruption, bending and invagination of the cell membranes, the contrast agents are then encapsulated into cytoplasm [19, 20] (Figure 3.3). The main advantage of the incubation labeling method is its simplicity, while its primary disadvantage is the long-time incubation that takes hours or days, depending on the types of cells, transfection reagents and MR contrast agents used. The long-time incubation may change the cellular properties and increase the potential of bacterial contamination, and thus FDA approval of transfection agents is required for clinical use. Although the transfection reagent, protamine sulfate, is available as a clinical grade formulation for reversing heparin toxicity, the fate and bioeffects following intracellular uptake may not necessarily be similar to the situation when presenting outside cells in blood plasma [21].

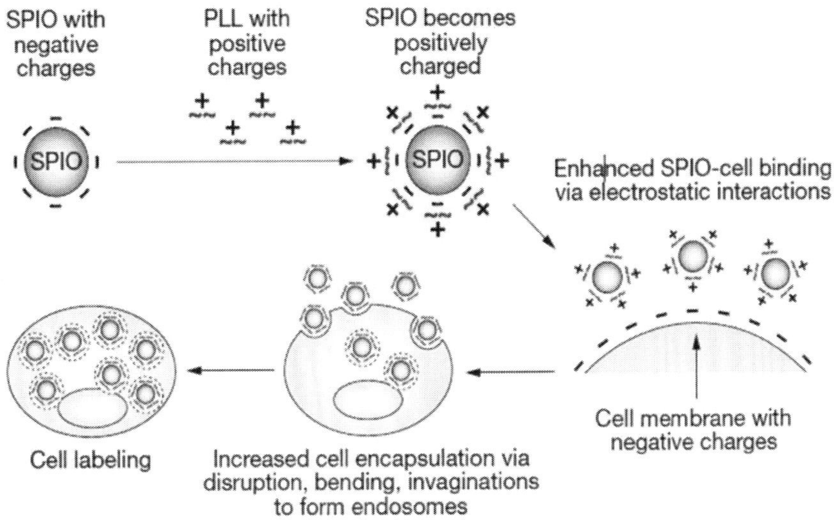

Figure 3.3. Direct magnetic cell labeling using the simple incubation approach. Superparamagnetic iron oxide (SPIO) particles carry a negative charge, but by coating the particles with a positively charged transfection reagent, such as poly-l-lysine (PLL), the SPIO particles become positive. Thus, the interaction between PLL-coated SPIO particles and cells is enhanced via electrostatic effect, which increases the cell uptake of SPIO particles via possible mechanisms of membrane disruption and bending as well as invagination. Reprinted, with permission, from [20].

Magnetoelectroporation

To overcome these problems associated with the simple incubation method, other advanced cell-labeling approaches have been developed, such as magnetoelectroporation (MEP) [21] and magnetosonoporation (MSP) [22]. The principle of MEP approach is that it uses an electrical pulse to shock cells, which increase permeability of cell membranes temporally, and thereby facilitate MRI contrast agents entering the cells (Figure 3.4). Using this approach, stem cells from mice, rats, and humans were successfully and instantly labelled with the FDA-approved formulation Feridex, without the need for adjunct transfection reagents or initiating cell cultures. Since MEP is harmful at higher voltages or pulse durations, the procedure is properly calibrated using a pulse of 130 V and 17 ms. The uptake of MR metals, such as iron, is in a pictogram range, which is comparable to values obtained using the simple incubation approach. MEP-labeled stem cells exhibit an unaltered viability, proliferation, and mitochondrial metabolic rate (Figure 3.5). Labeled mesenchymal stem cells (MSCs) and neural stem cells (NSCs) differentiate into adipogenic, osteogenic, and neural lineages in an identical fashion as unlabeled cells, while containing Feridex particles as demonstrated by double immunofluorescent staining [21]. MEP-labeled NSCs proliferate normally following intrastriatal transplantation, and can be readily detected by cellular MRI *in vivo*. This MEP approach offers two key advantages over the simple incubation method - no need for transfection agents and almost instant labeling of stem cells. However, the use of such high-voltage electrical pulse can kill cells and may affect the long-term viability of the labeled cells.

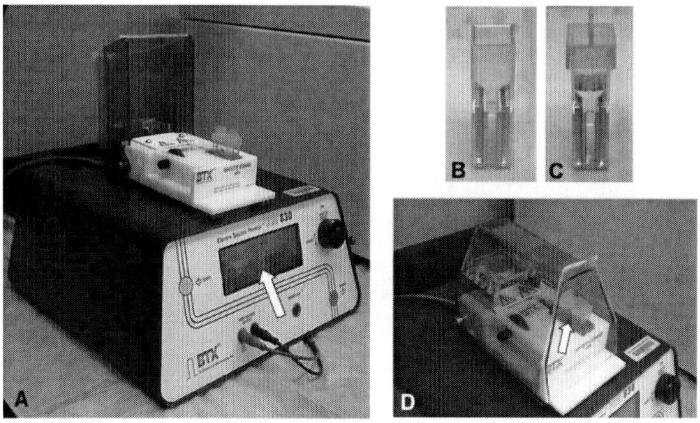

Figure 3.4. The magnetoelectroporation (MEP) instrument for direct MR cell labeling. (A) A photograph of the MEP instrument, on which the parameters for electroporation can be adjusted via the digital control panel (arrow). (B&C) Cuvettes with 3- or 5-mm cell-containing culture medium, and (D) the cuvette (arrow) are installed on the platform for electroporation.

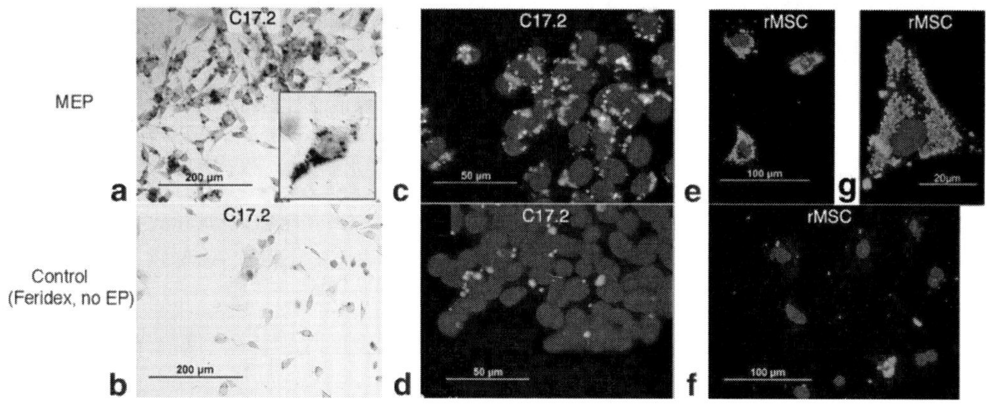

Figure 3.5. Fe uptake by MEP-treated cells. C17.2 mouse neural stem cells (a–d) and rat mesenchymal stem cells (e–g) are incubated with Feridex (2 mg Fe/mL) with (a, c, e, g) and without (b, d, f) electroporation (EP). Only MEP-treated cells show significant Feridex uptake as assessed by diaminobenzidine (DAB)-enhanced Prussian blue stain (a) and anti-dextran immunofluorescence (c, e). The higher magnification in (g) demonstrates Feridex-containing clusters with a measured diameter of 830 ± 350 nm. Reprinted, with permission, from [21].

Magnetosonoporation

Magnetosonoporation (MSP) is another advanced method for instant magnetic labeling of stem cells. Like electroporation, sonoporation is based on the cavitation effect of ultrasound that increases permeability of cell membranes [23-26], which thereby enables intracellular uptake of exogenous compounds, such as MRI contrast agents [22]. Moderated level of low-frequency ultrasound, ranging from 1 to 3 MHz, is known to be safe, as it has been widely applied in clinical applications such as physical therapy. Therefore, magnetosonoporation could be expected to be a safe, efficient, simple and cost-effective approach for direct magnetic labeling of stem cells, if the parameters are calibrated properly. To establish this instant magnetic cell labeling technique, a MSP labeling apparatus was developed that composed of a sterilized cell container and a clinically used therapeutic ultrasound generator (Richmar; Rich-Mar Co., Inola, OK) (Figure 3.6).

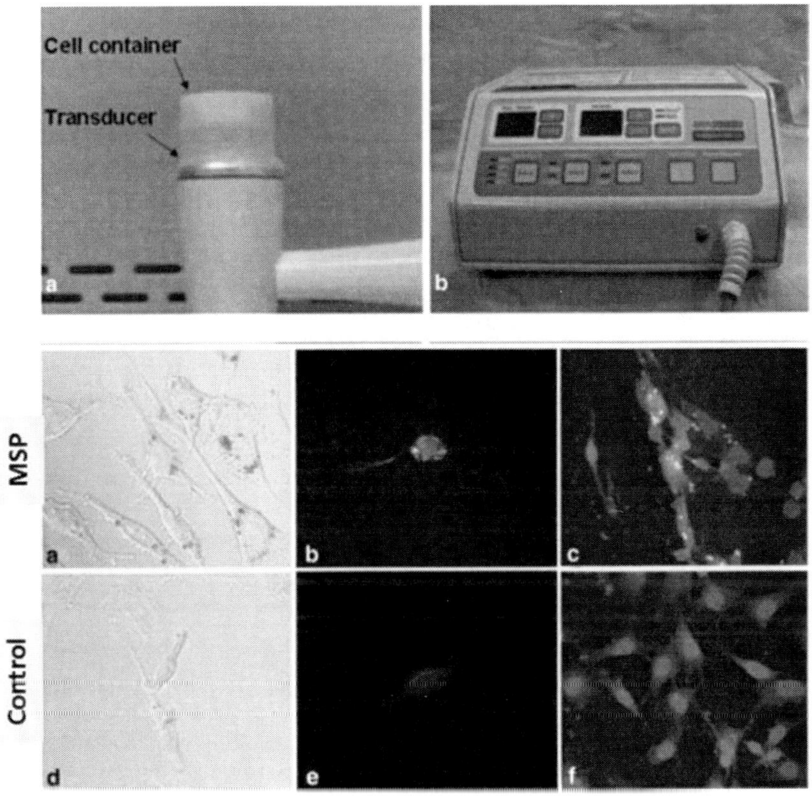

Figure 3.6. The upper panel: MSP-based cell labeling apparatus. (a) The cell labeling container, a sterilized plastic tube, is built on the top of the ultrasound transducer, and (b) the transducer is connected to a therapeutic ultrasound generator, which has a digital panel for the adjusting the output of ultrasonic energies. The lower panel: Confirmation of successful MSP/Feridex labeling of C17.2 neural stem cell. Upper row shows the cells labeled with Feridex using MSP, and the lower row shows the control cells without MSP treatment. (a) Prussian-blue staining of Feridex-labeled cells, showing successful cell labeling (blue dots) following MSP treatment, which are barely seen in the control group without MSP treatment (d). (b) Immunocytochemistry to detect dextran, a component of the coat of Feridex particles, showing successful cell labeling (green dots) following MSP treatment. (c) Double staining with beta-galactosidase for LacZ and anti-dextran for Feridex, demonstrating green-dotted dextran-coated Feridex in pink-colored LacZ cells. No such finding is seen in the control group without MSP treatment (e&f). Reprinted, with permission, from [22].

The cell container was made of a plastic tube and mounted on the top of the ultrasonic transducer. The transducer was connected to the ultrasound generator, capable of delivering ultrasound frequencies at 1 MHz or 3 MHz, intensities from 0.1 to 2 W/cm^2 with duty cycles of 10, 20, 30, 50, and 100%, and a pulse-repetition frequency of 100 Hz. Via the digital control panel of the ultrasound generator, the parameters of selected ultrasound energies can be precisely adjusted. Based on the MSP labeling apparatus, the optimal MSP protocol was obtained by performing a series of *in vitro* experiments using and comparing different MSP parameters (including various ultrasound intensities, duty cycles, ultrasound exposure times, and concentrations of MR contrast agents), in order to achieve both high cell viability and high intracellular uptake of MR contrast agents. The *in vitro* experiments demonstrated that the optimal MSP protocol was achieved at 20% duty cycle, 0.3 w/cm^2 ultrasound intensity, and 5-min exposure time for 1mg/mL Feridex [27]. Then, the safety of this MSP cell labeling approach was further confirmed by *in vitro* evaluation of the proliferation and differentiation of MSP-labeled and unlabeled neural stem cells, as well as *in vivo* evaluation of the migration of MSP-labeled neural stem cells to gliomas by using cellular MRI and subsequent histological confirmation [27] (Figure 3.7). These experiments demonstrate that MSP is a convenient, efficient, and safe direct magnetic cell labeling technique. However, the device described above is an "open" apparatus that may cause potential risk of cell contamination, and thus is not convenient for future clinical cell labeling or translational studies.

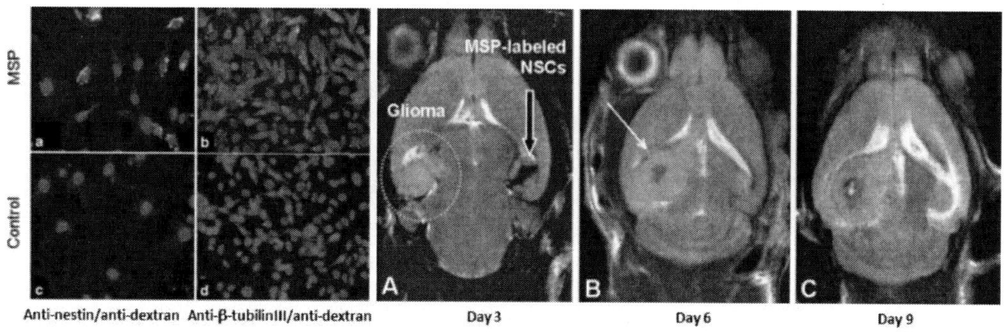

Figure 3.7. Left column: Stem cell differentiation after MSP-Feridex labeling. (a–d) neural stem-progenitor cells develop typical neuronal morphology and express neuronal protein nestin and beta-tubulin (pink colors) for both MSP-treated cells (a&b) and control cells (c&d). Dextran (green dots)-containing endosomes in MSP-treated groups are detected (a&b) due to the proliferation of neural stem cells and dilution of Feridex before terminal differentiation, which is not visualized in the control cell groups (c&d). Right column: *In vivo* MRI of the migration of MSP-labeled neural stem cells to gliomas in mice. (A) T2-weighted MRI demonstrates a glioma mass in the right hemisphere (circle) and MR signal voids at the site injected with MSP-treated, Feridex-labeled cells in the left hemisphere of the mouse brain. (B&C) At days 6 and 9 post-cell implantation, the area of signal void at cell-injected sites decreases, whereas hypointense areas within or surrounding the glioma masses (long arrow on B) is detected. Reprinted, with permission, from [27].

In order to translating MSP technique into clinical application, a "closed" MSP apparatus was subsequently designed and the feasibility of MSP-assisted stem cell labeling using focused ultrasound was validated by evaluating the proliferation, migration and differentiation of the magnetically labeled cells [28] (Figure 3.8). The *in vivo* MRI with histological confirmation demonstrated that MSP/SPIO-labeled neural stem cells could migrate from the transplantation side to the contralateral, glioma-bearing side of nude mice brains. All of these experimental results show that MSP-assisted cell labeling using focused ultrasound is a feasible technique and the "closed" device is feasible, convenient and safe for instant direct magnetic cell labeling and MRI cell tracking.

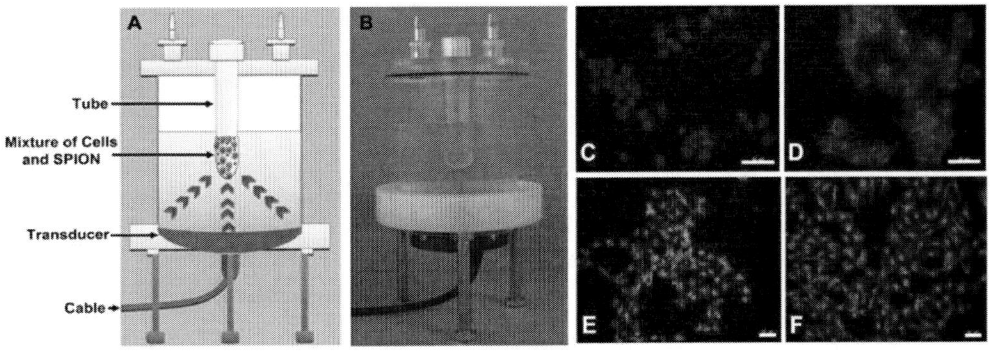

Figure 3.8. Design of "closed" MSP apparatus using focused ultrasound. Design (A) and photograph (B) of the MSP apparatus for convenient clinical applications. To validate the iron uptake, unlabeled (C) and MSP/SPIO-labeled cells (D) are stained by immunocytochemistry. Green fluorescence indicates the uptake of SPIO, which is coated by dextran and visualized with FITC-conjugated dextran antibody. (E-F) for neural differentiation, MSP-labeled cells are exposed to neurobasal medium containing 2% B-27 and 1% GlutaMAX. For astrocyte differentiation, cells are incubated in DMEM medium supplemented with 1% FBS, 1% N-2 supplement and 1% GlutaMAX. After 2 weeks, neuron-specific beta III tubulin (green) and astrocyte-specific glial fibrillary acidic protein (GFAP, red) are detected, respectively, by immunocytochemistry. Nucleoli are stained with 4',6-diamidino-2-phenylindole (DAPI, blue) and the images are merged using SPOT™ Imaging Solutions. Scale bars 50 μm. (C&D) Original magnification x 400. (E&F) Original magnification x 200. Reprinted, with permission, from [28].

Conclusion

In conclusion, direct magnetic cell labeling is one of the key steps for *in vivo* MRI of stem cells. Different MR contrast agents provide various applications on MRI of cell trafficking, depending on the target background, as well as MRI hardware and imaging techniques. Direct magnetic cell labeling techniques have been continuously developed to be more efficient, convenient and safe for future clinical translation of MRI-guided stem cell therapies.

References

[1] Weissman IL. Translating stem and progenitor cell biology to the clinic: barriers and opportunities. *Science* 2000;287(5457):1442-1446.

[2] Bulte JW, Douglas T, Witwer B, Zhang SC, Strable E, Lewis BK, et al. Magnetodendrimers allow endosomal magnetic labeling and in vivo tracking of stem cells. *Nat. Biotechnol.* 2001;19(12):1141-1147.

[3] Frank JA, Miller BR, Arbab AS, Zywicke HA, Jordan EK, Lewis BK, et al. Clinically applicable labeling of mammalian and stem cells by combining superparamagnetic iron oxides and transfection agents. *Radiology* 2003;228(2):480-487.

[4] Bulte JW, Kraitchman DL. Iron oxide MR contrast agents for molecular and cellular imaging. *NMR Biomed.* 2004;17(7):484-499.

[5] Daldrup-Link HE, Rudelius M, Metz S, Piontek G, Pichler B, Settles M, et al. Cell tracking with gadophrin-2: a bifunctional contrast agent for MR imaging, optical imaging, and fluorescence microscopy. *Eur. J. Nucl. Med. Mol. Imaging* 2004;31(9):1312-1321.

[6] Qiu B, Treuting P, Zhan X, Xie D, Frevert CW, Yang X. Dual transfer of GFP gene and MGd into stem-progenitor cells: toward in vivo MRI of stem cell-mediated gene therapy of atherosclerosis. *Acad. Radiol.* 2010;17(5):547-552.

[7] Woodburn K. Intracellular localization of the radiation enhancer motexafin gadolinium using interferometric Fourier fluorescence microscopy. *J. Pharmacol. Exp. Ther.* 2001;297(888-894.

[8] Chen J, Lanza GM, Wickline SA. Quantitative magnetic resonance fluorine imaging: today and tomorrow. *Wiley Interdiscip Rev. Nanomed. Nanobiotechnol.* 2(4):431-440.

[9] Partlow KC, Chen J, Brant JA, Neubauer AM, Meyerrose TE, Creer MH, et al. 19F magnetic resonance imaging for stem/progenitor cell tracking with multiple unique perfluorocarbon nanobeacons. *Faseb J.* 2007;21(8):1647-1654.

[10] Boehm-Sturm P, Mengler L, Wecker S, Hoehn M, Kallur T. In vivo tracking of human neural stem cells with 19F magnetic resonance imaging. *PLoS One* 6(12):e29040.

[11] Tc BL, T K, M W, A H, R E, U N, et al. Double-labeled Mesenchymal Stem Cells for 1H / 19F MR Imaging. *J. Stem Cells Regen Med.* 2007;2(1):88-89.

[12] Ruiz-Cabello J, Barnett BP, Bottomley PA, Bulte JW. Fluorine (19F) MRS and MRI in biomedicine. *NMR Biomed.* 24(2):114-129.

[13] Ward KM, Aletras AH, Balaban RS. A new class of contrast agents for MRI based on proton chemical exchange dependent saturation transfer (CEST). *J. Magn Reson* 2000;143(1):79-87.

[14] Khemtong C, Kessinger CW, Gao J. Polymeric nanomedicine for cancer MR imaging and drug delivery. *Chem. Commun.* (Camb) 2009;24):3497-3510.

[15] Woods M, Woessner DE, Sherry AD. Paramagnetic lanthanide complexes as PARACEST agents for medical imaging. *Chem. Soc. Rev.* 2006;35(6):500-511.

[16] Zhang S, Winter P, Wu K, Sherry AD. A novel europium(III)-based MRI contrast agent. *J. Am. Chem. Soc.* 2001;123(7):1517-1518.

[17] Hoehn M, Kustermann E, Blunk J, Wiedermann D, Trapp T, Wecker S, et al. Monitoring of implanted stem cell migration in vivo: a highly resolved in vivo magnetic resonance imaging investigation of experimental stroke in rat. *Proc. Natl. Acad. Sci. USA* 2002;99(25):16267-16272.

[18] Arbab AS, Yocum GT, Kalish H, Jordan EK, Anderson SA, Khakoo AY, et al. Efficient magnetic cell labeling with protamine sulfate complexed to ferumoxides for cellular MRI. *Blood* 2004;104(4):1217-1223.

[19] Bulte JW, Arbab AS, Douglas T, Frank JA. Preparation of magnetically labeled cells for cell tracking by magnetic resonance imaging. *Methods Enzymol.* 2004;386(275-299.

[20] Qiu B, Yang X. Molecular MRI of hematopoietic stem-progenitor cells: in vivo monitoring of gene therapy and atherosclerosis. *Nat. Clin. Pract. Cardiovasc. Med.* 2008;5(7):396-404.

[21] Walczak P, Kedziorek DA, Gilad AA, Lin S, Bulte JW. Instant MR labeling of stem cells using magnetoelectroporation. *Magn Reson Med.* 2005;54(4):769-774.

[22] Qiu B, Walczak P, Li X, Ruiz-Cabello J, Minoshima S, Bulte J, et al. Magnetosonoporation: Instant magnetic labeling of stem cells. *Magn Reson Med.* 2010;63(6):1437-1441.

[23] Liu J, Lewis TN, Prausnitz MR. Non-invasive assessment and control of ultrasound-mediated membrane permeabilization. *Pharm Res.* 1998;15(6):918-924.

[24] Han YW, Ikegami A, Chung P, Zhang L, Deng CX. Sonoporation is an efficient tool for intracellular fluorescent dextran delivery and one-step double-crossover mutant construction in Fusobacterium nucleatum. *Appl. Environ. Microbiol.* 2007;73(11):3677-3683.

[25] Schlicher RK, Radhakrishna H, Tolentino TP, Apkarian RP, Zarnitsyn V, Prausnitz MR. Mechanism of intracellular delivery by acoustic cavitation. *Ultrasound Med. Biol.* 2006;32(6):915-924.

[26] Zarnitsyn VG, Prausnitz MR. Physical parameters influencing optimization of ultrasound-mediated DNA transfection. *Ultrasound Med. Biol.* 2004;30(4):527-538.

[27] Xie D, Qiu B, Walczak P, Li X, Ruiz-Cabello J, Minoshima S, et al. Optimization of magnetosonoporation for stem cell labeling. *NMR Biomed.* 2010.

[28] Lei H, Nan X, Wang Z, Gao L, Xie L, Zou C, et al. Stem cell labeling with superparamagnetic iron oxide nanoparticles using focused ultrasound and magnetic resonance imaging tracking. *Journal of Nanoscience and Nanotechnology* 2014;14:1-8.

In: Magnetic Resonance Imaging of Stem Cell Applications ISBN: 978-1-63463-910-1
Editor: Xiaoming Yang

Chapter 4

Indirect Magnetic Labeling of Stem Cells

***Anna V. Naumova*[*,1,3,6] *and Charles E. Murry*[2,3,4,5,6]**

[1]Department of Radiology, University of Washington School of Medicine, Seattle, Washington, US
[2]Department of Pathology, University of Washington School of Medicine, Seattle, Washington, US
[3]Center for Cardiovascular Biology, University of Washington, Seattle, Washington, US
[4]Department of Bioengineering, University of Washington, Seattle, Washington, US
[5]Department of Medicine/Cardiology, University of Washington, Seattle, Washington, US
[6]Institute for Stem Cell and Regenerative Medicine, University of Washington, Seattle, Washington, US

Abstract

Stem cell-based therapy has the potential to become one of the major milestones in modern medicine, promising regeneration of organ structure and function. Longitudinal magnetic resonance imaging (MRI) studies of transplanted cells are important in providing functional endpoints (such as safety and efficacy) as well as insights into the biological mechanism of transplanted cells. To distinguish grafts from the host tissue with MRI, transplanted cells must be either labeled with exogenous MRI-visible particles (direct labeling) or genetically modified (indirect labeling) to express MRI-detectable probes. Direct cell labeling is the more common approach for MRI tracking of transplanted cell migration and homing. However, this approach suffers from label dilution as cells proliferate and false-positive MRI signal when particles are released from dead cells and captured by macrophages. Indirect (genetic) cell labeling via the gene-reporter approach, despite its lower MRI signal intensity, enables longitudinal

[*] Correspondence: Anna V. Naumova, PhD, (nav@uw.edu).

assessment of live transplanted cells. Several reporter genes have been developed for indirect MR labeling of stem cells, including ferritin, tyrosinase, β-galactosidase, MagA, and chemical exchange saturation transfer (CEST) reporters. This chapter focuses on indirect (genetic) magnetic cell labeling techniques and their applications in stem cell therapeutics.

Keywords: Indirect cell labeling, MRI, stem cells

Introduction

Non-invasive imaging is a valuable tool for assessment of safety and efficacy of stem cell-based therapy. It also helps to understand the behavior of transplanted cells, including cell survival, migration, differentiation, tumorgenicity, and immunogenicity [1, 2]. Different imaging modalities can be used to track transplanted cells in vivo. Among these are bioluminescence and fluorescence imaging, ultrasound (US), radionuclide imaging techniques such as single-photon emission computed tomography (SPECT) and positron emission tomography (PET), X-ray computed tomography (CT), and magnetic resonance imaging (MRI). Some imaging modalities are applicable for preclinical studies of transplanted cells on small animals only (for example, bioluminescence and fluorescence imaging); but low penetration depth precludes use of these imaging modalities in large animals and humans. Other imaging techniques are capable of cell tracking in large animals and humans (for example, US, SPECT, PET, MRI, and CT). Selection of the optimal imaging modality depends on the cellular processes that need to be studied, as well as the most desirable readouts. The brief characteristics of each imaging modality are represented in Table 4.1.

Table 4.1. Comparison of Imaging techniques for Cell Therapies (reprinted with permission from [3])

Imaging Modality	Spatial Resolution	Time	Limit: Cells	Labeling Strategy	Advantages	Disadvantages
Bioluminescence imaging (BLI) (preclinical only)	5–20 mm depending on depth of signal	seconds	$\sim 10^3$	reporter gene	cheap, simple, high throughput	small animals only, low resolution, only 2D images
Fluorescence tomography (FMT) (preclinical only)	2–3 mm	seconds to minutes	$\sim 10^6$	reporter gene, fluorescent dye	cheap, simple	low resolution, cells need to be close to surface
Ultrasound (US) (preclinical and clinical)	150 µm; –2 mm depending on depth	seconds to minutes	not well characterized	reporter gene, antibody with microbubble	cheap, relatively simple	limited 3D capabilities, low signal to noise ratio
Single-photon emission computed tomography (SPECT) (preclinical and *clinical*)	1–2 mm; *8–12 mm*	minutes	$\sim 10^5$	reporter gene, incubation with radiotracer	3D imaging	anatomic reference required, radioactive tracer required
Positron emission tomography (PET) (preclinical and *clinical*)	~1 mm; *4–6 mm*	seconds to minutes	$\sim 10^4$	reporter gene, incubation with radiotracer	3D imaging, high sensitivity	anatomic reference required, radioactive tracer required
Magnetic resonance tomography (MRI) (preclinical and *clinical*)	25–500 µm; *0.5–5 mm*	minutes to hours	$\sim 10^4$	internalization or surface labeling with nanoparticles or specific ions	3D imaging, good soft tissue contrast, no radiation, high resolution	very expensive, complicated
Computed tomography (CT) (preclinical and *clinical*)	<50 µm; *<1 mm*	seconds to minutes	not well characterized	internalization or surface labeling with nanoparticles	3D imaging, relatively cheap, high resolution	uses ionizing radiation

Fields in italics indicate parameters specific to clinical systems if they are different from preclinical systems.

In recent years, multimodality imaging has become widespread for cell tracking. It is based on co-registration of images obtained from different modalities, such as MRI/PET, PET/CT, and SPECT/CT. It combines highly sensitive/quantitative but low-resolution imaging modalities, such as PET and SPECT, with high-resolution anatomical images acquired with MRI or CT scanners.

Among imaging modalities, MRI stands out in cell tracking applications, because it provides high resolution anatomical images without restriction in penetration depth. MRI can be used for single cell tracking [4, 5] as well as for assessment of organ function (for example, heart contractility and brain function). MRI does not use ionizing irradiation, which makes this imaging modality especially valuable for longitudinal follow-up studies on the same patient. MRI contrast comes from magnetic polarization of hydrogen nuclei in water molecules. Since 70% of tissues in the body consist of water, MRI provides excellent soft tissue contrast. MRI contrast weighting techniques can detect areas of pathology (scar, inflammation) [6], volume loss [7], restrictive water diffusion [8, 9], chemical exchange within the macromolecular environment (CEST) [10-12], cellular death and inflammation [13-15], metabolite concentration [16-18], tissue perfusion [19-21], and vascularity [22-24].

Graft visualization remains challenging, because the new tissue constructed from the transplanted cells has insufficient endogenous contrast relative to the host. To discriminate transplanted cells from surrounding host tissues with MRI, scientists have developed cell labeling techniques, which can be divided into two categories: direct and indirect cell labeling. In this chapter, we provide an overview of the MRI cell labeling techniques with a primary focus on indirect (genetic) cell labeling and agents that are used for longitudinal MRI of transplanted cells.

Direct MR Cell Labeling

Direct cell labeling is a relatively simple and commonly used method for MRI tracking of transplanted cells. It requires the uptake of an exogenous contrast agent by the cell (Figure 4.1). Various exogenous MR contrast agents, such as superparamagnetic iron oxide nanoparticles (SPIOs) and paramagnetic contrast agents (e.g., manganese-based nanoparticles, perfluorocarbon nanoparticles, and gadolinium-loaded liposomes) allow detection of a single group of cells or cell clusters within target tissues [25-30]. Exogenous nanoparticle-based MR agents can be easily endocytosed by cells [31-33]. To facilitate the MR-agent uptake by cells, different transfection reagents [34, 35] are often used, or the cell surfaces need to be modified [36, 37]. Additionally, to increase the capability of MR agents to enter interested cells through cellular membranes, advanced MR labelling techniques, such as magnetoelectroporation and magnetosonoporation, have been developed [38-41] as described in the chapter 3. The main advantages of direct cell labeling are its relatively simple labeling approach and strong MRI signal from the highly concentrated imaging agent accumulated in the labeled cells. Disadvantages of this labeling approach include: (1) labeling agent dilution as cells divide, which therefore leads to the decrease and ultimate disappearance of MRI signals over time [42, 43]; (2) the incapability to distinguish live cells from dead cells, since labeled MR contrast agents can be released from dead cells and captured by macrophages (This false-positive result essentially generates macrophage imaging rather than transplanted cell imaging [43, 44]); and (3) difficulty on differentiation of hypointensities between pathological hemorrhage and the accumulation of these "negative" MR signals created by superparamagnetic irons of labeled cells, which can cause misinterpretation of MR images [45].

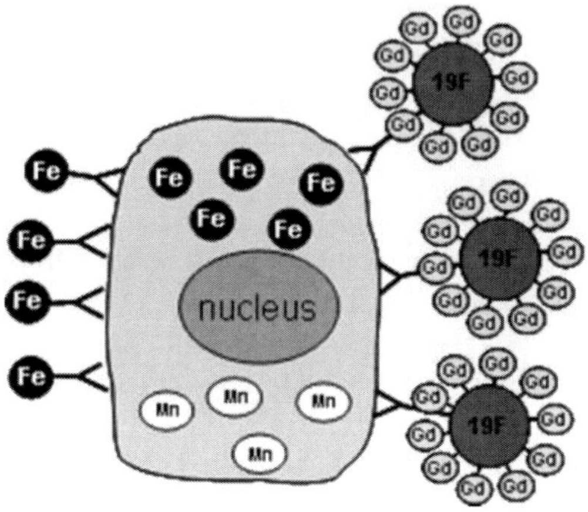

Figure 4.1. Direct cell labeling methods. Cells can be loaded with exogenous nanoparticles that contain MRI-detectable agents, such as gadolinium (Gd) iron oxide (Fe), manganese (Mn), or fluorine (^{19}F). Exogenous nanoparticles can be accumulated in the cytoplasm or attached onto the cell surface via specific antibody-receptor complex.

All these factors together result in incapability to reflect transplanted cell viability and quantity, as well as cellular and molecular functions of the transplanted cells at the targets. In addition, cellular toxicity is also a concern when MR contrast agents are used in high concentrations [46, 47]. Cell labeling efficiency as well as effect of labeling agent on cell viability, proliferation and differentiation must be verified for each individual cell type prior to transplantation. As a bottom line, particle-based approaches are well suited for short term studies of the initial retention of stem cells, but are not well suited for longer term studies of graft cell death, proliferation or migration.

Indirect MR Cell Labeling

Indirect (genetic) MR cell labeling is based on genetic modification of cells prior to their transplantation to express reporter genes encoding specific enzymes/proteins, which generate imaging signals with or without administration of MR probes (Figure 4.2).

Indirect cell labeling is a more complicated and time consuming technique, compared to direct cell labeling described above. Indirect cell labeling via genetic modification of transplanted cells requires (1) the correct choice of the gene promoter that functions in the specific stem cell type and does not silence over time as transplanted stem cells differentiate; (2) molecular cloning procedures; (3) successful cellular transfection by viral or non-viral gene vectors; and (4) selection of an adequate procedure for creating transgenic cell line expressing detectable level of imaging reporters.

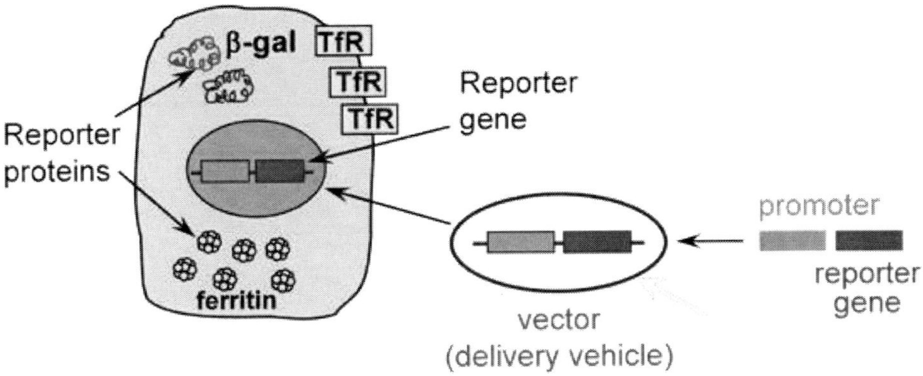

Figure 4.2. Indirect cell labeling techniques require genetic modification of cells prior to their transplantation. Molecular cloning and modification of cellular genome are required for efficient expression of reporter proteins in targeted cells. Examples of the MRI reporters shown in this schematic are the endogenous iron storage protein ferritin, the enzyme β-galactosidase (β-gal), and the transferrin receptor (TfR) located at the cellular membranes. After transplantation, the genetically modified cells can generate MRI signal without exogenous administration of a contrast agent (such as accumulation of endogenous iron in ferritin complexes) or after injection of target-specific MRI probes (for example, β-galactosidase-activated MRI probes).

The reporter gene and a promoter should be carefully chosen based on cell type and the specific research question. Choice of the vector or delivery vehicle will depend on the reporter gene size, transfection efficacy of the specific cell type, and regulatory issues (for example, restrictions on the viral gene transfer). A multidisciplinary team, consisting of molecular and stem cell biologists, as well as imaging specialists, is required for successful application of this technique.

The advantages of reporter gene-based indirect cell labeling include: (1) the reporter gene does not dilute out as cells divide, allowing longitudinal cell tracking after the cells arriving at the target; (2) the reporter gene is only expressed by viable cells [44, 48]; and (3) the reporter gene can be switched on and off under specific conditions, such as the stem cell differentiation into a particular phenotype [49, 50]. The primary disadvantage of reporter gene-based indirect cell labeling is its lower cellular signal intensity in comparison to direct cell imaging [44, 51].

In addition, this technique raises regulatory concerns on the potential that the gene integration may cause mutagenesis, immunogenic responses or oncogenic transformation. Advanced methods of genomic editing using zinc-finger nucleases (ZFN) [52, 53] and transcription activator-like effector nucleases (TALENs), as well as a system of clustered regularly interspaced short palindromic repeats (CRISPR) [54] may open new possibilities for wide implementation of reporter gene-based indirect cell labeling for future clinical MRI of stem cell applications.

Table 4.2 summarizes the advantages and disadvantages of direct and indirect approaches for cell labeling.

Table 4.2. Advantages and disadvantages of direct and indirect methods of MR cell labeling

	Direct MR cell labeling	Indirect MR cell labeling
Advantages	Well established technique; creation of strong MRI signal with easy detection; capability for MR tracking of transplanted cell migration to and homing at targets.	Gene expression closely related to cell viability; reporter genes dividing as cell division; MRI signals reflecting cell numbers; capability for longitudinal MRI following-up functions of grafted cells after their arriving at targets.
Disadvantages	Inability to distinguish live and dead cells; labeling dilution with cell division; inability to longitudinal follow up transplanted cells after their arriving at targets; difficulty in distinguishing MRI signal voids by superparamagnetic "negative" agents from hemosiderin deposits or hemorrhage; risk of cellular toxicity when using highly concentrated MR contrast agents.	Complicated modification of cell genome; weak MRI signal; potential restrictions in clinical applications due to use of viral vectors; potential alteration of cell potency by reporter genes, immunogenicity, and malignant transformation.

Reporter Genes for Indirect MR Cell labeling

Transferrin Receptor

Transferrin is a single-strand glycoprotein (~80kDa) containing two structurally similar metal-binding domains, which can very tightly bind circulating endogenous iron [55]. The transferrin receptor (TfR) is an endocytotic receptor that functions to internalize transferrin-iron complexes through receptor-mediated endocytosis, and is needed for importing iron into the cell. TfR can be highly expressed (several million copies per cell) on the cell membrane, and its expression is regulated in response to intracellular iron concentration [56, 57].

TfR was the first MRI reporter gene, proposed in 1996 [58]. Increase of iron concentration in cells via upregulation of TfR can generate MRI-detectable contrast [59, 60]. Fibroblasts overexpressing TfRs exhibit an approximately threefold increase in cellular iron content, yielding significant MRI signal in T2-weighted sequences at longer echo times [58]. Increase in TfR expression can be imaged by using superparamagnetic iron oxide–transferrin conjugates [59-63]. Figure 4.3 represents increased signal intensity in the tumor overexpressing TfR due to accumulation of Tf-MION [60].

Interestingly, several studies have shown that cell labeling with superparamagnetic iron oxide particles (SPIOs) without using a transfection agent could strengthen expression of TfR and ferritin genes [64-66]. One study described the feasibility of manganese labeling of murine hepatocytes via the TfR-dependent and/or -independent metal-transport pathways [67]. This method of cell labeling is based on the chemical similarities between manganese and iron (e.g., similarities on ionic radii, valence states – (II) and (III) – under physiological conditions, and binding affinities for transferrin). The results of this study demonstrate that Mn(III)-transferrin is an effective MRI contrast agent for MR labeling of murine hepatocytes.

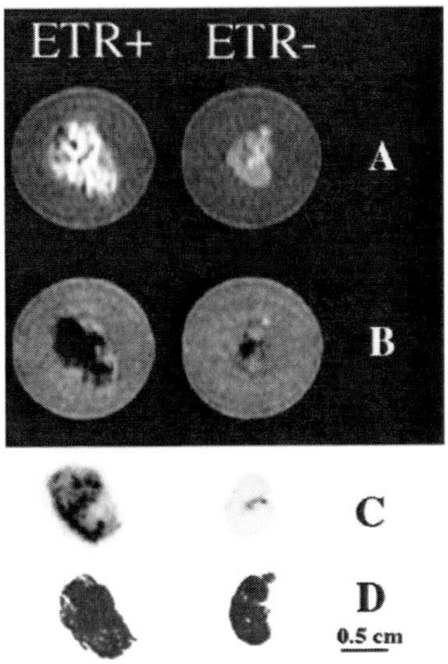

Figure 4.3. Ex vivo MRI detection of tumors overexpressing TfR (ETR+). (A) Increased signal intensity in the tumor in T1 weighed images due to Tf-MION accumulation. (B) Substantial decreased signal intensity within the ETR+ tumor in T2-weighted images. (C) Autoradiographs of tumors. (D) Corresponding hematoxylin-eosin–stained tumor sections show the viable solid tumor mass with no regions of necrosis. Reprinted, with permission, from [60].

Tyrosinase

Overexpression of tyrosinase is another approach in molecular imaging. Tyrosinase is a key enzyme in melanin production from tyrosine, and this enzyme alone is sufficient to promote melanin production in non-melanogenic cells [68, 69]. Tyrosinase catalyzes the hydroxylation of tyrosine-yielding dioxyphenylalanine (DOPA) and its subsequent oxidation to DOPAquinone. DOPAquinone is then converted into melanin. Melanin is a unique biopolymeric pigment found in animals and plants, and plays roles in coloration, photoprotection [70], and the scavenging of toxic substances, such as circulating metal ions [71]. The high affinity of melanin for a large variety of metal ions [72-77] has been used for cellular MRI [78-82].

It has been shown that overexpression of tyrosinase results in accumulation of melanin, which sequesters paramagnetic ions and thus generates imaging contrast in MRI and scintigraphy [69]. Recent reports described tyrosinase as a stand-alone reporter gene suitable for multimodality imaging, including photoacoustic imaging, MRI and positron emission tomography [83, 84] (Figure 4.4).

Mn(II)-based MRI/molecular Imaging responsive to the enzyme tyrosinase were described for the development of diagnostic probes to detect melanoma cancer [85]. There is also evidence that melanin can be cytotoxic at certain cytosolic concentrations unless sequestered within intracellular compartments such as melanosomes or lysosomes [86, 87].

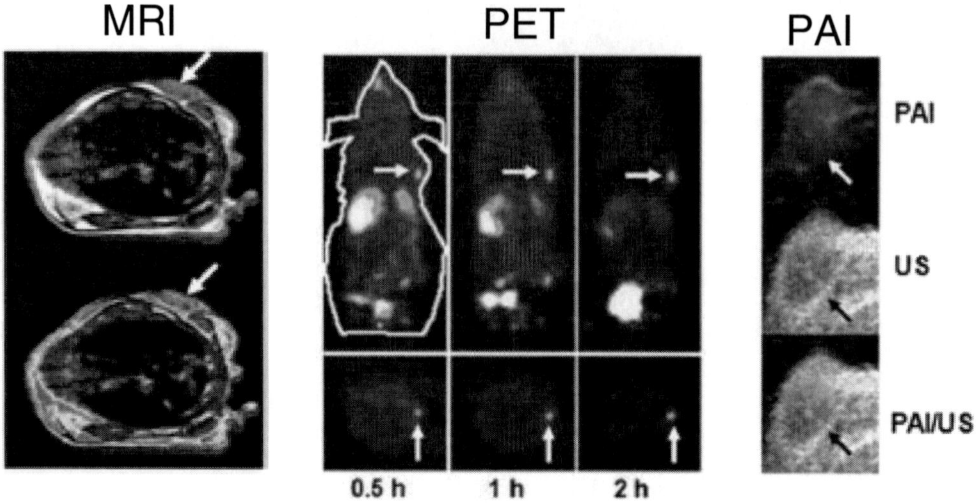

Figure 4.4. In vivo multimodality imaging of tumor bearing mice with magnetic resonance imaging (MRI), positron emission tomography (PET), and photoacoustic imaging (PAI). Human breast cancer cells (MCF-7) are transfected with a plasmid that encodes tyrosinase. Then, 1×10^{7} cells are inoculated subcutaneously in the shoulder of nude mice. Melanin targeted N-(2-(diethylamino)ethyl)-18F-5-fluoropicolinamide is used as a PET reporter probe. Reprinted, with permission, from [84].

β-Galactosidase

β-galactosidase (β-gal) is an essential enzyme in bacteria that catalyzes the hydrolysis of β-galactosides into monosacharaides. β-gal is encoded by a lacZ gene, which is essentially absent from normal eukaryotic cells, and therefore expression of lacZ is commonly used in molecular biology as a reporter marker. Eukariotic cells have a lysosomal version of β-gal that goes up during senscence and inflammation, giving some background signal. β-galactosidase-activated MRI contrast agents were synthesized to report on the physiological state or metabolic activity deep within living specimens. Newly synthesized compounds can be detected by increase in the R1 relaxivity on proton MRI [88-90] or by non-proton NMR techniques (such as ^{19}F-NMR) [91, 92], yielding bright MRI signal (zones of signal hyper-intensity). One example of a β-gal-specific MR compound is (1-(2-(b-galactopyranosyloxy)propyl)-4,7,10-tris(carboxymethyl)-1,4,7,10-tetraazacyclododecane) gadolinium(III), abbreviated as EgadMe, which was synthesized by Louie et al. [93] . EgadMe is enzymatically processed by β-galactosidase and can be switched between low-relaxivity (inactive) and high-relaxivity (active) states. Figure 4.5 demonstrates the use of EgadMe to follow β-galactosidase expression in living Xenopus laevis embryos [93]. Another study showed the use of ^{19}F-magnetic resonance spectroscopy in observing β-gal activity in cancer cells via chemical shift imaging (CSI) techniques [94]. Recently, some authors reported the feasibility of detecting β-gal activity specifically in tyrosinase expressing cells [95]. Enzymatic cleavage of a MR probe by β-gal can release a Gd–DOTA containing substrate for tyrosinase, which thus leads to the concept on incorporation of β-gal-based cellular MRI to melanin synthesis pathway, as described above.

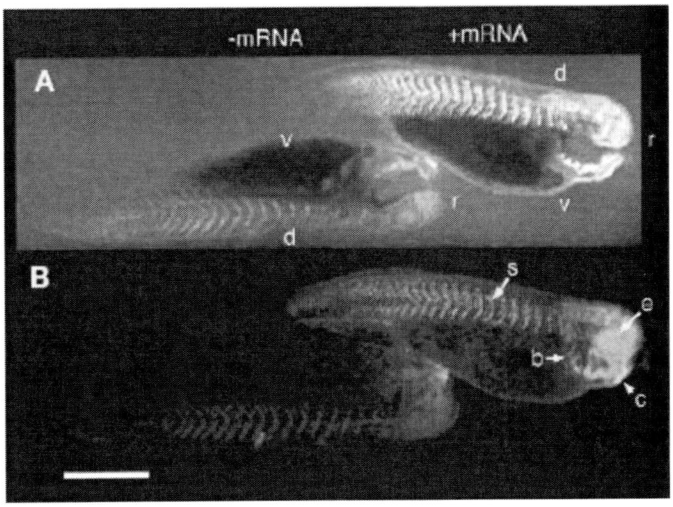

Figure 4.5. MRI detection of β -galactosidase mRNA expression in living X. laevis embryos. MR images of two embryos injected with EgadMe at the two-cell stages. (A) Unenhanced MR image. The embryo was also injected with β -gal mRNA, resulting in the higher intensity regions. (B) Pseudocolor rendering of same image in (A) with water made transparent. The image correction makes the possibility to recognize the eye, and brachial arches in the injected embryo: d, dorsal; v, ventral; r, rostral; e, eye; c, cement gland; s, somite; b, brachial arches. Scale bar = 1 mm. Reprinted, with permission, from [93].

MagA

MagA, a gene in magnetotactic bacteria known to be involved with production of magnetosomes, has been evaluated as a reporter gene for cellular MRI. Magnetotactic bacteria naturally synthesize intracellular magnetic structures, magnetosomes, which help to direct motility of the bacteria based on earth's magnetic field [96, 97].

Minor change: Letter 'a' was removed from the figure

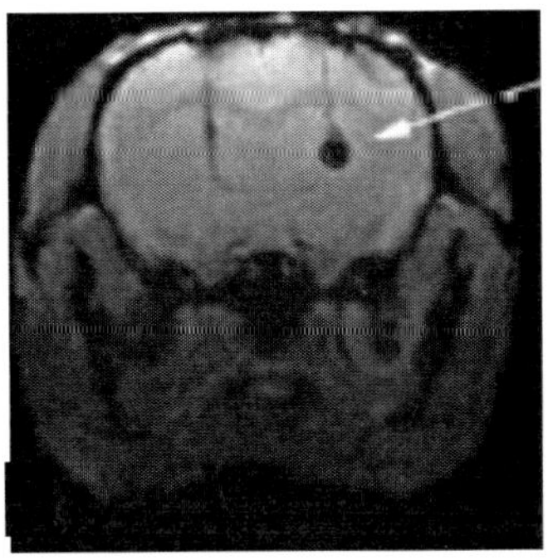

Figure 4.6. T2*-weighted MRI of mouse brain with transplanted 293FT cells transfected with lentivirus carrying magA genes. MagA-cells were neither induced nor incubated with iron supplement prior to transplantation. Reprinted, with permission, from [98].

It has been shown that MagA can be expressed in mammalian cells and its expression leads to the formation of magnetic nanoparticles that increase R2 relaxation and strongly attenuate MRI signal in a manner similar to ferritin imaging [98](Figure 4.6). MRI detection of Mag A expression has been shown in mouse neuroblastoma N2A cells [99], in human 293FT cell line [98], and both MagA and ferritin were expressed in MDA-MB-435 tumor cells [100]. Additional iron supplementation of MagA-expressing cells can further increase transverse relaxation rates compared to non-supplemented cells [100]. These results highlight the potential of magnetotactic bacterial gene expression to improve MRI cell tracking after their transplantation.

CEST

Chemical exchange saturation transfer (CEST) techniques use radiofrequency saturation pulses to detect molecules containing protons that exchange rapidly with water. Unique, genetically encoded, CEST-detectable amino acids and proteins (e.g., poly-L-arginine, lysine-rich protein and protamine) enabled imaging of transplanted cells by MRI in experimental models [12-14]. The contrast produced by CEST agents, unlike that produced by superparamagnetic metals, can be switched on and off by selectively irradiating (saturating) at the exchangeable proton resonance frequency. The proton exchange rate, and thus the generation of CEST contrast, depends strongly on pH [10, 14], which displays CEST signals that can report important biological events, such as death and inflammation of the transplanted cells with concurrent acidification of extracellular pH. CEST-detectable molecules have been proposed to function as nanosensors for identifying cell viability [15] (Figure 4.7).

The CEST-detectable molecules, such as poly-L-arginine and protamine, can be genetically encoded and used to identify the location of transplanted cells by cellular MRI [12]. A nonmetallic, biodegradable, lysine rich–protein reporter has been proposed as a CEST reporter recently [101].

To express lysine rich–protein in 9L rat glioma cells, eight synthetic oligonucleotides encoding lysine rich–protein were designed and cloned into a mammalian expression vector. CEST contrast has been achieved with frequency-selective targeting of amide protons of expressed lysine rich–protein in vitro as well as in vivo after transplantation of transgenic glioma cells into the mouse brain [101]. A novel reporter probe, 5-methyl-5,6-dihydrothymidine (5-MDHT), was described for detection of herpes simplex virus thymidine kinase (HSV-tk) expression with CEST imaging [102]; this opens up the possibility of using MRI for HSV-tk imaging. Recently, the exchange of amine protons from creatine with protons in bulk water was used to map myocardial creatine kinase metabolism in healthy and infarcted hearts (swine or sheep) in vivo in a clinical 3T scanner [18]. CEST signal based on creatine kinase proton exchange (CrEST) does not require any exogenous contrast agent and provides about two orders of magnitude with higher MRI sensitivity, compared to proton magnetic resonance spectroscopy. CrEST is expected to contribute to the early diagnosis of myocardial disorders (Figure 4.8).

The threshold for detection of CEST molecule-tagged cells ranges from 10^4-10^6 cells/voxel to distinguish the labeled cells using clinical MRI field strengths [103]. The main limitation of CEST imaging is the difficulty in distinguishing the reporter from intrinsic macromolecules.

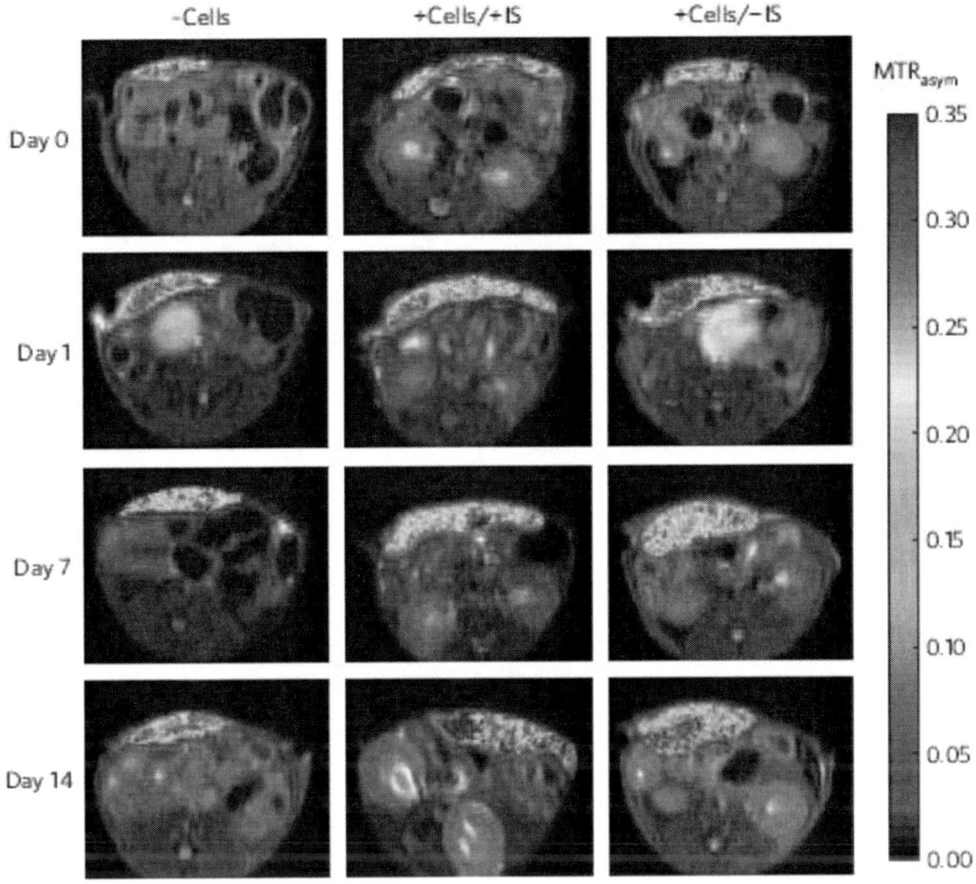

Figure 4.7. In vivo imaging of LipoCEST capsules containing hepatocytes subcutaneously transplanted in BALB/c mice. (- Cells) 2,500 empty LipoCEST capsules. (+Cells/ +IS) LipoCEST capsules containing hepatocytes while receiving immunosuppression. (+Cells/ -IS) LipoCEST capsules containing hepatocytes but no immunosuppression. Magnetization transfer-weighted overlays using a frequency offset of 2 ppm at days 0, 1, 7 and 14 after transplantation. Reprinted, with permission, from [15].

Ferritin

Ferritin, an endogenous iron storage protein, has been used as an MR gene reporter. The concept of using ferritin as an MRI reporter is based on its natural iron-sequestering function. Ferritin is a ubiquitously expressed metalloprotein, assembled out of 24 light and heavy subunits [104]. Ferritin is a globular protein that can be considered an "endogenous nanoparticle." It accumulates endogenous Fe(II) from the intracellular labile iron pool of the organism and stores Fe(II) as ferrihydrite (Fe(III)), which does not take part in the Fenton reaction, and therefore is not toxic [105-107]. If the intracellular level of ferritin is genetically altered, the higher number of ferritin complexes per cell causes higher iron accumulation, which thus directly affect MRI contrast [49, 108]. The use of the endogenous ferritin as a tool to visualize gene expression was described first in 2003 [109].

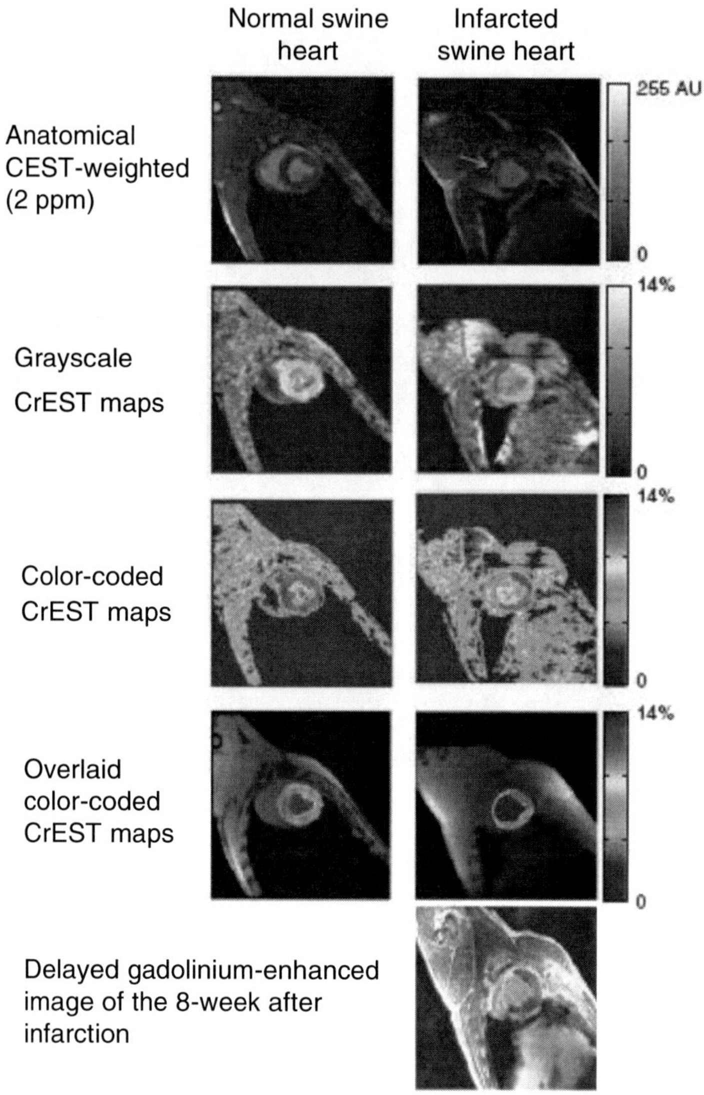

Figure 4.8. In vivo CrEST data from normal and infarcted swine myocardium. Reprinted, with permission, from [18].

The most sensitive MRI method for the detection of iron-accumulating cells is based on hypointense (i.e., dark or negative) contrast in so-called T2*-weighted MRI [51, 110, 111]. These images are based on modulations of T2* relaxation times.

Several studies have shown that ferritin overexpression increases intracellular iron content and transverse relaxation rates of tumor cells in vitro and in vivo [49, 112, 113]. Ferritin overexpression has been used for in vivo studies in the mouse brain [108, 114], utero of transgenic mice [115], and hepatocytes [116]. A ferritin shell is used in material science as a precursor for nano-composite particles as an effective MRI contrast agent for macrophage tracking [117] and for non-invasive imaging of atherosclerosis [118]. To date, several molecular biology approaches and different vectors have been used to overexpress ferritin, including adenoviral vector [108, 119], retroviral and lentiviral vectors [49, 112, 120, 121] and adeno-associated viral vectors [121], as well as different plasmid vectors [113, 122, 123].

Attempts have been made to validate the feasibility of using cellular MRI to detect cardiac grafts that overexpress ferritin in infarcted mouse hearts in vivo [44, 51, 124]. High heart rates in mice (500-600 beats per minute) present considerable challenges for imaging of cardiac grafts. Some authors have used two T2*-weighted imaging sequences to visualize cardiac grafts in the mouse hearts (Figure 4.9).

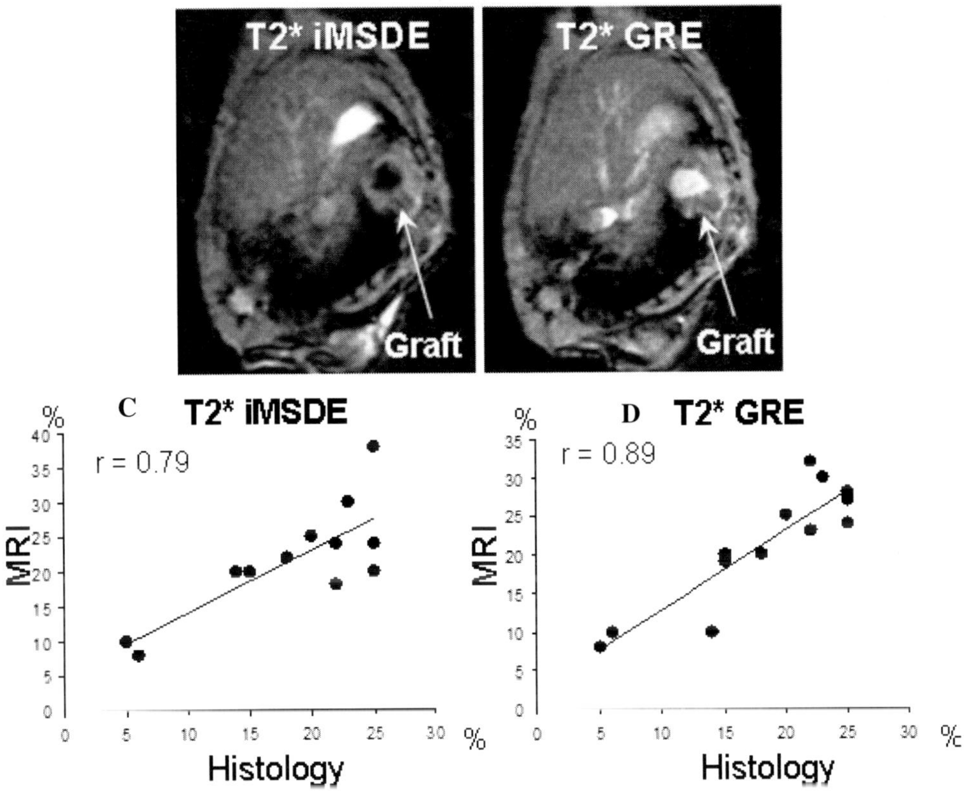

Figure 4.9. (A&B) MRI detection of ferritin-tagged graft in the infarcted mouse heart in T2* iMSDE and GRE pulse sequences and correlation of the graft size measurements by MRI and histology (C&D). Reprinted, with permission, from [51].

The first is the standard bright-blood cine gradient-echo (GRE) imaging sequence, which is an essential technique in the majority of cardiac imaging protocols. Based on the choice of the echo time (TE), this technique enables T2*-weighted imaging, which is beneficial for graft detection. The second technique is a new black-blood imaging method based on the motion-sensitized driven equilibrium (MSDE) preparation, which has been recently improved (iMSDE) [125]. In the iMSDE technique, the blood suppression effect is achieved via generating two consecutive spin echoes in the presence of flow-dephasing gradients, followed by restoring magnetization with a flip-back pulse. The key advantage of the iMSDE technique is its time efficiency, since the preparation period in MSDE requires short time. It also has been demonstrated that MSDE blood suppression is effective for elimination of slow-flow artifacts [126]. The iMSDE technique allows combination with a fast cardiac-gated cine GRE sequence, thus enabling black-blood imaging with T2*-weighted imaging. This study demonstrated that both black-blood and bright-blood T2*-weighted MRI sequences were sensitive for detection of transgenic grafts overexpressing ferritin. Quantification of MRI signal intensity changes showed a 30% reduction of signal intensity in ferritin-tagged areas in T2* bright-blood GRE images and 20% in T2* black-blood iMSDE images [51]. It has also been shown that MRI allows morphological graft size measurements with reasonable accuracy and precision (Figure 4.9). The bright-blood T2* GRE images provided the highest contrast-to-noise ratio and enables more precise graft size measurements [51]. However, this sequence frequently suffers from signal non-uniformity and voids in the ventricles caused by complex flow patterns. It is advisable, therefore, to use bright-blood T2*-weighted GRE images in combination with black-blood images, allowing reliable localization of the cardiac wall.

It is important to emphasize that no external iron supplementation is needed for ferritin-based MRI contrast. Changes in MRI signal intensity in graft areas are caused by redistribution and accumulation of endogenous iron in the overexpressed ferritin complexes of the genetically modified grafted cells [49, 51]. It has been shown that external iron supplementation may enhance ferritin-based MRI contrast [127].

The limitation of ferritin-based imaging of tissue grafts, which generally pertains to any cell labeling strategies based on "negative" contrast, is that the signal void caused by iron accumulation is difficult to be distinguished from hemosiderin depositions. In normal conditions, ferritin functions as a natural mechanism to sequester excess of iron intracellularly in a dispersed soluble form, which prevents elevation of hydroxyl-radical formation [106, 107, 128]. With further increases in cytosolic iron, ferritin is collected by lysosomes [129, 130], where the ferritin shell denatures [131] and the iron core aggregates in insoluble masses of hemosiderin for long-term storage [129, 130]. Under pathological conditions, the total amount of tissue iron may increase and iron can be deposited in hemosiderin, while the capacity of ferritin to store iron is overwhelmed [107, 128, 132]. Therefore, overexpression of ferritin in transplanted cells might have a protective effect based on the iron sequestration mechanism to prevent toxic effects of free iron. The challenge for imaging of ferritin-tagged grafts is to distinguish MRI signal changes between irons deposited in ferritin from hemosiderin. New technical approaches, such as analysis of non-monoexponential signal decay [133, 134] or phase-contrast imaging [135], may be helpful to distinguish the different sources of signal voids, though more research is necessary to identify the possibility of their applications in vivo.

Conclusion

Longitudinal repetitive magnetic resonance imaging of transplanted cells is extremely important for providing key functional endpoints as well as insights into mechanisms of biological actions. To distinguish grafted cells from the host tissue, cells must be labeled with exogenous particles (direct labeling) or genetically modified (indirect labeling) prior to their transplantation. Direct cell labeling is commonly used for MRI tracking of transplanted cell migration and homing. The direct labeling approach suffers from label dilution as cells proliferate and false-positive MRI signal when particles are released from dead cells and captured by macrophages. Indirect (genetic) cell labeling via the gene-reporter mechanism, despite its lower MRI signal intensity, enables longitudinal assessment of live transplanted cells.

References

[1] Naumova AV, Modo M, Moore A, Murry CE, Frank JA. Clinical imaging in regenerative medicine. *Nat. Biotechnol.* 2014;32(8):804-818.

[2] Nguyen PK, Lan F, Wang Y, Wu JC. Imaging: guiding the clinical translation of cardiac stem cell therapy. *Circ. Res.* 2011;109(8):962-979.

[3] Nguyen PK, Riegler J, Wu JC. Stem cell imaging: from bench to bedside. *Cell Stem Cell* 2014;14(4):431-444.

[4] Shapiro EM, Sharer K, Skrtic S, Koretsky AP. In vivo detection of single cells by MRI. *Magn. Reson. Med.* 2006;55(2):242-249.

[5] Himmelreich U, Dresselaers T. Cell labeling and tracking for experimental models using magnetic resonance imaging. *Methods* 2009;48(2):112-124.

[6] Dash R, Chung J, Ikeno F, Hahn-Windgassen A, Matsuura Y, Bennett MV, et al. Dual manganese-enhanced and delayed gadolinium-enhanced MRI detects myocardial border zone injury in a pig ischemia-reperfusion model. *Circ. Cardiovasc. Imaging* 2011;4(5):574-582.

[7] Mezer A, Yeatman JD, Stikov N, Kay KN, Cho NJ, Dougherty RF, et al. Quantifying the local tissue volume and composition in individual brains with magnetic resonance imaging. *Nat. Med.* 2013;19(12):1667-1672.

[8] Wedeen VJ, Hagmann P, Tseng WY, Reese TG, Weisskoff RM. Mapping complex tissue architecture with diffusion spectrum magnetic resonance imaging. *Magn. Reson. Med.* 2005;54(6):1377-1386.

[9] Sosnovik DE, Wang R, Dai G, Wang T, Aikawa E, Novikov M, et al. Diffusion spectrum MRI tractography reveals the presence of a complex network of residual myofibers in infarcted myocardium. *Circ. Cardiovasc. Imaging* 2009;2(3):206-212.

[10] Zhou J, Payen JF, Wilson DA, Traystman RJ, van Zijl PC. Using the amide proton signals of intracellular proteins and peptides to detect pH effects in MRI. *Nat. Med.* 2003;9(8):1085-1090.

[11] Zhou J, van Zijl PC. Defining an Acidosis-Based Ischemic Penumbra from pH-Weighted MRI. *Transl Stroke Res.* 2011;3(1):76-83.

[12] Bar-Shir A, Liu G, Chan KW, Oskolkov N, Song X, Yadav NN, et al. Human protamine-1 as an MRI reporter gene based on chemical exchange. *ACS Chem. Biol.* 2014;9(1):134-138.

[13] Ward KM, Aletras AH, Balaban RS. A new class of contrast agents for MRI based on proton chemical exchange dependent saturation transfer (CEST). *J. Magn. Reson.* 2000;143(1):79-87.

[14] van Zijl PC, Yadav NN. Chemical exchange saturation transfer (CEST): what is in a name and what isn't? *Magn. Reson. Med.* 2011;65(4):927-948.

[15] Chan KW, Liu G, Song X, Kim H, Yu T, Arifin DR, et al. MRI-detectable pH nanosensors incorporated into hydrogels for in vivo sensing of transplanted-cell viability. *Nat. Mater* 2013;12(3):268-275.

[16] Nelson SJ, Ozhinsky E, Li Y, Park I, Crane J. Strategies for rapid in vivo 1H and hyperpolarized 13C MR spectroscopic imaging. *J. Magn. Reson.* 2013;229(187-197.

[17] Zhu H, Barker PB. MR spectroscopy and spectroscopic imaging of the brain. *Methods Mol Biol* 2011;711(203-226.

[18] Haris M, Singh A, Cai K, Kogan F, McGarvey J, Debrosse C, et al. A technique for in vivo mapping of myocardial creatine kinase metabolism. *Nat. Med.* 2014;20(2):209-214.

[19] Naresh NK, Chen X, Roy RJ, Antkowiak PF, Annex BH, Epstein FH. Accelerated dual-contrast first-pass perfusion MRI of the mouse heart: Development and application to diet-induced obese mice. *Magn. Reson. Med.* 2014;

[20] Robbers LF, Nijveldt R, Beek AM, Hirsch A, van der Laan AM, Delewi R, et al. Cell therapy in reperfused acute myocardial infarction does not improve the recovery of perfusion in the infarcted myocardium: a cardiac MR imaging study. *Radiology* 2014;272(1):113-122.

[21] Kerwin WS, Naumova A, Storb R, Tapscott SJ, Wang Z. Mapping contrast agent uptake and retention in MRI studies of myocardial perfusion: case control study of dogs with Duchenne muscular dystrophy. *Int. J. Cardiovasc. Imaging* 2013;29(4):819-826.

[22] Kerwin WS, Zhao X, Yuan C, Hatsukami TS, Maravilla KR, Underhill HR, et al. Contrast-enhanced MRI of carotid atherosclerosis: dependence on contrast agent. *J. Magn. Reson. Imaging* 2009;30(1):35-40.

[23] Henningsson M, Greil GF, Burch M, Hussain T, Taylor AM, Muthurangu V, et al. Coronary magnetic resonance angiography in heterotopic heart transplant recipient. *Circulation* 2014;129(13):1453-1455.

[24] Bizino MB, Bonetti C, van der Geest RJ, Versluis MJ, Webb AG, Lamb HJ. High spatial resolution coronary magnetic resonance angiography at 7 T: comparison with low spatial resolution bright blood imaging. *Invest Radiol.* 2014;49(5):326-330.

[25] Arbab AS, Liu W, Frank JA. Cellular magnetic resonance imaging: current status and future prospects. *Expert Rev. Med. Devices* 2006;3(4):427-439.

[26] Partlow KC, Chen J, Brant JA, Neubauer AM, Meyerrose TE, Creer MH, et al. 19F magnetic resonance imaging for stem/progenitor cell tracking with multiple unique perfluorocarbon nanobeacons. *FASEB J.* 2007;21(8):1647-1654.

[27] Zhen Z, Xie J. Development of manganese-based nanoparticles as contrast probes for magnetic resonance imaging. *Theranostics* 2012;2(1):45-54.

[28] Dahnke H, Schaeffter T. Limits of detection of SPIO at 3.0 T using T2 relaxometry. *Magn. Reson. Med.* 2005;53(5):1202-1206.

[29] Thu MS, Bryant LH, Coppola T, Jordan EK, Budde MD, Lewis BK, et al. Self-assembling nanocomplexes by combining ferumoxytol, heparin and protamine for cell tracking by magnetic resonance imaging. *Nat. Med.* 2012;18(3):463-467.

[30] Gutova M, Frank JA, D'Apuzzo M, Khankaldyyan V, Gilchrist MM, Annala AJ, et al. Magnetic resonance imaging tracking of ferumoxytol-labeled human neural stem cells: studies leading to clinical use. *Stem Cells Transl. Med.* 2013;2(10):766-775.

[31] Shapiro EM, Skrtic S, Sharer K, Hill JM, Dunbar CE, Koretsky AP. MRI detection of single particles for cellular imaging. *Proc. Natl. Acad. Sci. USA* 2004;101(30):10901-10906.
[32] Hinds KA, Hill JM, Shapiro EM, Laukkanen MO, Silva AC, Combs CA, et al. Highly efficient endosomal labeling of progenitor and stem cells with large magnetic particles allows magnetic resonance imaging of single cells. *Blood* 2003;102(3):867-872.
[33] Yeh TC, Zhang W, Ildstad ST, Ho C. Intracellular labeling of T-cells with superparamagnetic contrast agents. *Magn. Reson. Med.* 1993;30(5):617-625.
[34] Arbab AS, Yocum GT, Kalish H, Jordan EK, Anderson SA, Khakoo AY, et al. Efficient magnetic cell labeling with protamine sulfate complexed to ferumoxides for cellular MRI. *Blood* 2004;104(4):1217-1223.
[35] Frank JA, Miller BR, Arbab AS, Zywicke HA, Jordan EK, Lewis BK, et al. Clinically applicable labeling of mammalian and stem cells by combining superparamagnetic iron oxides and transfection agents. *Radiology* 2003;228(2):480-487.
[36] Tannous BA, Grimm J, Perry KF, Chen JW, Weissleder R, Breakefield XO. Metabolic biotinylation of cell surface receptors for in vivo imaging. *Nat. Methods* 2006;3(5):391-396.
[37] So PW, Kalber T, Hunt D, Farquharson M, Al-Ebraheem A, Parkes HG, et al. Efficient and rapid labeling of transplanted cell populations with superparamagnetic iron oxide nanoparticles using cell surface chemical biotinylation for in vivo monitoring by MRI. *Cell Transplant* 2010;19(4):419-429.
[38] Walczak P, Kedziorek DA, Gilad AA, Lin S, Bulte JW. Instant MR labeling of stem cells using magnetoelectroporation. *Magn. Reson. Med.* 2005;54(4):769-774.
[39] Walczak P, Ruiz-Cabello J, Kedziorek DA, Gilad AA, Lin S, Barnett B, et al. Magnetoelectroporation: improved labeling of neural stem cells and leukocytes for cellular magnetic resonance imaging using a single FDA-approved agent. *Nanomedicine* 2006;2(2):89-94.
[40] Qiu B, Xie D, Walczak P, Li X, Ruiz-Cabello J, Minoshima S, et al. Magnetosonoporation: instant magnetic labeling of stem cells. *Magn. Reson. Med.* 2010;63(6):1437-1441.
[41] Xie D, Qiu B, Walczak P, Li X, Ruiz-Cabello J, Minoshima S, et al. Optimization of magnetosonoporation for stem cell labeling. *NMR Biomed.* 2010;23(5):480-484.
[42] Walczak P, Kedziorek DA, Gilad AA, Barnett BP, Bulte JW. Applicability and limitations of MR tracking of neural stem cells with asymmetric cell division and rapid turnover: the case of the shiverer dysmyelinated mouse brain. *Magn. Reson. Med.* 2007;58(2):261-269.
[43] Terrovitis J, Stuber M, Youssef A, Preece S, Leppo M, Kizana E, et al. Magnetic resonance imaging overestimates ferumoxide-labeled stem cell survival after transplantation in the heart. *Circulation* 2008;117(12):1555-1562.
[44] Naumova AV, Balu N, Yarnykh VL, Reinecke H, Murry CE, Yuan C. Magnetic Resonance Imaging Tracking of Graft Survival in the Infarcted Heart: Iron Oxide Particles Versus Ferritin Overexpression Approach. *J. Cardiovasc. Pharmacol. Ther.* 2014;19(4):358-367.
[45] van den Bos EJ, Baks T, Moelker AD, Kerver W, van Geuns RJ, van der Giessen WJ, et al. Magnetic resonance imaging of haemorrhage within reperfused myocardial

infarcts: possible interference with iron oxide-labelled cell tracking? *Eur. Heart J.* 2006;27(13):1620-1626.
[46] Schafer R, Kehlbach R, Muller M, Bantleon R, Kluba T, Ayturan M, et al. Labeling of human mesenchymal stromal cells with superparamagnetic iron oxide leads to a decrease in migration capacity and colony formation ability. *Cytotherapy* 2009;11(1):68-78.
[47] Kostura L, Kraitchman DL, Mackay AM, Pittenger MF, Bulte JW. Feridex labeling of mesenchymal stem cells inhibits chondrogenesis but not adipogenesis or osteogenesis. *NMR Biomed.* 2004;17(7):513-517.
[48] Li Z, Suzuki Y, Huang M, Cao F, Xie X, Connolly AJ, et al. Comparison of reporter gene and iron particle labeling for tracking fate of human embryonic stem cells and differentiated endothelial cells in living subjects. *Stem Cells* 2008;26(4):864-873.
[49] Cohen B, Dafni H, Meir G, Harmelin A, Neeman M. Ferritin as an endogenous MRI reporter for noninvasive imaging of gene expression in C6 glioma tumors. *Neoplasia* 2005;7(2):109-117.
[50] Haenebalcke L, Goossens S, Naessens M, Kruse N, Farhang Ghahremani M, Bartunkova S, et al. Efficient ROSA26-based conditional and/or inducible transgenesis using RMCE-compatible F1 hybrid mouse embryonic stem cells. *Stem Cell Rev.* 2013;9(6):774-785.
[51] Naumova AV, Yarnykh VL, Balu N, Reinecke H, Murry CE, Yuan C. Quantification of MRI signal of transgenic grafts overexpressing ferritin in murine myocardial infarcts. *NMR Biomed.* 2012;25(10):1187-1195.
[52] Urnov FD, Miller JC, Lee YL, Beausejour CM, Rock JM, Augustus S, et al. Highly efficient endogenous human gene correction using designed zinc-finger nucleases. *Nature* 2005;435(7042):646-651.
[53] Wang Y, Zhang WY, Hu S, Lan F, Lee AS, Huber B, et al. Genome editing of human embryonic stem cells and induced pluripotent stem cells with zinc finger nucleases for cellular imaging. *Circ. Res.* 2012;111(12):1494-1503.
[54] Ding Q, Regan SN, Xia Y, Oostrom LA, Cowan CA, Musunuru K. Enhanced efficiency of human pluripotent stem cell genome editing through replacing TALENs with CRISPRs. *Cell Stem Cell* 2013;12(4):393-394.
[55] Aisen P, Enns C, Wessling-Resnick M. Chemistry and biology of eukaryotic iron metabolism. *Int. J. Biochem. Cell Biol.* 2001;33(10):940-959.
[56] Aisen P. Transferrin, the transferrin receptor, and the uptake of iron by cells. *Met. Ions Biol. Syst.* 1998;35(585-631.
[57] Thorstensen K, Romslo I. The role of transferrin in the mechanism of cellular iron uptake. *Biochem. J.* 1990;271(1):1-9.
[58] Koretsky A, Lin Y, Schorle H, R. J. Genetic control of MRI contrast by expression of the transferrin receptor. in ISMRM Proceedings. 1996. New York.
[59] Moore A, Basilion JP, Chiocca EA, Weissleder R. Measuring transferrin receptor gene expression by NMR imaging. *Biochim. Biophys. Acta* 1998;1402(3):239-249.
[60] Moore A, Josephson L, Bhorade RM, Basilion JP, Weissleder R. Human transferrin receptor gene as a marker gene for MR imaging. *Radiology* 2001;221(1):244-250.
[61] Bulte JW, Zhang S, van Gelderen P, Herynek V, Jordan EK, Duncan ID, et al. Neurotransplantation of magnetically labeled oligodendrocyte progenitors: magnetic

resonance tracking of cell migration and myelination. *Proc. Natl. Acad. Sci. USA* 1999;96(26):15256-15261.

[62] Kayyem JF, Kumar RM, Fraser SE, Meade TJ. Receptor-targeted co-transport of DNA and magnetic resonance contrast agents. *Chem. Biol.* 1995;2(9):615-620.

[63] Hogemann D, Josephson L, Weissleder R, Basilion JP. Improvement of MRI probes to allow efficient detection of gene expression. *Bioconjug Chem.* 2000;11(6):941-946.

[64] Schafer R, Kehlbach R, Wiskirchen J, Bantleon R, Pintaske J, Brehm BR, et al. Transferrin receptor upregulation: in vitro labeling of rat mesenchymal stem cells with superparamagnetic iron oxide. *Radiology* 2007;244(2):514-523.

[65] Pawelczyk E, Frank JA. Transferrin receptor expression in iron oxide-labeled mesenchymal stem cells. *Radiology* 2008;247(3):913; author reply 914-915.

[66] Pawelczyk E, Arbab AS, Pandit S, Hu E, Frank JA. Expression of transferrin receptor and ferritin following ferumoxides-protamine sulfate labeling of cells: implications for cellular magnetic resonance imaging. *NMR Biomed.* 2006;19(5):581-592.

[67] Sotak CH, Sharer K, Koretsky AP. Manganese cell labeling of murine hepatocytes using manganese(III)-transferrin. *Contrast Media Mol. Imaging* 2008;3(3):95-105.

[68] Krumholz A, Vanvickle-Chavez SJ, Yao J, Fleming TP, Gillanders WE, Wang LV. Photoacoustic microscopy of tyrosinase reporter gene in vivo. *J. Biomed. Opt.* 2011;16(8):080503.

[69] Weissleder R, Simonova M, Bogdanova A, Bredow S, Enochs WS, Bogdanov A, Jr. MR imaging and scintigraphy of gene expression through melanin induction. *Radiology* 1997;204(2):425-429.

[70] Jimbow K, Quevedo WC, Jr., Fitzpatrick TB, Szabo G. Some aspects of melanin biology: 1950-1975. *J. Invest Dermatol.* 1976;67(1):72-89.

[71] Larsson BS. Interaction between chemicals and melanin. *Pigment Cell Res.* 1993;6(3):127-133.

[72] Sarna T, Hyde JS, Swartz HM. Ion-exchange in melanin: an electron spin resonance study with lanthanide probes. *Science* 1976;192(4244):1132-1134.

[73] Sarna T, Duleba A, Korytowski W, Swartz H. Interaction of melanin with oxygen. *Arch. Biochem. Biophys.* 1980;200(1):140-148.

[74] Sarna T, Froncisz W, Hyde JS. Cu2+ probe of metal-ion binding sites in melanin using electron paramagentic resonance spectroscopy. II. Natural melanin. *Arch. Biochem. Biophys.* 1980;202(1):304-313.

[75] Sarna T, Sealy RC. Photoinduced oxygen consumption in melanin systems. Action spectra and quantum yields for eumelanin and synthetic melanin. *Photochem. Photobiol.* 1984;39(1):69-74.

[76] Potts AM, Au PC. The affinity of melanin for inorganic ions. *Exp. Eye Res.* 1976;22(5):487-491.

[77] Bahbouth E, Siwek B, De Pauw-Gillet MC, Sabbioni E, Bassleer R. Effects of trace metals on mouse B16 melanoma cells in culture. *Biol. Trace Elem Res.* 1993;36(2):191-201.

[78] Enochs WS, Hyslop WB, Bennett HF, Brown RD, 3rd, Koenig SH, Swartz HM. Sources of the increased longitudinal relaxation rates observed in melanotic melanoma. An in vitro study of synthetic melanins. *Invest Radiol.* 1989;24(10):794-804.

[79] Enochs WS, Petherick P, Bogdanova A, Mohr U, Weissleder R. Paramagnetic metal scavenging by melanin: MR imaging. *Radiology* 1997;204(2):417-423.

[80] DeJordy JO, Bendel P, Horowitz A, Salomon Y, Degani H. Correlation of MR imaging and histologic findings in mouse melanoma. *J. Magn. Reson. Imaging* 1992;2(6):695-700.

[81] Isiklar I, Leeds NE, Fuller GN, Kumar AJ. Intracranial metastatic melanoma: correlation between MR imaging characteristics and melanin content. *AJR Am. J. Roentgenol.* 1995;165(6):1503-1512.

[82] Alfke H, Stoppler H, Nocken F, Heverhagen JT, Kleb B, Czubayko F, et al. In vitro MR imaging of regulated gene expression. *Radiology* 2003;228(2):488-492.

[83] Paproski RJ, Forbrich AE, Wachowicz K, Hitt MM, Zemp RJ. Tyrosinase as a dual reporter gene for both photoacoustic and magnetic resonance imaging. *Biomed. Opt. Express* 2011;2(4):771-780.

[84] Qin C, Cheng K, Chen K, Hu X, Liu Y, Lan X, et al. Tyrosinase as a multifunctional reporter gene for Photoacoustic/MRI/PET triple modality molecular imaging. *Sci. Rep.* 2013;3(1490.

[85] Rolla GA, Tei L, Fekete M, Arena F, Gianolio E, Botta M. Responsive Mn(II) complexes for potential applications in diagnostic Magnetic Resonance Imaging. *Bioorg. Med. Chem.* 2011;19(3):1115-1122.

[86] Pawelek JM, Murray M. Increase in melanin formation and promotion of cytotoxicity in cultured melanoma cells caused by phosphorylated isomers of L-dopa. *Cancer Res.* 1986;46(2):493-497.

[87] Pawelek JM, Lerner AB. 5,6-Dihydroxyindole is a melanin precursor showing potent cytotoxicity. *Nature* 1978;276(5688):626-628.

[88] Hanaoka K, Kikuchi K, Terai T, Komatsu T, Nagano T. A Gd3+-based magnetic resonance imaging contrast agent sensitive to beta-galactosidase activity utilizing a receptor-induced magnetization enhancement (RIME) phenomenon. *Chemistry* 2008;14(3):987-995.

[89] Chang YT, Cheng CM, Su YZ, Lee WT, Hsu JS, Liu GC, et al. Synthesis and characterization of a new bioactivated paramagnetic gadolinium(III) complex [Gd(DOTA-FPG)(H2O)] for tracing gene expression. *Bioconjug. Chem.* 2007;18(6):1716-1727.

[90] Moats RA, Fraser SE, T M. A ''smart'' magnetic resonance imaging agent that reports on specific enzyme activity. *Angew Chem. Intl. Edn. Engl.* 1997;36(726-728.

[91] Cui W, Otten P, Li Y, Koeneman KS, Yu J, Mason RP. Novel NMR approach to assessing gene transfection: 4-fluoro-2-nitrophenyl-beta-D-galactopyranoside as a prototype reporter molecule for beta-galactosidase. *Magn. Reson. Med.* 2004;51(3):616-620.

[92] Yu J, Liu L, Kodibagkar VD, Cui W, Mason RP. Synthesis and evaluation of novel enhanced gene reporter molecules: detection of beta-galactosidase activity using 19F NMR of trifluoromethylated aryl beta-D-galactopyranosides. *Bioorg. Med. Chem.* 2006;14(2):326-333.

[93] Louie AY, Huber MM, Ahrens ET, Rothbacher U, Moats R, Jacobs RE, et al. In vivo visualization of gene expression using magnetic resonance imaging. *Nat. Biotechnol.* 2000;18(3):321-325.

[94] Kodibagkar VD, Yu J, Liu L, Hetherington HP, Mason RP. Imaging beta-galactosidase activity using 19F chemical shift imaging of LacZ gene-reporter molecule 2-fluoro-4-nitrophenol-beta-D-galactopyranoside. *Magn. Reson. Imaging* 2006;24(7):959-962.

[95] Arena F, Singh JB, Gianolio E, Stefania R, Aime S. beta-Gal gene expression MRI reporter in melanoma tumor cells. Design, synthesis, and in vitro and in vivo testing of a Gd(III) containing probe forming a high relaxivity, melanin-like structure upon beta-Gal enzymatic activation. *Bioconjug Chem.* 2011;22(12):2625-2635.

[96] Blakemore R. Magnetotactic bacteria. *Science* 1975;190(4212):377-379.

[97] Bazylinski DA, Frankel RB. Magnetosome formation in prokaryotes. *Nat. Rev. Microbiol.* 2004;2(3):217-230.

[98] Zurkiya O, Chan AW, Hu X. MagA is sufficient for producing magnetic nanoparticles in mammalian cells, making it an MRI reporter. *Magn. Reson. Med.* 2008;59(6):1225-1231.

[99] Goldhawk DE, Lemaire C, McCreary CR, McGirr R, Dhanvantari S, Thompson RT, et al. Magnetic resonance imaging of cells overexpressing MagA, an endogenous contrast agent for live cell imaging. *Mol. Imaging* 2009;8(3):129-139.

[100] Sengupta A, Quiaoit K, Thompson RT, Prato FS, Gelman N, Goldhawk DE. Biophysical features of MagA expression in mammalian cells: implications for MRI contrast. *Front Microbiol.* 2014;5(29.

[101] Gilad AA, McMahon MT, Walczak P, Winnard PT, Jr., Raman V, van Laarhoven HW, et al. Artificial reporter gene providing MRI contrast based on proton exchange. *Nat. Biotechnol.* 2007;25(2):217-219.

[102] Bar-Shir A, Liu G, Greenberg MM, Bulte JW, Gilad AA. Synthesis of a probe for monitoring HSV1-tk reporter gene expression using chemical exchange saturation transfer MRI. *Nat. Protoc.* 2013;8(12):2380-2391.

[103] Ahrens ET, Bulte JW. Tracking immune cells in vivo using magnetic resonance imaging. *Nat. Rev. Immunol.* 2013;13(10):755-763.

[104] Theil EC. Ferritin: structure, gene regulation, and cellular function in animals, plants, and microorganisms. *Annu. Rev. Biochem.* 1987;56(289-315.

[105] Valko M, Morris H, Cronin MT. Metals, toxicity and oxidative stress. *Curr. Med. Chem.* 2005;12(10):1161-1208.

[106] Crichton RR, Wilmet S, Legssyer R, Ward RJ. Molecular and cellular mechanisms of iron homeostasis and toxicity in mammalian cells. *J. Inorg. Biochem.* 2002;91(1):9-18.

[107] Arosio P, Levi S. Ferritin, iron homeostasis, and oxidative damage. *Free Radic. Biol. Med.* 2002;33(4):457-463.

[108] Genove G, DeMarco U, Xu H, Goins WF, Ahrens ET. A new transgene reporter for in vivo magnetic resonance imaging. *Nat. Med.* 2005;11(4):450-454.

[109] Ahrens E, Contrast agents for magnetic resonance imaging and methods related thereto., 2003, Patent application: USPTO US. p. 0219385.

[110] Baksi AJ, Pennell DJ. T2* imaging of the heart: methods, applications, and outcomes. *Top Magn. Reson. Imaging* 2014;23(1):13-20.

[111] Taylor BA, Loeffler RB, Song R, McCarville ME, Hankins JS, Hillenbrand CM. Automated T(2) * measurements using supplementary field mapping to assess cardiac iron content. *J. Magn. Reson. Imaging* 2013;38(2):441-447.

[112] Kim HS, Cho HR, Choi SH, Woo JS, Moon WK. In vivo imaging of tumor transduced with bimodal lentiviral vector encoding human ferritin and green fluorescent protein on a 1.5T clinical magnetic resonance scanner. *Cancer Res.* 2010;70(18):7315-7324.

[113] Ono K, Fuma K, Tabata K, Sawada M. Ferritin reporter used for gene expression imaging by magnetic resonance. *Biochem. Biophys. Res. Commun.* 2009;388(3):589-594.
[114] Vande Velde G, Raman Rangarajan J, Vreys R, Guglielmetti C, Dresselaers T, Verhoye M, et al. Quantitative evaluation of MRI-based tracking of ferritin-labeled endogenous neural stem cell progeny in rodent brain. *Neuroimage* 2012;62(1):367-380.
[115] Cohen B, Ziv K, Plaks V, Israely T, Kalchenko V, Harmelin A, et al. MRI detection of transcriptional regulation of gene expression in transgenic mice. *Nat. Med.* 2007;13(4):498-503.
[116] Ziv K, Meir G, Harmelin A, Shimoni E, Klein E, Neeman M. Ferritin as a reporter gene for MRI: chronic liver over expression of H-ferritin during dietary iron supplementation and aging. *NMR Biomed.* 2010;23(5):523-531.
[117] Uchida M, Terashima M, Cunningham CH, Suzuki Y, Willits DA, Willis AF, et al. A human ferritin iron oxide nano-composite magnetic resonance contrast agent. *Magn. Reson. Med.* 2008;60(5):1073-1081.
[118] Terashima M, Uchida M, Kosuge H, Tsao PS, Young MJ, Conolly SM, et al. Human ferritin cages for imaging vascular macrophages. *Biomaterials* 2011;32(5):1430-1437.
[119] Iordanova B, Robison CS, Ahrens ET. Design and characterization of a chimeric ferritin with enhanced iron loading and transverse NMR relaxation rate. *J. Biol. Inorg. Chem* 2010;15(6):957-965.
[120] Liu J, Cheng EC, Long RC, Yang SH, Wang L, Cheng PH, et al. Noninvasive monitoring of embryonic stem cells in vivo with MRI transgene reporter. *Tissue Eng. Part C Methods* 2009;15(4):739-747.
[121] Vande Velde G, Rangarajan JR, Toelen J, Dresselaers T, Ibrahimi A, Krylychkina O, et al. Evaluation of the specificity and sensitivity of ferritin as an MRI reporter gene in the mouse brain using lentiviral and adeno-associated viral vectors. *Gene Ther.* 2011;18(6):594-605.
[122] Deans AE, Wadghiri YZ, Bernas LM, Yu X, Rutt BK, Turnbull DH. Cellular MRI contrast via coexpression of transferrin receptor and ferritin. *Magn. Reson. Med.* 2006;56(1):51-59.
[123] Aung W, Hasegawa S, Koshikawa-Yano M, Obata T, Ikehira H, Furukawa T, et al. Visualization of in vivo electroporation-mediated transgene expression in experimental tumors by optical and magnetic resonance imaging. *Gene Ther.* 2009;16(7):830-839.
[124] Naumova AV, Reinecke H, Yarnykh V, Deem J, Yuan C, Murry CE. Ferritin overexpression for noninvasive magnetic resonance imaging-based tracking of stem cells transplanted into the heart. *Mol Imaging* 2010;9(4):201-210.
[125] Wang J, Yarnykh VL, Yuan C. Enhanced image quality in black-blood MRI using the improved motion-sensitized driven-equilibrium (iMSDE) sequence. *J. Magn. Reson. Imaging* 2010;31(5):1256-1263.
[126] Wang J, Yarnykh VL, Hatsukami T, Chu B, Balu N, Yuan C. Improved suppression of plaque-mimicking artifacts in black-blood carotid atherosclerosis imaging using a multislice motion-sensitized driven-equilibrium (MSDE) turbo spin-echo (TSE) sequence. *Magn. Reson. Med.* 2007;58(5):973-981.
[127] Feng Y, Liu Q, Zhu J, Xie F, Li L. Efficiency of ferritin as an MRI reporter gene in NPC cells is enhanced by iron supplementation. *J. Biomed. Biotechnol.* 2012;2012(434878.

[128] Arosio P, Levi S. Cytosolic and mitochondrial ferritins in the regulation of cellular iron homeostasis and oxidative damage. *Biochim. Biophys. Acta* 2010;1800(8):783-792.
[129] De Domenico I, Ward DM, Kaplan J. Specific iron chelators determine the route of ferritin degradation. *Blood* 2009;114(20):4546-4551.
[130] Iancu TC. Ferritin and hemosiderin in pathological tissues. *Electron Microsc. Rev.* 1992;5(2):209-229.
[131] Miyazaki E, Kato J, Kobune M, Okumura K, Sasaki K, Shintani N, et al. Denatured H-ferritin subunit is a major constituent of haemosiderin in the liver of patients with iron overload. *Gut* 2002;50(3):413-419.
[132] Harrison PM, Arosio P. The ferritins: molecular properties, iron storage function and cellular regulation. *Biochim. Biophys. Acta* 1996;1275(3):161-203.
[133] Jensen JH, Chandra R. Theory of nonexponential NMR signal decay in liver with iron overload or superparamagnetic iron oxide particles. *Magn. Reson. Med.* 2002;47(6):1131-1138.
[134] Wu EX, Kim D, Tosti CL, Tang H, Jensen JH, Cheung JS, et al. Magnetic resonance assessment of iron overload by separate measurement of tissue ferritin and hemosiderin iron. *Ann. N Y Acad. Sci.* 2010;1202(115-122.
[135] Mills PH, Ahrens ET. Enhanced positive-contrast visualization of paramagnetic contrast agents using phase images. *Magn. Reson. Med.* 2009;62(5):1349-1355.

In: Magnetic Resonance Imaging of Stem Cell Applications ISBN: 978-1-63463-910-1
Editor: Xiaoming Yang

Chapter 5

Strategies for Delivery of Stem Cells

Sandeep Vaidya* and Manjiri Dighe
Division of Interventional Radiology, Department of Radiology,
University of Washington School of Medicine, Seattle, Washington, US

Abstract

In recent years, research advancement in stem cell therapy has been rapid. Accordingly, general clinical, scientific, and public attention to the application of stem cell therapy has been substantial. Promises are great, most notably with regard to the application of stem cell therapy for diseases that are currently difficult to treat or incurable such as Parkinson disease or diabetes mellitus.

Targeted stem cells offer great potential as therapeutic agents. For any systemically administered agent to have clinical efficacy it must first circulate through the systemic vasculature, exit from vascular space, traverse the interstitium and enter or affect the target or substrate in large enough quantities. At each of these steps there are barriers, related to anatomy and physiology, which hinder delivery of the therapeutics throughout the entire target. Interventional radiologists may circumvent these barriers using imaging guidance for delivery.

In the context of Interventional Radiology, "targeted delivery" of an agent may encompass image-guided local delivery, such as intraarterial and percutaneous intratumoral deliveries. In addition, there is a potential role for the interventionists to create engraftment territory and increase engraftment bed fertility with controlled intentional tissue destruction (e.g., by means of thermal ablation) that might precede stem cell administration. This chapter focuses on different types of interventional approaches for local delivery of stem cells.

Keywords: Active targeting, interventional radiology, image-guided interventions, stem cells, stem cell therapy

* Corresponding author: Sandeep Vaidya, MD, Division of Interventional Radiology, Department of Radiology, University of Washington School of Medicine, Seattle, Washington, US (svaidya@uw.edu).

Introduction

The field of stem cell therapy aims to use the properties and physical characteristics of these cells for the diagnosis and treatment of diseases at the molecular level [1, 2]. Rapidly evolving imaging technologies are being utilized for targeted anatomic and molecular imaging as well as for treatment of tumors and other pathologies.

Stem cell based therapeutics, allowing specific delivery to molecular targets, are being developed for many pathologies. Targeted stem cell-based therapies offer significant improvements in efficacy, particularly as anti-neoplastic agents. However, it is necessary to understand biology and the barriers to the delivery of these agents imposed by the microvasculature and microenvironment so as to better understand the possible potential and limitations of targeted imaging and therapeutics. In the context of Interventional Radiology, "targeted delivery" of an agent may encompass image-guided local delivery, such as intraarterial and percutaneous intratumoral deliveries, direct targeting of organ vasculature or interstitium delivery, as well as creation of engraftment territory and increase of engraftment bed fertility. These approaches may also be utilized to circumvent barriers to the systemic intravenous delivery of the agent.

These technologies will likely have important applications in all areas of radiology. Furthermore, Interventional Radiologists will have a role in the localized targeted delivery of stem cells to circumvent potential toxicities and optimize delivery and efficacy. Moreover, stem cell therapy will likely affect the clinical care of patients with a number of disease entities treated by Interventional Radiologists [3, 4]. The Society of Interventional Radiology Interventional Oncology Task Force vision statement suggested that by 2015 there should be improved integration of current image-guided oncologic technologies with new developments in genomics, proteomics, molecular imaging, and nanotechnology [5].

Targeted Stem Cell Applications and Approaches in Interventional Radiology

An increasing number of therapeutics are being developed, which might indirectly or directly affect the practice of Interventional Radiology. Clearly, interventionists should have a pivotal role in targeted stem cell delivery to certain organs such as the pancreas, liver, or kidney. Interventionists' participation may overcome some of the challenges that are currently associated with stem cell homing and trafficking. In particular, selective and direct stem cell release to the target organ by means of transcatheter intraarterial delivery may overcome potential mechanical barriers such as caused by liver cirrhosis and fibrosis that have been postulated to exist for nonselective stem cell delivery techniques. In this context, recipient organ perfusion with donor cells "via a radiologically placed catheter" has been recommended. In a recent clinical study, hepatic regeneration could be enhanced with portal venous infusion of bone marrow–derived stem cells into portal vein branches before portal vein embolization and partial hepatectomy.

An additional relevant parameter with regard to stem cell engraftment success is the target area receptiveness for stem cells after their administration. Depending on the type of target organ and stem cell type that is used, infliction of acute organ injury is known to be necessary for cell uptake and differentiation, the former of which is triggered by the release of certain key cytokines [6]. Ablating and devascularizing dysfunctional tissue by means of radiofrequency (RF) ablation creates periablational hyperemia and/or ingrowing granulation tissue, which may then provide a vascular environment that allows for highly efficient stem cell trafficking to the selected target area and subsequent stem cell engraftment. In addition, the role of devascularization of dysfunctional tissue through transarterial catheter embolization could be explored. Both techniques (i.e., RF ablation and transarterial catheter embolization) may be followed by subsequent targeted cell delivery to improve stem cell trafficking efficiency when compared to peripheral intravenous cell administration [7-10].

Different approaches for delivery of stem cells have been proposed and studied in research settings. The approach varies with the disease entity naturally and below is a brief overview of the various types of approaches based on disease pattern. Details of each approach in terms of technical discussion and risks and benefits of the actual procedure itself are beyond the scope of this chapter.

Peripheral Arterial Disease

The first report in 2002 demonstrated the safety and efficacy of intramuscular injection of bone marrow cells in patients with chronic limb ischemia and significantly improved anklebrachial pressure indexes, transcutaneous oxygen pressures, and pain-free walking times while reducing rest pain. Both intramuscular injection of cells, intra-arterial injection, or the combination of both have been reported as effective ways to administer stem cell therapy. With intramuscular injection, local depots of stem cells are created in the ischemic muscle, which augment neovascularization by facilitating cell-to-cell contact and then cell transdifferentiation. However, survival of the stem cells may be reduced since the depots are laid down in an ischemic environment. With intra-arterial administration, stem cells travel to the border zone of ischemia in the nutrient- and oxygen-rich circulation, thus providing a favorable environment for survival and engraftment, but cell uptake from the circulation to the ischemic tissue may be limited [11]. Recently, some scientists have developed a novel approach in this regards. It involves enclosing stem cells in an alginate capsule or "bubble" made from seaweed that contains stem cells, creating factors to recruit the regenerating blood vessels. This is still being worked upon.

Parkinson's Disease

A very interesting and more elegant approach is stem cell–mediated delivery of glial cell line–derived neurotropic factor, a protein that promotes dopaminergic neuron preservation and differentiation. This type of stem cell use as a vehicle for gene therapy has resulted in glial cell line–derived neurotropic factor expression in vivo and led to prolonged neuron survival as well as functional improvement [12].

Notably, intraarterial catheter-directed administration of adult stem cells into the posterior circulation has recently been presented as a beneficial and efficient way of improving symptoms in patients with Parkinson disease in a clinical trial encompassing 47 patients [13, 14].

Stroke

Bone marrow–derived—specifically mesenchymal stem cells—and human umbilical cord blood stem cells have been tested for potential therapeutic applications in stroke. Multiple studies have demonstrated functional outcome improvement after intravenous, intracerebral, or intraarterial stem cell application. There has also been one clinical trial in which the study group received mesenchymal stem cells intravenously after middle cerebral artery infarction and showed improved functional recovery compared to a control group during 1-year follow-up [15].

Intrastriatal injections (directly into the globus pallidus/putamen) for stroke have been tried. All these approaches are experimental and being studied. No long term data is available understandably.

Multiple Sclerosis

Intraventricular administration of neural progenitor cells in Multiple Sclerosis (MS) has been attempted. MS is an inflammatory autoimmune disease that may be characterized by a progressive or relapsing course. Autologous bone marrow–derived stem cells have been found most suitable for stem cell–based therapy for this and have been most successful at an early stage of the disease and if performed as nonmyeloablative therapy [9, 10, 16].

Diabetes Mellitus

Cell-based therapy, compared to pancreas transplant, is more elegant, more cost effective, and less invasive. Various target areas and delivery routes of stem cell injection have been explored (percutaneous intrasplenic, subcapsular renal, intra-omental, subcutaneous, and into the celiac artery).

Direct intraportal venous delivery has emerged as the technically most feasible, least complicated, and most efficient way of islet cell delivery even though occurrence of bleeding complications as well as portal vein thrombosis that is apparently related to intraprocedural increases in portal venous pressure have been described [17, 18].

Disc Disease

Degenerated intervertebral discs (IVDs) are a significant contributor to low back pain, and effective therapies for this entity are lacking. Novel stem cell therapies have shown great promise for the regeneration and biological repair of degenerated IVDs, and may represent a promising alternative.

Percutaneously transplanting human mesenchymal stem cells (MSCs) under image guidance into models of degenerated IVDs in which a 25-gauge needle was advanced to the middle one-third of the IVD using a 22-guage coaxial system under fluoroscopic guidance and approximately 100,000 radiolabeled (I-124 FIAU) MSCs has been proposed and presented [19].

Myocardial Infarction

There is currently an ongoing trial to assess the safety and efficacy of injecting autologous bone marrow stem cells intra-coronary arterially after intervention for acute myocardial ischemia. This was built on the idea described earlier about targeting myocardial cells using micro-bubbles [20, 21].

Conclusion

Rapidly emerging stem cell therapy offers great promise for advances in most medical fields including Diagnostic and Interventional Radiology. A large number of multifunctional imaging and therapeutic agents are in various stages of development. While there are significant potential benefits, toxicities and physiologic barriers to the delivery of these agents may exist. Image-guided local delivery may circumvent these barriers resulting in improved delivery and efficacy with reduced toxicity. Hence the Interventional Radiologists will have a greater role to play as these therapies mature. The approach for targeting for the interventionists will depend on the disease entity and hence can be a wide spectrum each with a specific target. In addition, there is a role also in increasing the stem cell deposition in the target area by causing tissue ischemia for better cell trafficking [8].

References

[1] Ratner M, Ratner D. Size Matters. In: Ratner M, Ratner D, ed. *Nanotechnology.* 1rd ed. Upper Saddle River, New Jersey: Bemard Goodwin, 2003; 11-18.

[2] Kim BY, Rutka JT, Chan WC. Nanomedicine. *N. Engl. J. Med.* 2010;363(25):2434-2443.

[3] Power S, Slattery MM, Lee MJ. Nanotechnology and its relationship to interventional radiology. *Part I: imaging. Cardiovasc Intervent Radiol* 2011;34(2):221-226.

[4] Power S, Slattery MM, Lee MJ. Nanotechnology and its relationship to interventional radiology. *Part II: Drug Delivery, Thermotherapy, and Vascular Intervention. Cardiovasc Intervent Radiol* 2011;34(4):676-690.

[5] Nikolic B, Faintuch S, Goldberg SN, Kuo MD, Cardella JF. Stem cell therapy: a primer for interventionalists and imagers. *J. Vasc Interv. Radiol.* 2009;20(8):999-1012.

[6] Ahmed M, Monsky WE, Girnun G, Lukyanov A, D'Ippolito G, Kruskal JB, et al. Radiofrequency thermal ablation sharply increases intratumoral liposomal doxorubicin accumulation and tumor coagulation. *Cancer Res* 2003;63(19):6327-6333.

[7] Goldberg SN, Bonn J, Dodd G, Dupuy D, Geschwind JH, Hicks M, et al. Society of Interventional Radiology Interventional Oncology Task Force: interventional oncology research vision statement and critical assessment of the state of research affairs. *J. Vasc. Interv Radiol.* 2005;16(10):1287-1294.

[8] Ahmed M, Lukyanov AN, Torchilin V, Tournier H, Schneider AN, Goldberg SN. Combined radiofrequency ablation and adjuvant liposomal chemotherapy: effect of chemotherapeutic agent, nanoparticle size, and circulation time. *J. Vasc. Interv. Radiol.* 2005;16(10):1365-1371.

[9] Burt RK, Cohen B, Rose J, Petersen F, Oyama Y, Stefoski D, et al. Hematopoietic stem cell transplantation for multiple sclerosis. *Arch. Neurol.* 2005;62(6):860-864.

[10] Uccelli A, Zappia E, Benvenuto F, Frassoni F, Mancardi G. Stem cells in inflammatory demyelinating disorders: a dual role for immunosuppression and neuroprotection. *Expert Opin Biol. Ther* 2006;6(1):17-22.

[11] Sprengers RW, Moll FL, Verhaar MC. Stem cell therapy in PAD. *Eur. J. Vasc. Endovasc Surg.* 2010;39(Suppl 1):S38-S43.

[12] Behrstock S, Ebert A, McHugh J, Vosberg S, Moore J, Schneider B, et al. Human neural progenitors deliver glial cell line-derived neurotrophic factor to parkinsonian rodents and aged primates. *Gene Ther* 2006;13(5):379-388.

[13] Brazzini A CR, Gallardo A, et al. Intraarterial autologous implant of adult stem cell for patients with Parkinson's disease (abstr). *J. Vasc. Interv. Radiol.* 2008;19(suppl 2):S111.

[14] Brazzini A, Cantella R, De la Cruz A, Yupanqui J, Leon C, Jorquiera T, et al. Intraarterial autologous implantation of adult stem cells for patients with Parkinson disease. *J. Vasc Interv Radiol.* 2010;21(4):443-451.

[15] Bang OY, Lee JS, Lee PH, Lee G. Autologous mesenchymal stem cell transplantation in stroke patients. *Ann. Neurol.* 2005;57(6):874-882.

[16] Pluchino S, Quattrini A, Brambilla E, Gritti A, Salani G, Dina G, et al. Injection of adult neurospheres induces recovery in a chronic model of multiple sclerosis. *Nature* 2003;422(6933):688-694.

[17] Owen RJ, Ryan EA, O'Kelly K, Lakey JR, McCarthy MC, Paty BW, et al. Percutaneous transhepatic pancreatic islet cell transplantation in type 1 diabetes mellitus: radiologic aspects. *Radiology* 2003;229(1):165-170.

[18] Casey JJ, Lakey JR, Ryan EA, Paty BW, Owen R, O'Kelly K, et al. Portal venous pressure changes after sequential clinical islet transplantation. *Transplantation* 2002;74(7):913-915.

[19] J.D. Prologo DC, A. Sattar, L.W. Yuan, N. Tenley, D. Hart, Z. Love, Z. Lee. Percutaneous image-guided transplantation of human mesenchymal stem cells for the treatment of symptomatic degenerated intervertebral discs. *J. Vasc. Interv. Radiol.* 2012;23(suppl 3):S3-S4.

[20] Wollert KC, Meyer GP, Lotz J, Ringes-Lichtenberg S, Lippolt P, Breidenbach C, et al. Intracoronary autologous bone-marrow cell transfer after myocardial infarction: the BOOST randomised controlled clinical trial. *Lancet* 2004;364(9429):141-148.

[21] Villanueva FS, Jankowski RJ, Klibanov S, Pina ML, Alber SM, Watkins SC, et al. Microbubbles targeted to intercellular adhesion molecule-1 bind to activated coronary artery endothelial cells. *Circulation* 1998;98(1):1-5.

SECTION II. APPLICATIONS

In: Magnetic Resonance Imaging of Stem Cell Applications ISBN: 978-1-63463-910-1
Editor: Xiaoming Yang

Chapter 6

Magnetic Resonance Imaging of Stem Cell Application in Neurology

Antje Arnold, Miroslaw Janowski and Piotr Walczak*
The Russell H. Morgan Department of Radiology and Radiological Science;
Division of MR Research, Institute for Cell Engineering,
Johns Hopkins University School of Medicine, Baltimore, Maryland, US

Abstract

Stem cell-based therapy for diseases of the central nervous system is an attractive approach and frequently the only viable therapeutic option. Tremendous progress in the field of regenerative medicine and stem cell biology, identification of new therapeutic cells and expanding evidence about therapeutic utility of stem cells in various neurological diseases has already led to the exciting translation of this approach into clinical scenario. However, it has to be emphasized that without the ability to monitor the transplanted cells non-invasively and interrogating cell status in patients, interpretation and optimization of cell therapies would be extremely difficult. Consequently, over the last two decades there was a significant effort towards developing cellular imaging tools and these efforts effected in quite an impressive repertoire of imaging methods suitable for detection of transplanted cells, monitoring their biodistribution, migration, and functional integration. Several imaging modalities are now available for imaging cells with MRI being by far the most frequently applied for both preclinical and clinical studies. In this chapter, we describe various aspects of MRI cell tracking including available contrast agents, reporter genes, advantages and challenges related to each specific imaging technic, and will provide examples of applications of MRI cell tracking in neurological field with animal models as well as first pioneering clinical trials.

Keywords: MRI; stem cells, transplantation, cell tracking, cell labeling, neurology

* Corresponding author: Piotr Walczak, MD, PhD, The Russell H. Morgan Department of Radiology and Radiological Science; Division of MR Research, Institute for Cell Engineering, Johns Hopkins University School of Medicine, Broadway Research Building Rm 649, 733 N Broadway, Baltimore, Maryland, US. E-mail: pwalcza1@jhu.edu.

Introduction

One of the most important aspects of stem cell-based therapy is to ensure the safety and efficacy of the cell transplantation procedure. Due to the complexity of the central nervous system, the safety aspects of cell-based therapy of neurological disorders are of even greater significance. In addition, therapeutic outcomes in cell transplantation are highly dependent on proper biodistribution, survival, proliferation, and migration of the transplanted cells, while these parameters require careful optimization.

It is now well recognized that the use of novel cellular imaging technologies can help to achieve these goals. Serial imaging helps to define optimal cell administration routes, and monitor cell status without the need for biopsy, which, in the brain, is impractical and can lead to serious side effects (e.g., intracranial hemorrhage, seizures, or stroke). Imaging modalities such as fluorescence or bioluminescence imaging, positron emission tomography (PET), single-photon emission computed tomography (SPECT), computed tomography (CT), and magnetic resonance imaging (MRI) can be used to visualize transplanted pre-labeled cells (Figure 6.1) [1]. Because of the limited tissue penetration, fluorescence and bioluminescence is only used in the preclinical setting for imaging of small animals. The disadvantage of PET and SPECT is the reliance on radioactivity and probes with a very short half-life. MRI is a relatively expensive imaging technique, but offers a variety of advantages, including high resolution imaging capacity, three-dimensional (3D) imaging, no radiation, non-invasiveness, and the option for whole-body imaging. The benefits of MRI clearly outweigh the drawbacks, rendering it the imaging modality of choice for many indications. Indeed, MRI has been successfully used for stem cell tracking, including extensive use in preclinical studies [2, 3] and, recently, also in clinical trials [4].

While MRI cell-tracking provides unique and important information about transplanted cells, at this stage of development, it is important to know the specifics of the disease system very well, as some processes typical of a specific disease course may negatively affect the reliability of the information obtained by imaging. It is prudent to validate pre-clinical cell-tracking outcomes for each application with post-mortem histological analysis not only to reveal information about the cell status, but also to assess processes that may interfere with imaging, including local inflammation, rejection processes, or hemorrhaging. Various cellular MR imaging contrast mechanisms and several contrast agents have now been validated and are effectively used for cell-tracking, offering a variety of advantages and disadvantages. These unique features should be carefully considered when selecting a cellular imaging strategy, and these will be discussed in this chapter.

Cell Labeling Techniques

Although there have been attempts to identify specific endogenous contrast for cell detection, [6] to acquire specific and reliable information about transplanted cells it is currently necessary to specifically tag the cells using a contrast agent or a reporter gene. That provides the necessary contrast to identify transplanted cells in animals or specific organs long after their transplantation. This can be accomplished with molecular contrast agents or by engineering the target cells through transduction or transfection of specific reporter genes.

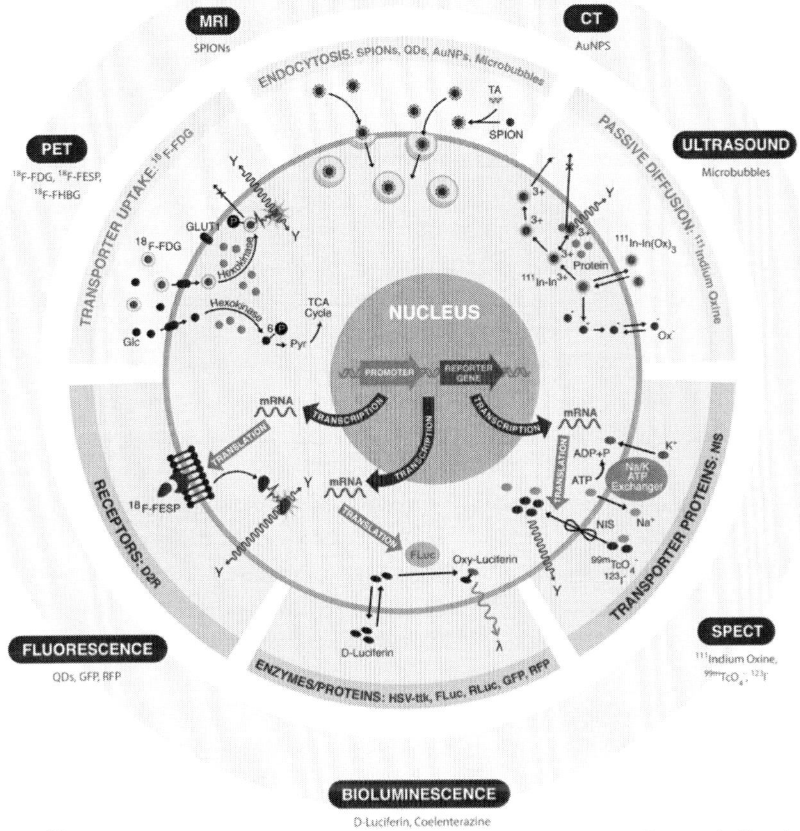

Abbreviations: ^{18}F-FDG, 18F-fluorodeoxyglucose; 18F-FESP, 3-(20 [18F]-fluoroethyl)-spiperone; ^{18}F-FHBG, 9-(4-18Ffluoro-3-[hydroxymethyl]butyl) guanine; Glc, glucose; GLUT1, glucose transport type 1; Pyr, pyruvate; TCA, tricarboxylic acid cycle; TA, transfection agents; SPIONs, superparamagnetic iron oxide nanoparticles; QDs, quantum dots; AuNPs, gold nanoparticles; ^{111}In-ox, indium oxine; Asp, aspartic acid; Ser, serine; NIS, sodium iodide symporter; I, iodine; ^{99m}TcO4$^-$, technetium pertechnetate; D2R, dopamine 2 receptor; HSV-ttk, herpes simplex virus truncated thymidine kinase; FLuc, firefly luciferase; RLuc, renilla luciferase; GFP, green fluorescent protein; RFP, red fluorescent protein; PET, positron emission tomography; MRI, magnetic resonance imaging; CT, computed tomography; FLI, fluorescence imaging; BLI, bioluminescence imaging; SPECT, single-photon emission computed tomography. Reprinted, with permission, from [5].

Figure 6.1. Cell Labeling Strategies and Detectors for Stem Cell Imaging. For direct labeling (in green), cells are incubated with imaging probes that enter the cell via transporter uptake (i.e., ^{18}F-FDG, ^{18}F-FESP, and ^{18}F-FHBG), endocytosis (i.e., SPIONs, QDs, AuNPs, and microbubbles), or passive diffusion (i.e., ^{111}In-ox). In reporter gene imaging (in blue), cells are transfected or transduced with the reporter gene construct. Transcription of the reporter gene under the control of a promoter, followed by translation of its mRNA, leads to accumulation of different reporter proteins, such as receptors (i.e., D2R), enzymes/proteins (HSVtk, FLuc, RLuc, GFP, and RFP), and transporter proteins (NIS). Introduction of a reporter gene probe (i.e., ^{18}F-FESP, D-luciferin, coelenterazine) results in signal generation. Labeled cells are detected by imaging systems such as PET, MRI, CT, ultrasound, FLI, BLI, and SPECT.

Utilization of a reporter gene has many advantages (which will be discussed later); however, as a general rule sensitivity is much lower compared to contrast agents. An additional concern is the requirement for genome modification and the risk of altering gene function. Consequently, cell-tracking based on contrast agents is applied more frequently, including for all clinical applications [4]. To date, the most frequently used cell-tracking agents are various formulations of superparamagnetic iron oxide nanoparticles (SPION); however, new classes of agents that facilitate hot-spot imaging, such as ^{19}F emulsions, [7] are emerging as an attractive option. With the ample choice of MR contrast mechanisms and available contrast agents, the optimal protocol should be selected after a series of validation tests with target cells, including the assessment of direct toxicity and the effect on the specific functional aspect of the cells of interest (differentiation, production of trophic factors, or neurotransmitters, etc.). Prior to transplantation and imaging, target cells must be properly labeled with a contrast agent. Over the years, different techniques have been developed to label cells for MRI, [8-13] with different advantages and disadvantages that should be considered, and which will be discussed below.

Phagocytic cells are naturally capable of internalizing particles via endocytosis, as demonstrated for the *in vivo* labeling of liver macrophages (Kupffer cells) with SPION [14], or labeling of phagocytes in lymph nodes with injected ultra-small paramagnetic iron oxide nanoparticles (USPION) [14-16]. Based on the phagocytic activity of these certain cell types, a simple *in vitro* incubation with SPION or USPION is sufficient to internalize the contrast agent. Even non-phagocytic cells, like MSCs, could internalize magnetic agents over a non-specific endocytic pathway after two to three days incubation time [17]. Obviously, for non-phagocytic cells, the uptake of contrast agents is less straightforward and depends on the relative concentration of magnetic agent and cultured cells, the size of nanoparticles, the incubation time, and the type of coating [18]. In line with the data for MSCs and fibroblasts [18], even for neural progenitor cells (NPC), a two-day incubation with SPIONs (Feridex®) leads to almost 100% efficient labeling of the cells [19]. But, an extensive labeling time could lead to cell death or excessive toxicity in case of sensitive cells. To shorten the incubation time and increase labeling efficiency, the cellular internalization of iron oxide nanoparticles could be enhanced through complexation with a transfection agent. Transfection with commercially available transfection reagents or calcium chloride is a well-established molecular biology procedure by which to transfer nucleic acids (e.g., DNA, RNA) into cells. Based on this method, SPIONs and transfection agents form a positive charged complex during the incubation time. The newly formed transfection complex can be absorbed by the negatively charged cell membrane and initiate the endocytosis pathway. In line with the complexation method, it has been shown that improved magnetic labeling can be achieved by use of negatively charged molecules, like dendrimers [10, 20]. For the clinical applications of stem cells, one concern that needs to be addressed is related to a potentially toxic microenvironment due to prolonged incubation with contrast agents, leading to oxidative stress, induction of apoptosis, or altered differentiation [21-24]. One technique that may minimize the incubation time is electroporation. Through a short electrical impulse, the cell membrane is reversibly perforated and macromolecules or particles can enter the cells. Magnetoelectroporation for intracellular labeling has been successfully used to image stem cells [25] and glioma [26]. For the opportunity to alter the transplanted microenvironment through the establishment of cell cultures, intracellular labeling by electroporation is the method of choice for the labeling of primary stem cells.

Contrast Agents

Among available contrast agents for MRI cell-tracking are iron oxide nanoparticles [27], fluorine compounds [7], gadolinium chelates [28], manganese oxide [26], and chemical exchange saturation transfer (CEST) agents [29]. The first two are the most promising for immediate application and those will be described in more detail.

Iron Oxide Nanoparticles

Iron oxide nanoparticles have been used extensively in preclinical studies that have confirmed their overall good safety profile and strong MRI contrast due to shortening the T2 relaxation time [30]. For example, **SPIONs** are internalized safely and persist in neural stem cells [27, 31] and glial-restricted progenitor cells [32].

The main compounds of SPIONs are the magnetic iron oxide core and a protective, biocompatible coating, providing further possibilities for particle modifications and therapeutic support. Examples of such modifications include receptors, enzymes, small molecules, antibodies, additional fluorochromes, or nucleic acids (Figure 6.2). One of the major advantages of SPIONs is that they are biologically safe [33] and actually are believed to safely degrade through the endogenous iron recycling pathways when released from dying cells. Neural stem cells can be heavily-labeled with SPIONs and remain viable without affecting their proliferative capacity [34]. The feasibility of imaging transplanted SPION-labeled cells has been shown in a number of studies [35, 36].

Nevertheless, the use of iron oxide for cell-labeling has some disadvantages. The hypointense MRI signal characteristic for this contrast agent is not necessarily specific, as it can be confused with microhemorrhages, labeled cell debris, and iron oxide particles internalized by local macrophages or microglia [31].

Fluorine (^{19}F)

Fluorine (^{19}F) as a contrast agent has the important advantage that it is practically absent in the human body; thus, ^{19}F imaging can be used for imaging with almost no background. Another advantage of this method is that, during the same imaging session, both anatomical and ^{19}F images can be acquired and superimposed [37], providing data in a quantitative manner [38]. While the signal-to-noise ratio (SNR) of ^{19}F is about 89% that of ^{1}H, per nucleus, the fluorine-based contrast agent requires a very high density of ^{19}F nuclei, similar to that of ^{1}H density in tissues [39].

This has been accomplished by synthesizing fluorine compounds from hydrocarbons through the exchange of ^{1}H to ^{19}F nuclei [40]. Good biocompatibility of ^{19}F agents is evidenced by the long-term use of fluorocarbons as an X-ray contrast agent [41], or as a blood substitute [42]. While perfluorocarbon is a very promising contrast agent for "hot-spot" MRI, its utility is still limited by the low sensitivity of the method [43], requiring a significant amount of cells for *in vivo* imaging [44].

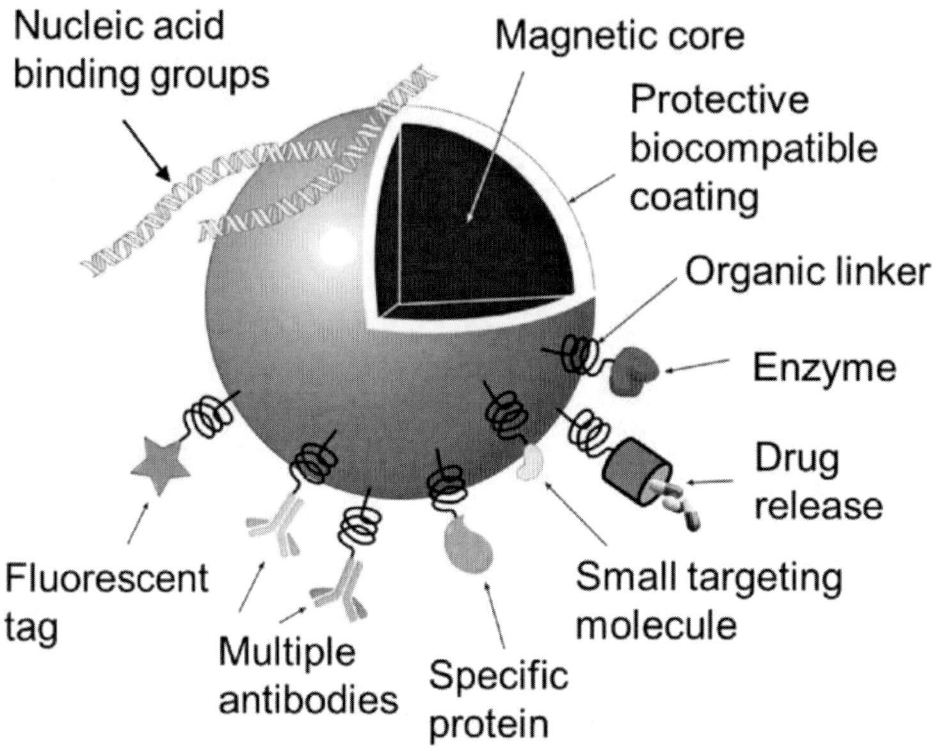

Courtesy by Jenkins et al., Molecular and Cellular Therapies 2014.

Figure 6.2. Schematic diagram illustrating possible magnetic nanoparticle features. Iron oxides (typically magnetite, Fe3O4, or maghemite, γ-Fe2O3) provide contrast for MRI and confer 'superparamagnetism' to the final particle. A protective biocompatible coating may be functionalized to carry drugs, cell-targeting molecules, fluorophores for histological detection, and/or nucleic acids for gene delivery.

Reporter Genes

Imaging cells labeled with contrast agents can be complicated by dilution of the agent due to cell division [45]. This problem can be solved through the use of cells engineered to express reporter genes. Reporter genes are available as viral or non-viral vectors, which are designed to integrate into the genome of the target cells for permanent or long-term expression. The advantage of using a reporter gene technique for cell-tracking includes the specificity of the molecular imaging signal generation linked to cell viability, and replenishment of the contrast following cell division. It also offers the possibility to use a specific promoter sequence linking the expression of the reporter gene with specific biological processes, such as cell differentiation, a feature frequently used in fluorescent microscopy [46]. To date, several different categories of reporter genes have been developed, including proteins that increase the internal accumulation in cells of iron, such as ferritin [47], or artificial proteins, such lysine-rich protein, a chemical exchange saturation transfer (CEST) reporter [48]. While proteins based on an increased accumulation of iron share some of the disadvantages ascribed to iron oxide nanoparticles, such as unspecific uptake by phagocytes following cell death, with CEST reporters the signal is highly specific. With this technique, the nuclear magnetic resonance frequency, which can be manipulated with a radiofrequency pulse, selectively tags and detects the reporter protein [49]. With this method, engineered cells can be specifically detected and separated from non-transfected cells in the brain [49]. These techniques based on reporter genes are already becoming an important tool for preclinical cell therapy studies; however, their clinical application will require extensive testing to ensure safety.

Preclinical Neurological Applications for MRI Cell-Tracking

MRI cell-tracking is frequently utilized in preclinical studies on small and large animals to help verify the accuracy and efficiency of stem cell transplantation. It has been shown that the use of SPION is efficient in tracking the migration, engraftment, and differentiation of cells for up to six weeks post-transplantation. Cells labeled with SPION (9 nm size) [50] can be detected after transplantation, with a high-field scanner (17.6T), almost as single cells *in vitro* and around 100 cells *in vivo* [50]. With larger, micron-sized iron oxide particles (MPIO, 1.63μm), it is possible to detect single cells [51]. The detection sensitivity is particularly important when cells migrate or proliferate after transplantation, effectively leading to less contrast agent per imaging voxel. There are several reports of successful longitudinal cellular MRI studies that were able to demonstrate the distribution of cells over time [28, 52-54]. An example of an application for MR cell-tracking and cell-based therapy is in animal model of multiple sclerosis [2]. In a rat experimental autoimmune encephalomyelitis (EAE) model, MRI cell-tracking was successfully implemented, and when MD-100-labeled neurospheres were transplanted into the ventricles of EAE rats at the peak of their disease, migration into white matter structures could be observed on the MR images, and the MRI data correlated well with histologically detected cells. Another longitudinal study in chronic EAE mice demonstrated that the distance of cell migration correlated well with the clinical severity of disease and with the number of microglia in white matter tracts [55].

In another study, magnetodendrimer-labeled oligodendrocyte progenitors were transplanted into neonatal dysmeylinated rats, and MRI cell-tracking enabled *in vivo* detection of cells for up to six weeks [10]. Stroke is an example of another neurological brain disorder that is of great interest in regenerative medicine, and that application also requires non-invasive verification of cell biodistribution by non-invasive means, such as MRI.

Indeed, it has been shown, with high-resolution MRI, that ESC-derived stem cells transplanted into the contralateral hemisphere migrate toward the stroke lesion. The extensive migratory behavior, which correlated with biodistribution detected by MRI, was confirmed by fluorescent microscopy [52]. Another example of trans-hemisphere migration was shown when gadolinium/rhodamine-labeled neural progenitors were injected in the contralateral hemisphere, with cells infiltrating the penumbra of the lesion [28]. Migration of SPIO-labeled neural stem cells toward stroke in a rat model could also be visualized with MRI following administration of cells into the cerebrospinal fluid via an intracisternal injection [56].

MRI cell-tracking has also been effectively applied to monitor cell trafficking toward brain tumors. The process of gradual tumor infiltration with transplanted microsphere-labeled neural stem cells has been shown over time using high-resolution MRI [57]. Neural stem cells were also labeled with FDA-approved ferumoxytol and transplanted through intracerebral or intravenous injection into mice with demonstrated targeting toward glioma [58]. Spinal cord injury (SCI) is another neurological disease where cell therapy, and cell-tracking, has been actively pursued. Monitoring the migration of iron oxide-labeled olfactory ensheathing cells (OECs) with MRI has been successful when cells were grafted into the intact rat spinal cord [54]; however, when the spinal cords were injured by transection, the interpretation of grafted cell biodistribution was severely confounded by local hemorrhaging. Of note, however, when a less severe, contusion model of spinal cord injury has been used, transplanted magnetically labeled cells were successfully visualized with MRI [59].

Targeting of large lesions or cell therapy of diseases with disseminated or global pathology, such as multiple sclerosis or amyotrophic lateral sclerosis, requires efficient cell delivery strategies with cells that can reach vast portions of the central nervous system. One attractive cell delivery strategy is intraarterial injection. For this approach, monitoring of cell trafficking is of paramount importance to assure both efficacy and safety. The successful application of MRI cell-tracking to monitor intraarterial injection has been reported in several rodent [3, 60] and canine [61] stroke model studies (Figure 6.3).

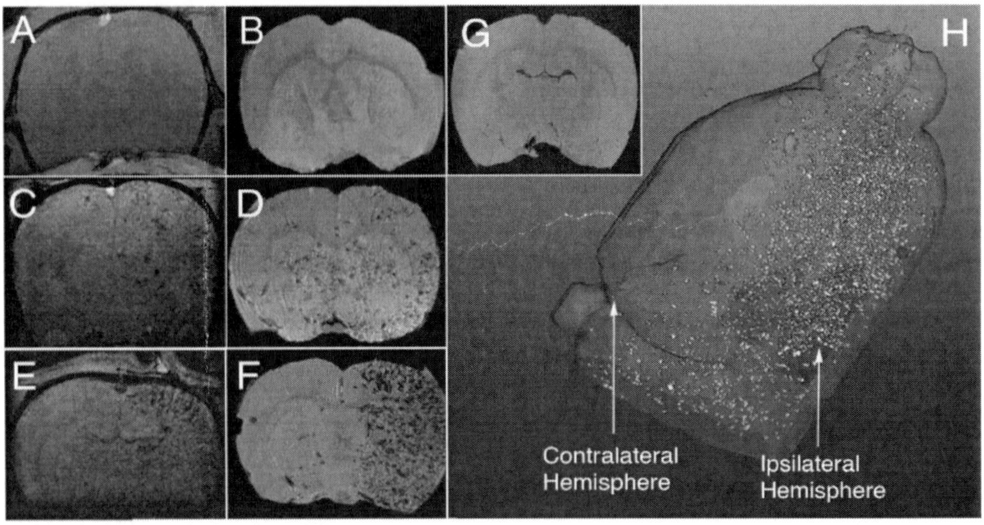

Reprinted with permission from [3].

Figure 6.3. MRI tracking of intraarterially injected stem cells. MR images of intracerebral cell engraftment after IA (A–F, H) and IV (G) injection. MSCs appear as hypointense spots on T2*-weighted images. A, *In vivo* and (B) *ex vivo* MR images of an animal corresponding to the black line in Figure 6.2. No brain engraftment can be observed. *In vivo* (C) and *ex vivo* (D) a moderate brain engraftment can be seen, with some cells entering the other hemisphere. *In vivo* (E) and *ex vivo* (F) MR images show a massive engraftment, but the cell distribution is limited to the right hemisphere perfused by the right carotid artery used for injection. G, No engraftment could be detected after IV injection. H, 3D reconstruction of cellular distribution in the brain of the example shown in E and F. Cells distributed widely throughout the right brain hemisphere, with a prevalence for the area directly fed by the right internal carotid artery; the territory of the anterior and posterior cerebral arteries also exhibit significant engraftment. Very few cells were detected in the contralateral (left) hemisphere, suggesting that cells did not circulate systemically before arriving at their final location.

Although transplanted iron oxide-labeled cells can be detected *in vivo* with MRI, long-term tracking using this agent is complicated by several factors, including local hemorrhaging or persistence of contrast after cell death, as reported for mismatched intracerebral neural stem cell allograft rejection [31]. One interesting strategy that, at least in part, addresses the disadvantages of iron oxide is the use of fluorine compounds. The very low content of this element in the human body enables background-free imaging. In a preclinical study, human neural stem cells were labeled with perfluoropolyether (PFPE, perfluorocarbon = PFC), which can be detected with ^{19}F MRI [62]. *In vivo* MRI successfully detected transplanted cells and imaging findings were confirmed by immunohistochemistry. Notably, ^{19}F labeling did not lead to any toxicity or phenotype changes.

Several other studies reported the successful detection of transplanted neural stem cells with ^{19}F MRI [62, 63]. Beyond neurological indications, perfluoropolyether nanoparticles have also been successfully used to track dendritic cells [64] or pancreatic islets [65].

Although ^{19}F has some advantages over iron oxides, there are still unresolved issues and clear disadvantages inherent to the imaging of cells loaded with any contrast agent. These disadvantages include dilution of the contrast agent during cell division, and lack of information about cell viability or function. Therefore, obtaining useful information about transplanted cells over longer post-transplantation periods is difficult. The ideal solution to this problem would be an MR reporter gene, with signal produced only in the viable cells. As outlined in previous section, there are significant interest and progress in this field [47, 49, 66, 67]; however, the sensitivity of imaging with these reporter genes is lower compared to that of cell labeling with iron oxide nanoparticles or fluorine. Thus, the detection of small numbers of transplanted neural stem cells with MRI reporter genes remains challenging.

Clinical Neurological Applications of MRI Cell-Tracking

The first reported clinical application of MRI cell-tracking in neurological disease was in Shanghai, China, with two traumatic brain injury patients treated with autologous neural stem cells isolated from the removed brain fragments following emergency neurosurgery [26]. Neural stem cells were labeled with ferumoxides and stereotactically injected near the area of brain injury. Gradient-echo MR images obtained at a 3 Tesla scanner showed dynamic changes in hypointensity over time, and these changes were attributed to movement of the neural stem cells from the injection site to the border zone of the lesion. The hypointense signal was detectable for a period of seven weeks, when it completely disappeared, possibly due to further migration and dispersion of cells or cell proliferation that diluted the contrast agent to undetectable levels. The second brain trauma patient in that study received unlabeled cells and served as a control, showing an absence of hypointensities. This study indicated the feasibility of cell detection in a clinical setting; however, that the hypointense signals were due to hemorrhaging, as shown in other trauma-related lesions, cannot be excluded.

In another clinical study, cells were labeled with magnetic particles (Dynal beads) used to label and sort CD34+ bone marrow stem cells. Ten patients with chronic spinal cord injury received magnetic bead-labeled bone marrow stem cells, and six patients acting as controls received beads without cells. All injections were into the spinal cord by lumbar puncture.

Serial MR images revealed migration of labeled cells toward the site of injury, and such a pattern was not observed in the patients who received injections of beads only. There were no safety concerns reported in this study; however, there is considerable ethical concern about the use of non-biodegradable contrast agents, particularly about their implantation without stem cells for control groups of patients.

Recently, another report described utilization of MRI cell-tracking in a pediatric global cerebral ischemia patient treated with autologous umbilical cord blood-derived stem cells [68]. Cells were labeled with Feridex and injected into the lateral ventricle. Longitudinal MR imaging showed that the cells, rather than circulating with the cerebrospinal fluid, settled toward the posterior ventricular horns (Figure 6.4). Follow-up of the patient up to 33 months post-transplantation revealed no detrimental effects related to the therapy, and evidence of modest neurological improvement.

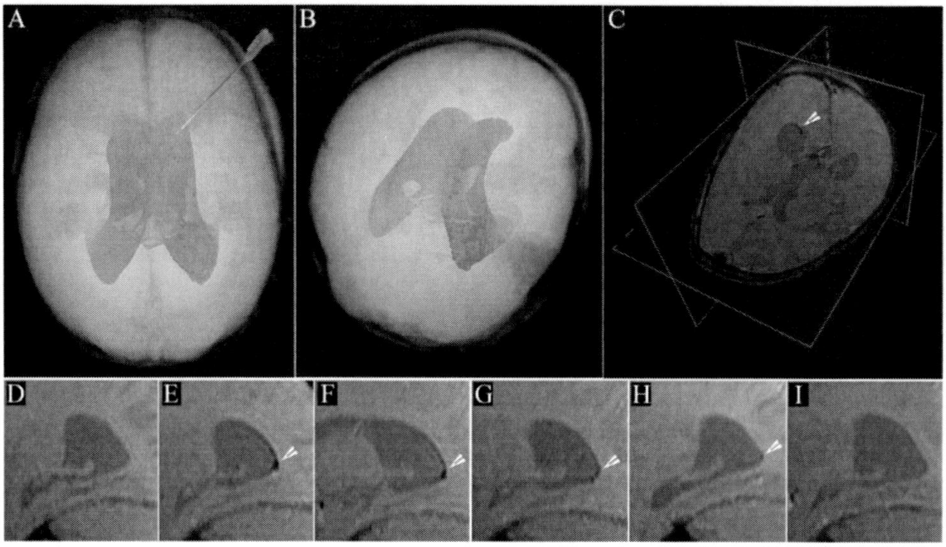

Reprinted, with permission, from [68].

Figure 6.4. Imaging of SPION-labeled autologous cord blood-derived cells in a patient with global cerebral ischemia. (A) Volume-rendering of MRI data obtained 24 hours post-transplantation. Semi-automatic segmentation is based on pixel intensity, showing the projection of the ventricular system (green) and the distribution of the SPION signal from the transplanted cells within the occipital horn of the right ventricle (red). Note the supine configuration of the head, corresponding to positioning during surgery. The route and trajectory of cell transplantation via the frontal horn is represented by the needle. (B) Postero-superior view of the patient's head, emphasizing the location of the hypointense SPION signal from autologous cord blood-derived cells transplanted within the occipital horn. (C) T2*-weighted image, with an orthogonal view, centered on the cellular SPION signal in the occipital horn (white arrowhead). (D–I) Sagittal T2*-weighted MRI scans showing a longitudinal dispersion of the SPION signal within the occipital horn (white arrowheads); (D) pre-transplantation; (E) 24 hours post transplantation (PT); (F) seven days PT; (G) two months PT; (H) four months PT; and (I) 33 months PT.

Conclusion

Stem cell-based therapy for diseases of the central nervous system is an attractive approach and frequently the only viable therapeutic option. Over the last two decades there was a significant effort towards developing cellular imaging tools and these efforts effected in quite an impressive repertoire of imaging methods suitable for detection of transplanted cells, monitoring their biodistribution, migration, and functional integration.

MRI cell tracking is the most frequently applied for both preclinical and clinical studies of stem cell applications in neurological field with animal models as well as pioneering clinical trials.

This work has been supported by MSCRFII-0193; MSCRFII0052 and NIH/NINDS R01NS076573

References

[1] Walczak, P., Bulte, J. W. The role of noninvasive cellular imaging in developing cell-based therapies for neurodegenerative disorders. *Neurodegener. Dis.* 2007;4(4):306-313.

[2] Bulte, J. W., Ben-Hur, T., Miller, B. R., Mizrachi-Kol, R., Einstein, O., Reinhartz, E., et al. MR microscopy of magnetically labeled neurospheres transplanted into the Lewis EAE rat brain. *Magn. Reson. Med.* 2003;50(1):201-205.

[3] Walczak, P., Zhang, J., Gilad, A. A., Kedziorek, D. A., Ruiz-Cabello, J., Young, R. G., et al. Dual-modality monitoring of targeted intraarterial delivery of mesenchymal stem cells after transient ischemia. *Stroke* 2008;39(5):1569-1574.

[4] Bulte, J. W. In vivo MRI cell tracking: clinical studies. *AJR Am. J. Roentgenol.* 2009; 193(2):314-325.

[5] Nguyen, P. K., Riegler, J., Wu, J. C. Stem cell imaging: from bench to bedside. *Cell Stem Cell* 2014;14(4):431-444.

[6] Chung, Y. L., El Akabawy, G., So, P. W., Solanky, B. S., Leach, M. O., Modo, M. Profiling metabolite changes in the neuronal differentiation of human striatal neural stem cells using 1H-magnetic resonance spectroscopy. *Neuroreport* 2013;24(18):1035-1040.

[7] Hitchens, T. K., Ye, Q., Eytan, D. F., Janjic, J. M., Ahrens, E. T., Ho, C. 19F MRI detection of acute allograft rejection with in vivo perfluorocarbon labeling of immune cells. *Magn. Reson. Med.* 2011;65(4):1144-1153.

[8] Bulte, J. W., Zhang, S., van Gelderen, P., Herynek, V., Jordan, E. K., Duncan, I. D, et al. Neurotransplantation of magnetically labeled oligodendrocyte progenitors: magnetic resonance tracking of cell migration and myelination. *Proc. Natl. Acad. Sci. US* 1999; 96(26):15256-15261.

[9] Lewin, M., Carlesso, N., Tung, C. H., Tang, X. W., Cory, D., Scadden, D. T., et al. Tat peptide-derivatized magnetic nanoparticles allow in vivo tracking and recovery of progenitor cells. *Nat. Biotechnol.* 2000;18(4):410-414.

[10] Bulte, J. W., Douglas, T., Witwer, B., Zhang, S. C., Strable, E., Lewis, B. K., et al. Magnetodendrimers allow endosomal magnetic labeling and in vivo tracking of stem cells. *Nat. Biotechnol.* 2001;19(12):1141-1147.

[11] Frank, J. A., Zywicke, H., Jordan, E. K., Mitchell, J., Lewis, B. K., Miller, B., et al. Magnetic intracellular labeling of mammalian cells by combining (FDA-approved) superparamagnetic iron oxide MR contrast agents and commonly used transfection agents. *Academic Radiology* 2002;9 Suppl. 2:S484-487.

[12] Arbab, A. S., Bashaw, L. A., Miller, B. R., Jordan, E. K., Bulte, J. W., Frank, J. A. Intracytoplasmic tagging of cells with ferumoxides and transfection agent for cellular magnetic resonance imaging after cell transplantation: methods and techniques. *Transplantation* 2003;76(7):1123-1130.

[13] Hinds, K. A., Hill, J. M., Shapiro, E. M., Laukkanen, M. O., Silva, A. C., Combs, C. A., et al. Highly efficient endosomal labeling of progenitor and stem cells with large magnetic particles allows magnetic resonance imaging of single cells. *Blood* 2003;102 (3):867-872.

[14] Reimer, P., Tombach, B. Hepatic MRI with SPIO: detection and characterization of focal liver lesions. *Eur. Radiol.* 1998;8(7):1198-1204.

[15] Modo, M., Hoehn, M., Bulte, J. W. Cellular MR imaging. *Mol. Imaging* 2005;4(3):143-164.

[16] Weinmann, H. J., Ebert, W., Misselwitz, B., Schmitt-Willich, H. Tissue-specific MR contrast agents. *Eur. J. Radiol.* 2003;46(1):33-44.

[17] Jendelova, P., Herynek, V., DeCroos, J., Glogarova, K., Andersson, B., Hajek, M., et al. Imaging the fate of implanted bone marrow stromal cells labeled with superparamagnetic nanoparticles. *Magnetic Resonance in Medicine* 2003;50(4):767-776.

[18] Boutry, S., Brunin, S., Mahieu, I., Laurent, S., Vander Elst, L., Muller, R. N. Magnetic labeling of non-phagocytic adherent cells with iron oxide nanoparticles: a comprehensive study. *Contrast Media Mol. Imaging* 2008;3(6):223-232.

[19] Chen, C. C., Ku, M. C., D MJ, Lai, J. S., Hueng, D. Y., Chang, C. Simple SPION incubation as an efficient intracellular labeling method for tracking neural progenitor cells using MRI. *PLoS One* 2013;8(2):e56125.

[20] Wilhelm, C., Billotey, C., Roger, J., Pons, J. N., Bacri, J. C., Gazeau, F. Intracellular uptake of anionic superparamagnetic nanoparticles as a function of their surface coating. *Biomaterials* 2003;24(6):1001-1011.

[21] Arbab, A. S., Wilson, L. B., Ashari, P., Jordan, E. K., Lewis, B. K., Frank, J. A. A model of lysosomal metabolism of dextran coated superparamagnetic iron oxide (SPIO) nanoparticles: implications for cellular magnetic resonance imaging. *Nmr. in Biomedicine* 2005;18(6):383-389.

[22] Dokka, S., Toledo, D., Shi, X., Castranova, V., Rojanasakul, Y. Oxygen radical-mediated pulmonary toxicity induced by some cationic liposomes. *Pharm. Res.* 2000; 17(5):521-525.

[23] Hunter, A. C. Molecular hurdles in polyfectin design and mechanistic background to polycation induced cytotoxicity. *Adv. Drug Deliv. Rev.* 2006;58(14):1523-1531.

[24] Singh, N., Jenkins, G. J., Asadi, R., Doak, S. H. Potential toxicity of superparamagnetic iron oxide nanoparticles (SPION). *Nano Rev.* 2010;1:5358.

[25] Walczak, P., Kedziorek, D. A., Gilad, A. A., Lin, S., Bulte, J. W. Instant MR labeling of stem cells using magnetoelectroporation. *Magn. Reson. Med.* 2005;54(4):769-774.

[26] Gilad, A. A., Walczak, P., McMahon, M. T., Na, H. B., Lee, J. H., An, K., et al. MR tracking of transplanted cells with "positive contrast" using manganese oxide nanoparticles. *Magn. Reson. Med.* 2008;60(1):1-7.

[27] Bulte, J. W. M., Zhang, S. C., van Gelderen, P., Herynek, V., Jordan, E. K., Janssen, C. H. C., et al. Magnetically labeled glial cells as cellular MR contrast agents. *Academic Radiology* 2002;9:S148-S150.

[28] Modo, M., Mellodew, K., Cash, D., Fraser, S. E., Meade, T. J., Price, J., et al. Mapping transplanted stem cell migration after a stroke: a serial, in vivo magnetic resonance imaging study. *Neuroimage* 2004;21(1):311-317.

[29] Chan, K. W., Liu, G., Song, X., Kim, H., Yu, T., Arifin, D. R., et al. MRI-detectable pH nanosensors incorporated into hydrogels for in vivo sensing of transplanted-cell viability. *Nat. Mater.* 2013;12(3):268-275.

[30] Sykova, E., Jendelova, P., Herynek, V. Magnetic resonance imaging of stem cell migration. *Methods Mol. Biol.* 2011;750:79-90.

[31] Berman, S. C., Galpoththawela, C., Gilad, A. A., Bulte, J. W., Walczak, P. Long-term MR cell tracking of neural stem cells grafted in immunocompetent versus immunodeficient mice reveals distinct differences in contrast between live and dead cells. *Magn. Reson. Med.* 2011;65(2):564-574.

[32] Janowski, M., Lyczek, A., Engels, C., Xu, J., Lukomska, B., Bulte, J. W., et al. Cell size and velocity of injection are major determinants of the safety of intracarotid stem cell transplantation. *J. Cereb. Blood Flow Metab.* 2013;33(6):921-927.

[33] Kedziorek, D. A., Kraitchman, D. L. Superparamagnetic iron oxide labeling of stem cells for MRI tracking and delivery in cardiovascular disease. *Methods Mol. Biol.* 2010; 660:171-183.

[34] Engberink, R. D. O., van der Pol, S. M. A., Dopp, E. A., de Vries, H. E., Blezer, E. L. A. Comparison of SPIO and USPIO for in vitro labeling of human monocytes: MR detection and cell function. *Radiology* 2007;243(2):467-474.

[35] Bulte, J. W., Kraitchman, D. L. Monitoring cell therapy using iron oxide MR contrast agents. *Curr. Pharm. Biotechnol.* 2004;5(6):567-584.

[36] Bult, J. W., Kraitchman, D. L. Iron oxide MR contrast agents for molecular and cellular imaging. *NMR Biomed.* 2004;17(7):484-499.

[37] Bulte, J. W. Hot spot MRI emerges from the background. *Nat. Biotechnol.* 2005;23(8): 945-946.

[38] Srinivas, M., Heerschap, A., Ahrens, E. T., Figdor, C. G., de Vries, I. J. (19)F MRI for quantitative in vivo cell tracking. *Trends Biotechnol.* 2010;28(7):363-370.

[39] Ruiz-Cabello, J., Barnett, B. P., Bottomley, P. A., Bulte, J. W. Fluorine (19F) MRS and MRI in biomedicine. *NMR Biomed.* 2011;24(2):114-129.

[40] Haszeldine, R. N. Synthesis of fluorocarbons, perfluoroalkyl iodides, bromides and chlorides, and perfluoroalkyl grignard reagents. *Nature* 1951;167(4239):139-140.

[41] Long, D. M., Liu, M. S., Szanto, P. S., Alrenga, P. Initial observations with a new x-ray contrast agent--radiopaque perfluorocarbon. *Rev. Surg.* 1972;29(1):71-76.

[42] Tremper, K. K., Lapin, R., Levine, E., Friedman, A., Shoemaker, W. C. Hemodynamic and oxygen transport effects of a perfluorochemical blood substitute, fluosol-DA (20%). *Crit. Care Med.* 1980;8(12):738-741.

[43] Chen, J., Lanza, G. M., Wickline, S. A. Quantitative magnetic resonance fluorine imaging: today and tomorrow. *Wiley Interdiscip. Rev. Nanomed. Nanobiotechnol.* 2010; 2(4):431-440.

[44] Partlow, K. C., Chen, J., Brant, J. A., Neubauer, A. M., Meyerrose, T. E., Creer, M. H., et al. 19F magnetic resonance imaging for stem/progenitor cell tracking with multiple unique perfluorocarbon nanobeacons. *FASEB J.* 2007;21(8):1647-1654.

[45] Arbab, A. S., Bashaw, L. A., Miller, B. R., Jordan, E. K., Lewis, B. K., Kalish, H., et al. Characterization of biophysical and metabolic properties of cells labeled with superparamagnetic iron oxide nanoparticles and transfection agent for cellular MR imaging. *Radiology* 2003;229(3):838-846.

[46] Jiang, H., Duchala, C. S., Awatramani, R., Shumas, S., Carlock, L., Kamholz, J., et al. Proteolipid protein mRNA stability is regulated by axonal contact in the rodent peripheral nervous system. *J. Neurobiol.* 2000;44(1):7-19.

[47] Genove, G., DeMarco, U., Xu, H., Goins, W. F., Ahrens, E. T. A new transgene reporter for in vivo magnetic resonance imaging. *Nat. Med.* 2005;11(4):450-454.

[48] Zhou, J. Y., Wilson, D. A., Sun, P. Z., Klaus, J. A., van Zijl, P. C. M. Quantitative description of proton exchange processes between water and endogenous and exogenous agents for WEX, CEST, and APT experiments. *Magnetic Resonance in Medicine* 2004;51(5):945-952.

[49] Gilad, A. A., McMahon, M. T., Walczak, P., Winnard, P. T., Jr., Raman, V., van Laarhoven, H. W., et al. Artificial reporter gene providing MRI contrast based on proton exchange. *Nat. Biotechnol.* 2007;25(2):217-219.

[50] Stroh, A., Faber, C., Neuberger, T., Lorenz, P., Sieland, K., Jakob, P. M., et al. In vivo detection limits of magnetically labeled embryonic stem cells in the rat brain using high-field (17.6 T) magnetic resonance imaging. *Neuroimage* 2005;24(3):635-645.

[51] Shapiro, E. M., Sharer, K., Skrtic, S., Koretsky, A. P. In vivo detection of single cells by MRI. *Magn. Reson. Med.* 2006;55(2):242-249.

[52] Hoehn, M., Kustermann, E., Blunk, J., Wiedermann, D., Trapp, T., Wecker, S., et al. Monitoring of implanted stem cell migration in vivo: A highly resolved in vivo magnetic resonance imaging investigation of experimental stroke in rat. *Proceedings of the National Academy of Sciences of the United States of America* 2002;99(25):16267-16272.

[53] Jendelova, P., Herynek, V., Urdzikova, L., Glogarova, K., Kroupova, J., Andersson, B., et al. Magnetic resonance tracking of transplanted bone marrow and embryonic stem cells labeled by iron oxide nanoparticles in rat brain and spinal cord. *J. Neurosci. Res.* 2004;76(2):232-243.

[54] Lee, I. H., Bulte, J. W., Schweinhardt, P., Douglas, T., Trifunovski, A., Hofstetter, C., et al. In vivo magnetic resonance tracking of olfactory ensheathing glia grafted into the rat spinal cord. *Exp. Neurol.* 2004;187(2):509-516.

[55] Ben-Hur, T., van Heeswijk, R., Einstein, O., Aharonovitch, M., Xue, R., Frost, E. E., et al. In vivo MR tracking of magnetically labeled neural spheres transplanted in chronic EAE mice: relation between cell migration and inflammation. *Magn. Reson. Med. In Press.*

[56] Zhang, Z. G., Jiang, Q., Zhang, R., Zhang, L., Wang, L., Zhang, L., et al. Magnetic resonance imaging and neurosphere therapy of stroke in rat. *Ann. Neurol.* 2003; 53 (2): 259-263.

[57] Zhang, Z., Jiang, Q., Jiang, F., Ding, G., Zhang, R., Wang, L., et al. In vivo magnetic resonance imaging tracks adult neural progenitor cell targeting of brain tumor. *Neuroimage* 2004;23(1):281-287.

[58] Gutova, M., Frank, J. A., D'Apuzzo, M., Khankaldyyan, V., Gilchrist, M. M., Annala, A. J., et al. Magnetic resonance imaging tracking of ferumoxytol-labeled human neural stem cells: studies leading to clinical use. *Stem Cells Transl. Med.* 2013;2(10):766-775.

[59] Urdzikova, L., Jendelova, P., Glogarova, K., Burian, M., Hajek, M., Sykova, E. Transplantation of bone marrow stem cells as well as mobilization by granulocyte-colony stimulating factor promotes recovery after spinal cord injury in rats. *Journal of Neurotrauma* 2006;23(9):1379-1391.

[60] Gorelik, M., Orukari, I., Wang, J., Galpoththawela, S., Kim, H., Levy, M., et al. Use of MR cell tracking to evaluate targeting of glial precursor cells to inflammatory tissue by exploiting the very late antigen-4 docking receptor. *Radiology* 2012;265(1):175-185.

[61] Lu, S. S., Liu, S., Zu, Q. Q., Xu, X. Q., Yu, J., Wang, J. W., et al. In vivo MR imaging of intraarterially delivered magnetically labeled mesenchymal stem cells in a canine stroke model. *PLoS One* 2013;8(2):e54963.

[62] Boehm-Sturm, P., Mengler, L., Wecker, S., Hoehn, M., Kallur, T. In vivo tracking of human neural stem cells with 19F magnetic resonance imaging. *PLoS One* 2011;6(12): e29040.

[63] Ruiz-Cabello, J., Walczak, P., Kedziorek, D. A., Chacko, V. P., Schmieder, A. H., Wickline, S. A., et al. In vivo "hot spot" MR imaging of neural stem cells using fluorinated nanoparticles. *Magn. Reson. Med.* 2008;60(6):1506-1511.

[64] Ahrens, E. T., Flores, R., Xu, H., Morel, P. A. In vivo imaging platform for tracking immunotherapeutic cells. *Nat. Biotechnol.* 2005;23(8):983-987.

[65] Barnett, B. P., Ruiz-Cabello, J., Hota, P., Ouwerkerk, R., Shamblott, M. J., Lauzon, C., et al. Use of perfluorocarbon nanoparticles for non-invasive multimodal cell tracking of human pancreatic islets. *Contrast Media Mol. Imaging* 2011;6(4):251-259.

[66] Weissleder, R., Moore, A., Mahmood, U., Bhorade, R., Benveniste, H., Chiocca, E. A., et al. In vivo magnetic resonance imaging of transgene expression. *Nat. Med.* 2000; 6 (3):351-355.

[67] Bar-Shir, A., Liu, G., Greenberg, M. M., Bulte, J. W., Gilad, A. A. Synthesis of a probe for monitoring HSV1-tk reporter gene expression using chemical exchange saturation transfer MRI. *Nat. Protoc.* 2013;8(12):2380-2391.

[68] Janowski, M., Walczak, P., Kropiwnicki, T., Jurkiewicz, E., Domanska-Janik, K., Bulte, J. W., et al. Long-term MRI cell tracking after intraventricular delivery in a patient with global cerebral ischemia and prospects for magnetic navigation of stem cells within the CSF. *PLoS One* 2014;9(2):e97631.

In: Magnetic Resonance Imaging of Stem Cell Applications
Editor: Xiaoming Yang
ISBN: 978-1-63463-910-1

Chapter 7

Magnetic Resonance Imaging of Stem Cell Application in Liver

Weitao Ye[1], Changhong Liang*[1] and Bin Zhou[2]
[1]Department of Radiology, Guangdong General Hospital, Guangzhou,Guangdong, China
[2]Department of Radiology, the Third Affiliated Hospital, Sun Yat-sen University, Guangzhou, Guangdong, China

Abstract

Stem cell therapy offers promising perspectives in the treatment of endstaged liver diseases. Magnetic resonance imaging (MRI) has emerged as a practical and non-invasive tool for real-time tracking of transplanted stem cells, and it is becoming reality with transition from preclinical researches to clinical trials. Superparamagnetic iron oxide(SPIO) is the major labeling contrast agent for MRI of stem cell therapy in liver diseases. In this chapter, we focus on typical MRI findings of stem cell transplantation in liver, which are characterized by decreased signal intensity at the implanted site on T2/T2*-weighted images due to susceptibility effect of SPIO-labeled stem cells that shortens T2* and T2 relaxation times. We also describe recent advances on basic research in this field, for example, optimization of transplantation procedure based on the anatomical and functional information with MRI. Finally, we discuss the limitations and challenges on MRI of stem cell application in liver diseases.

Keywords: Magnetic resonance imaging, liver, stem cell therapy

*Corresponding author: Changhong Liang, MD, (cjr.lchh@vip.163.com).

Introduction

Liver cirrhosis with chronic liver failure is the consequences of a spectrum of chronic liver injury(e.g., viral hepatitis, steatohepatitis, autoimmune hepatitis, etc.), and is ranked as one of the top leading causes of death worldwide [1]. To date, liver transplantation has been the primary treatment of choice for liver cirrhosis and chronic liver failure [2]. However, the scarcity of donor livers has become a major issue in liver transplantation. Currently, stem cell therapy in the liver is gaining special interest because it requires only a certain number of stem cells(e.g., mesenchymal stem cells), which possess the capability of stem cell differentiation into liver-like cells with certain hepatic functions[3]. Unlike surgical transplantation of the whole organ, stem cell therapy of liver diseases is less drastic, technically simpler, and more cost-effective as a single donor liver can provide sufficient derived stem cells to multiple recipient patients [2, 3].

Recent efforts on exploration of stem cell therapy of liver diseases have greatly advanced the innovative strategy with its promising future, even though it still requires some time for transition of this technology from preclinical research to clinical practice. To ensure the efficacy of the stem cell therapies, several critical issues remain to be addressed: 1) the optimum type of stem cells that are effective for treatment of liver diseases; 2) the preferred cell administration approaches, timing of cell transplantation, and optimum dosage of transplanted cells;and 3) the method of choice to qualitatively and quantitatively track and assess the process of homing, engraftment, interaction with the local microenvironment and differentiation of transplanted stem cells at the targets [4-6].

With the assistance of fluorescent dyes or other biomechanical materials, it has become possible for histology to determine the location of the transplanted donor cells and distinguish them from the endogenous cells [7]. However, histology examinations require harvested tissue samples from invasive approaches via either surgery, biopsy, or autopsy[8], which is impractical for repeatedly monitoring of migration and fate of the transplanted cells. To solve this problem, great efforts and advances have been made in developing cellular imaging techniques, which enable non-invasive and real-time tracking of the transplanted stem cells in vivo.The core of these cellular imaging techniques is to label the cells of interest with a specific imaging contrast agent [9], fluorescent dye [10] or so-called "reporter gene" [11, 12], which lead to amplified changes of image contrast. Optical imaging (e.g., bioluminescence and fluorescence imaging) [11] and nuclear medicine [13] (e.g., single photon emission computed tomography (SPECT) and positron emission tomography (PET)) are two representative techniques. Optical imaging requires either administration of exogenous fluorophores or genetic modification of targets [14], which is rather complicated with high cost [7]. In addition, successful application of optical imaging is limited to superficially-sited or near-surface organs as a consequence of high light absorption and scattering in the tissues [14]. With different labeling methods, nuclear medicine offers metabolism imaging, receptor imaging and antibody imaging, as well as gene expression imaging [7], with its high sensitivity in detection of the isotopes. However, the risk of ionizing radiation and lack of anatomical background limit the widespread use of nuclear medicine for stem cell therapy [14].

To date, magnetic resonance imaging (MRI) is considered the most promising cellular imaging technique. Owning to its high spatial and temporal resolution capabilities, cellular

MRI offers favorable anatomical information with a satisfactory soft tissue contrast [8]. Most importantly, there is no ionizing radiation with MR scanning, which ensures the repeated performance of real-time tracking and monitoring of transplanted cells in vivo without need of any invasive procedures [2, 15]. For in vivo cellular MRI of the liver, the special labeling of transplanted cells is essential.

Superparamagnetic Iron Oxides

An ideal cell labeling material must be intrinsically biocompatible, non-toxic and does not interfere with normal physiological activities or biochemical reactions of the stem cells [6]. Although several other kinds of contrast agents have been under investigation [16, 17], superparamagnetic iron oxides(SPIO) has emerged as the most intensively applicable labeling material due to its "blooming effect" (described below) on MRI, being intuitive enough to meet the clinical requirement [3, 18, 19]. SPIO particles are usually covered with a layer of low-molecular-weight polymers or dendrimers [8], such as dextran [20] or other polysaccharide, in order to allow further biochemical modification, improve their biocompatibility, increase the labeling efficiency, and prevent the particles from aggregation [20-23].

According to their sizes, SPIO can be classified as standard SPIO (SSPIO, 40-150mm), ultrasmall SPIO (USPIO, ~20-40mm), monocrystalline iron oxide nanoparticles (MION, 15-20mm), and very small iron oxide particles(VSIOP, core size 3-4mm, total size ~5-7mm) [22, 23]. SPIOs have different properties of various sizes, surface charges and hydrophilicity. In general, SPIOsat a larger hydrodynamic diameter with an ionic and hydrophobic surface tend to be easily eliminated from the blood stream by phagocytic cells, compared to SPIOs at a smaller hydrodynamic diameter with neutral and hydrophilic surface [23]. To date, commercially available US FDA-approved SSPIO particles include Endorem and Feridex, both of which have a dextran-coating [22]. A major concern regarding the SPIO is whether it has any negative effect on the growth, function, viability, proliferation and differentiation of the transplanted stem cells. Theoretically, the core of the SPIO is taken up by phagocytic cells and degraded by the lysosome, followed by integration into the iron storage pool or deposition in the liver as ferritin and/or hemosiderin [23, 24]. Therefore, these biological processes should make SPIO be not toxic unless an iron overload occurs. However, some researchers have reported the iron salts as catalysts of oxygen radical reactions that promotes lipid peroxidation and the formation of hydroxyl radicals that is superoxide-dependent [25]. Some authors found that the presence of SPIOs may lead to partially retarded development of embryo bodies, but had minimum effects on the self-renewal of mouse embryonic stem cells [24]. One study reported SPIOs playing a deviation role in cell differentiation, which is characterized by inhibition of chondrogenesis and promotion of neurogenesis with no significant influence on adipogenesis or osteogenesis [26]. In addition, one study demonstrates that SPIOs do not disturb the differentiation of mesenchymal stem cells into the hepatocytes or the expression of albumin [19]. Overall, these characteristics, including the variable sizes with different properties, the allowance for modification of their coatings, favorable biocompatibility and its intuitive signal properties, make SPIO a promising contrast agent for tracking of stem cells with MRI [23].

Cell Labeling Methods

To incorporate these labeling agents into the cells, special measures must be taken to enhance the internalization or endocytosis because of the poor phagocytic capacity of stem cells [18].

A series of labeling methods have been developed to facilitate the noninvasive visualization of the implanted stem cells on MRI. Direct labeling is considered as the most straight-forward method to improve the insufficient uptake of SPIOs [6]. By modification of these anionic nanoparticles with cationic transfection agents, such as poly-L-lysine(PLL) [3], lipofectamine [27], protamine sulfate etc., the neutrally charged SPIOs can be internalized more efficiently(e.g., almost 100% efficiency with PLL [20]) through incubation with the cells. Megnetoelectroporation (MEP) is another approach to induce a large amount of endocytosis within a few minutes using low voltage pulses [6, 28]. However, for both labeling techniques, there are several major concerns: 1) The signal intensity may gradually be undetectable as the cells proliferate, which leads to dilution of the contrast agents; 2) It remains unclear whether the signal of SPIOs is from the living stem cells, dead cells or macrophages that cleared the debris of the dead labeled cells; and 3) The hypointensity of SPIO-labeled cells may be confounded by hemorrhage, air or other causes of hypointensity on MRI [5, 6, 29].

Solutions to some of these issues has been attempted by developing an in situ labeling technique using magnetic iron microbeads, which is coupled with a special antibody against an antigen uniquely found on human hepatic progenitors —the epithelial cell adhesion molecule (EpCAM) [2]. This specific receptor-mediated cell labeling method allows long-term and continuous tracking of the stem cells by multiple injections of the microbeads without loss of the signals. Furthermore, it ensures that the signals on MRI are from the transplanted cells at the targets.

Some researchers attempted to address the problem of SPIO dilution by transfecting the stem cells with a reporter gene, which enables stable expression of a specific receptor, protein, enzyme, etc., which enhances visualization of the transplanted stem cells in vivo [6, 12].

This method can effectively avoid the dilution of the contrast agents within the progeny cells and ensure the origin of the signals from the living stem cells at the target. However, at this moment the reporter gene-based cell labeling techniques are not feasible in clinical settings due to their complicated manipulations and the increased risk of generating tumorsvia such approaches [2].

In order to distinguish the implanted stem cells from other confounding factors of hypointensity on MRI, some authors used MnO nanoparticles [16], which is a positive contrast agent on T1-weighted MR imaging. However, the biocompatibility of this labeling agent has yet to be optimized. Developments of other cell labeling techniques are underway, including modification of the coating of SPIOs [19, 30], using magnetodendrimers [31], or application of HIV-derived TAT proteinas a transduction agent [32].

Manifestations of MRI

The signal changes of stem cells labeled with SPIOs on MRI images can be explained by the effect of SPIOs on the dephasing of protons in a magnetic field. The homing or migration of stem cells may result in local accumulation of SPIOs at the target, which distorts the surrounding magnetic field and strongly interferes with the T1 relaxation and T2 relaxation of the adjacent protons—also known as the susceptibility effect [19, 23]. The R1, R2 and R2* relaxivities, defined as the reciprocal of T1, T2 and T2* relaxation times, are closely associated with the core diameter of SPIOs. SPIOs with a larger core diameter prove to have a higher R1, R2 or R2* relaxivity [23], Thus, the T1, T2* and T2 relaxation times are dramatically shortened with SPIOs, characterized by a hypointense signal on T2- or T2*-weighted images and a hyperintense signal on T1-weighted images [22].

However, most studies have found that the R1 effect is negligible and only the R2/R2* effects are strong enough to be detected. This phenomenon is explained by a reduced sensitivity when the SPIOs are internalized by cells, and the inner sphere dipole-dipole interactions of SPIOs become less efficient so that only the susceptibility effect from the outer sphere of SPIOs is evident [6]. One study compared the R2 and R2* values and found that the R2* effect was 30 times stronger than the R2 effect [33].

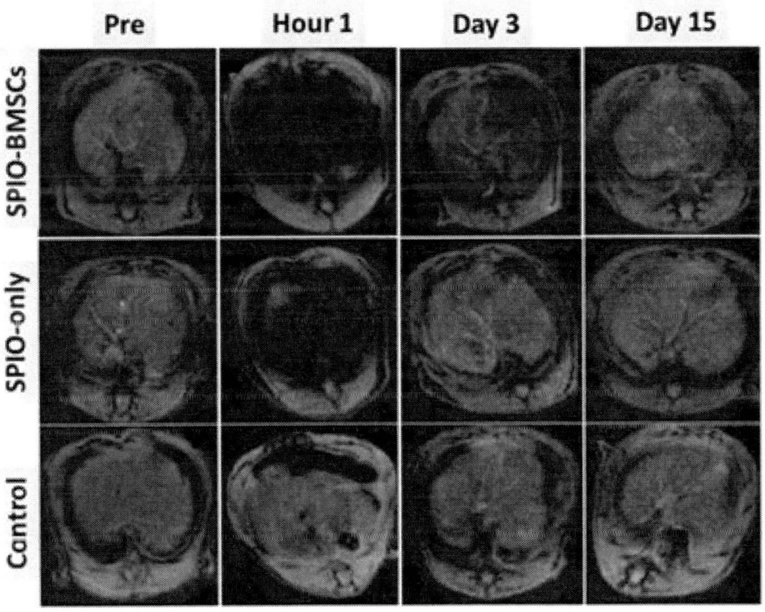

Figure 7.1. T2*-weighted MR imaging of the rodent liver. MRI findings of rodent models of CCl_4-induced liver fibrosis after SPIO-labeled bone marrow stem cells (BMSCs), SPIO or unlabeled BMSCs (control) were intravenously administered. MR imaging of the liver was performed before and after the labeled cell injection (1 h, Days 3 and 15). The liver signal intensities (SI) for both study groups with SPIO-labeled bone marrow stem cells and SPIOs only dramatically decreased at 1 h post labeled cell injection, and recovered to the pretreatment levels at Days 3 and 15, respectively. In the control group, the liver SI demonstrated no significant difference at the tested time points.Reprinted, with permission, from [35].

In addition, the signal changes in T2*-weighted images seem to be more significant due to the well-known "blooming effect", which describes that the hypointense area on T2*-weighted images usually extends well outside the actual size caused by the substantial susceptibility effect. As a result, T2*-weighted sequence is the most intensively used in MRI of SPIO-labeled stem cells.

Efforts have been made to investigate the dynamic image findings on T2*-weighted MRI. The results varied among different studies as various endpoints were examined. As a general principle, signal intensity of the transplanted cells in the liver on T2*-weighted MRI should substantially decrease during the first 1-24 hours and then present a gradual return to the initial level within 2-4 weeks[15, 18, 29, 34, 35](Figures 7.1 & 7.2). These decreased signal intensities have been proved to be consistent with the histologic findings of Prussian blue-positive cells at the same target sites[29]. Several reasons may contribute to the return of the signal intensity, including: 1) The labeled stem cells mobilize out of the liver; 2) Cell division leads to redistribution of SPIOs within the progeny cells; 3) Ischemia or hypoxia in the liver may decrease the number of SPIO-labeled stem cells; and 4) Immune rejection may result in cell death [15, 19].

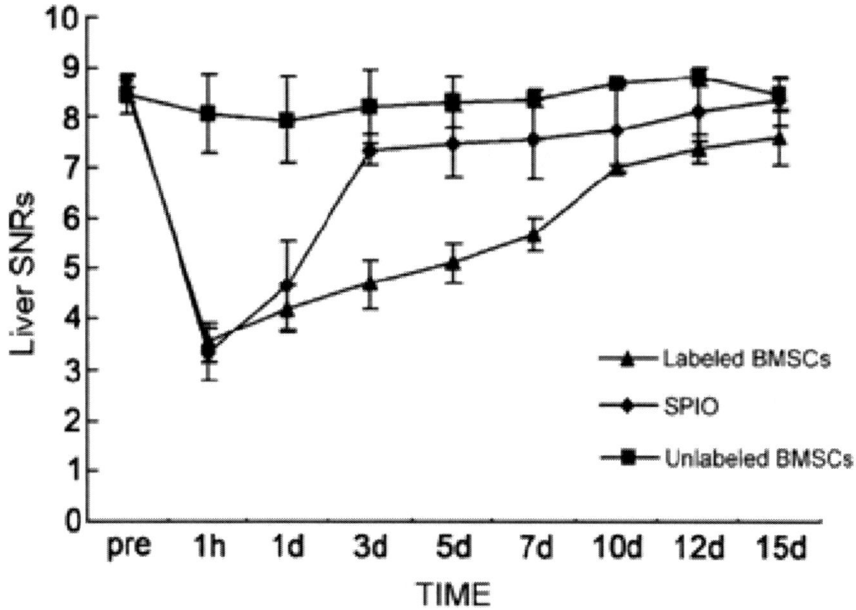

Figure 7.2. Graph compares liver signal-to-noise ratios (SNRs) among the SPIO-labeled bone marrow-derived stem cells (BMSC), SPIO-only and unlabeled BMSC groups. Rats with CCl_4-induced liver fibrosis received intravascular administration of SPIO-labeled BMSCs, SPIO or unlabeled BMSCs. MR imaging of the livers was performed before and after cell transplantation. The liver SNRs of the BMSC-labeled and SPIO groups are significantly lower than those of pretreatment at 1 h (P=.001 and P=.000, respectively) and 1 day (P=.011 and P=.019, respectively). At Day 3 liver SNR of the SPIO group returns to the pretreatment level, while liver SNR in the BMSC-labeled group remains at a considerably lower level for 12 days (P<.05, versus the level before). Reprinted, with permission, from [35].

Recent Progress in MRI of Stem Cell Application in Liver

Currently, MRI is the main imaging tool in non-invasive assessmentof cell transplantation in liver, with regards to the numbers of cells required, the optimum site of cell administration, as well as the therapeutic time window [22]. For example, MRI has been used to compare the efficacies of cell transplantation among different administration routes by monitor the distribution of transplanted stem cells in livers, which is directly related to cell homing efficiency and thereby potential cell therapeutic benefits [29]. To date, several possible cell transplantation routes for liver have been evaluated with MRI assessments, including 1) injection ofstem cells through a vascular route, such as the portal vein, hepatic artery, or peripheral vein; 2) intrasplenic injection of the stem cells; 3) local injection of the stem cells into the hepatic parenchyma; and 4) ectopic cell implantation, such as intraperitoneal implantation [18, 36]. According to post-transplantation MRI analysis, the vascular route via either the portal vein or hepatic artery seems to be the effective method of choice, compared to that via the peripheral vein that is less efficient [29]. However, a few studies showed that although the vascular administration route through the portal vein or hepatic artery allows a more diffused distribution of the cells throughout the liver on MRI, there is a high risk of vascular embolization caused by cell clots, and the transplanted cells may also distribute to the extrahepatic organs such as lungs and kidneys for unknown reasons [2, 33, 36]. The intrasplenic route requires a small number of transplanted cells with less possibility of vascular embolization as the stem cells migrate slowly to the liver [18]. Local implantation of the stem cells seems providing better therapeutic effects on focal lesions(e.g., ischemia) instead of diffuse liver diseases, due to limited migration rate of the implanted cells at a few millimeters per week [15, 33]. As for intraperitoneal implantation, insufficient metabolism usually results in inevitable hepatic cell necrosis [36].

MRI is an excellent tool for monitoring of cell distribution in the liver. Some studies show that MRI can clearly display the transplanted stem cells that are either trapped in hepatic sinusoids or later incorporated to periportal area of hepatic parenchyma when transplanting the cells via the intraportal approach. MRI findings suggest that the intraportal approach is an appropriate way for cell therapy of hepatic sinusoidal diseases or diseases affecting the portal veins. In addition, the studies also found that stem cells can be also attracted to the injured (or diseased) sites of the liver, which is considered as a consequence of the "active recruitment" by these sites [19, 33, 34]. Overall, by providing essential information such as when and where the stem cells migrate in vivo, and how long they remain detectable at the targets, MRI, combined with SPIO-labeled stem cells, acts as a useful tool for determining a preferred cell transplantation route and assisting decision-making with regard to the appropriate cell therapy of liver diseases.

Limitations and Challenges

Cellular MRI of SPIO-labeled stem cells has several disadvantages, such as dilution of SPIOs as cells differentiate and difficulty in distinguishing hypointense signals generated by the labeled stem cells migrated to the target or by the nature structures of the anatomic background around the target. A major challenge in current cellular MRI of stem cell application in liver is to quantify the number of transplanted stem cellsin vivo. Although one study demonstrated that R2* value was linearly proportional to the iron load of labeled cells in vitro [33], it is a complicated task to determine the number of stem cells in vivo based on R2* measurement because R2* value is often influenced by random noise caused by either air-tissue interfaces or respiratory and bowel motions. Moreover, the iron load within the cells is variable and the baseline R2* values may be different among patients [33]. Another challenge for cellular MRI of the liver is its limitation in detecting the survival and functional information of the implanted cells at the targets. Some authors found that the apparent diffusion coefficient (ADC) value could be used in evaluation of hepatic injury repair after transplantation of allogeneic mononuclear bone marrow cells [37]. However, this study was performed without using SPIO-based cellular MRI [38]. Thus, future efforts on cellular MRI are warranted to provide more quantitative and functional information about the transplanted stem cells in liver targets, which should impact the improvement of stem cell therapy for liver diseases.

Acknowledgments

The authors are grateful to Elsevier for the permission of reprinting two figures in this chapter. We also acknowledge Zaiyi Liu, MD for his advice on preparation of this work.

References

[1] Heidelbaugh JJ, Bruderly M. Cirrhosis and chronic liver failure: part I. Diagnosis and evaluation. *American family physician*. 2006;74(5):756-762.

[2] McClelland R, Wauthier E, Tallheden T, Reid LM, Hsu E. In situ labeling and magnetic resonance imaging of transplanted human hepatic stem cells. *Molecular imaging and biology : MIB : the official publication of the Academy of Molecular Imaging*. 2011 Oct;13(5):911-922.

[3] Shi X-L. Magnetically labeled mesenchymal stem cells after autologous transplantation into acutely injured liver. *World Journal of Gastroenterology*. 2010;16(29):3674.

[4] Nyolczas N, Charwat S, Posa A, Hemetsberger R, Pavo N, Hemetsberger H, et al. Tracking the migration of cardially delivered therapeutic stem cells in vivo: state of the art. *Regenerative medicine*. 2009 May;4(3):407-422.

[5] Lee Z, Dennis JE, Gerson SL. Imaging Stem Cell Implant for Cellular-Based Therapies. *Experimental Biology and Medicine*. 2008;233(8):930-940.

[6] Kraitchman DL, Bulte JWM. Imaging of stem cells using MRI. *Basic Research inCardiology*. 2008;103(2):105-113.

[7] Yan L, Han Y, He Y, Xie H, Liu J, Zhao L, et al. Cell tracing techniques in stem cell transplantation. *Stem cell reviews*. 2007 Dec;3(4):265-269.

[8] Shan L. FluidMAG iron nanoparticle-labeled mesenchymal stem cells for tracking cell homing to tumors.*Molecular Imaging and Contrast Agent Database* (MICAD). Bethesda MD2004.

[9] Iyer M, Barrio JR, Namavari M, Bauer E, Satyamurthy N, Nguyen K, et al. 8-[18F] Fluoropenciclovir: an improved reporter probe for imaging HSV1-tk reporter gene expression in vivo using PET. *Journal of Nuclear Medicine*. 2001;42(1):96-105.

[10] Stelter L, Pinkernelle JG, Michel R, Schwartländer R, Raschzok N, Morgul MH, et al. Modification of aminosilanizedsuperparamagnetic nanoparticles: feasibility of multimodal detection using 3T MRI, small animal PET, and fluorescence imaging. *Molecular Imaging and Biology*. 2010;12(1):25-34.

[11] Bhaumik S, Gambhir S. Optical imaging of Renilla luciferase reporter gene expression in living mice. *Proceedings of the National Academy of Sciences*. 2002;99(1):377-382.

[12] Cohen B, Ziv K, Plaks V, Israely T, Kalchenko V, Harmelin A, et al. MRI detection of transcriptional regulation of gene expression in transgenic mice. *Nature medicine*. 2007;13(4):498-503.

[13] Kang JH, Chung J-K. Molecular-genetic imaging based on reporter gene expression. *Journal of Nuclear Medicine*. 2008;49(Suppl 2):164S-179S.

[14] Pastor CM. Tracking mesenchymal stem cells in the liver by magnetic resonance imaging. *Journal of Hepatology*. 2005;43(5):915-916.

[15] Son KR. MRI of magnetically labeled mesenchymal stem cells in hepatic failure model. *World Journal of Gastroenterology*. 2010;16(44):5611.

[16] Gilad AA, Walczak P, McMahon MT, Na HB, Lee JH, An K, et al. MR tracking of transplanted cells with "positive contrast" using manganese oxide nanoparticles. *Magnetic Resonance in Medicine*. 2008;60(1):1-7.

[17] Hsiao JK, Tsai CP, Chung TH, Hung Y, Yao M, Liu HM, et al. Mesoporous silica nanoparticles as a delivery system of gadolinium for effective human stem cell tracking. *Small*. 2008;4(9):1445-1452.

[18] Kim TH, Kim JK, Shim W, Kim SY, Park TJ, Jung JY. Tracking of transplanted mesenchymal stem cells labeled with fluorescent magnetic nanoparticle in liver cirrhosis rat model with 3-T MRI. *Magnetic resonance imaging*. 2010 Sep;28(7):1004-1013..

[19] Ju S, Teng GJ, Lu H, Jin J, Zhang Y, Zhang A, et al. In vivo differentiation of magnetically labeled mesenchymal stem cells into hepatocytes for cell therapy to repair damaged liver. *Investigative radiology*. 2010 Oct;45(10):625-633.

[20] Zhang H. Iron oxide nanoparticles-poly-L-lysine complex. *Molecular Imaging andContrast Agent Database* (MICAD). Bethesda MD2004.

[21] Shan L. Magnetic iron microbeads coupled with HEA-125 monoclonal antibody against epithelial cell adhesion molecule. *Molecular Imaging and Contrast Agent Database (MICAD)*. Bethesda MD2004.

[22] Kubinová Š, Syková E. Nanotechnologies in regenerative medicine. *MinimallyInvasive Therapy & Allied Technologies*. 2010;19(3):144-156.

[23] Ittrich H, Peldschus K, Raabe N, Kaul M, Adam G. Superparamagnetic Iron Oxide Nanoparticles in Biomedicine: Applications and Developments in Diagnostics and Therapy. *RöFo - Fortschritte auf demGebiet der Röntgenstrahlen und der bildgebendenVerfahren*. 2013;185(12):1149-1166.

[24] Krejci J, Pachernik J, Hampl A, Dvorak P. In vitro labelling of mouse embryonic stem cells with SPIO nanoparticles. *General physiology and biophysics*. 2008 Sep;27(3):164-173..
[25] Gutteridge JM, Rowley DA, Halliwell B. Superoxide-dependent formation of hydroxyl radicals and lipid peroxidation in the presence of iron salts. Detection of 'catalytic' iron and anti-oxidant activity in extracellular fluids. *The Biochemical journal*. 1982 Sep 15;206(3):605-609.
[26] Kostura L, Kraitchman DL, Mackay AM, Pittenger MF, Bulte JW. Feridex labeling of mesenchymal stem cells inhibits chondrogenesis but not adipogenesis or osteogenesis. *NMR in Biomedicine*. 2004;17(7):513-517.
[27] Park B-H, Jung J-C, Lee G-H, Kim T-J, Lee Y-J, Kim J-Y, et al. Comparison of labeling efficiency of different magnetic nanoparticles into stem cell. *Colloids and Surfaces A: Physicochemical and Engineering Aspects*. 2008;313:145-149.
[28] Engberink RD, van der Pol SM, Walczak P, van der Toorn A, Viergever MA, Dijkstra CD, et al. Magnetic resonance imaging of monocytes labeled with ultrasmallsuperparamagnetic particles of iron oxide using magnetoelectroporation in an animal model of multiple sclerosis. *Molecular imaging*. 2010 Oct;9(5):268-277.
[29] Zhong Y, Tang Z, Xu R, Lin N, Deng M, Fang H, et al. Effect of transplantation route on stem cell migration to fibrotic liver of rats via cellular magnetic resonance imaging. *Cytotherapy*. 2013;15(10):1266-1274.
[30] Shan L. Poly(N,N-dimethylacrylamide)-coated maghemite nanoparticles for labeling and tracking mesenchymal stem cells. Molecular Imaging and Contrast Agent Database (MICAD). Bethesda MD2004.
[31] Bulte JW, Douglas T, Witwer B, Zhang S-C, Strable E, Lewis BK, et al. Magnetodendrimers allow endosomal magnetic labeling and in vivo tracking of stem cells. *Nature biotechnology*. 2001;19(12):1141-1147.
[32] Josephson L, Tung C-H, Moore A, Weissleder R. High-efficiency intracellular magnetic labeling with novel superparamagnetic-Tat peptide conjugates. *Bioconjugate chemistry*. 1999;10(2):186-191.
[33] Bos C, Delmas Y, Desmouliere A, Solanilla A, Hauger O, Grosset C, et al. In vivo MR imaging of intravascularly injected magnetically labeled mesenchymal stem cells in rat kidney and liver. *Radiology*. 2004 Dec;233(3):781-789.
[34] Chen XW, Zhu DJ, Ju YL, Zhou SF. Therapeutic effect of transplanting magnetically labeled bone marrow stromal stem cells in a liver injury rat model with 70%-hepatectomy. *Medical science monitor : international medical journal of experimental and clinical research*. 2012 Oct;18(10):BR375-382..
[35] Zhou B, Shan H, Li D, Jiang Z-B, Qian J-S, Zhu K-S, et al. MR tracking of magnetically labeled mesenchymal stem cells in rats with liver fibrosis. *Magnetic resonance imaging*. 2010;28(3):394-399.
[36] Ju S, Teng GJ, Lu H, Zhang Y, Zhang A, Chen F, et al. In vivo MR tracking of mesenchymal stem cells in rat liver after intrasplenic transplantation. *Radiology*. 2007 Oct;245(1):206-215.

[37] Shang QL, Xiao EH, Zhou QC, Luo JG, Wu HJ. Pathological and MR-DWI study of the acute hepatic injury model after stem cell transplantation. *World journal of gastroenterology : WJG*. 2011 Jun 21;17(23):2821-2828.
[38] Taouli B, Koh D-M. Diffusion-weighted MR imaging of the liver. *Radiology*. 2010;254(1):47.

In: Magnetic Resonance Imaging of Stem Cell Applications ISBN: 978-1-63463-910-1
Editor: Xiaoming Yang

Chapter 8

Magnetic Resonance Imaging of Stem Cell Application in Oncology

Mariangela Sottili, Chiara Gerini and Monica Mangoni*
Radiotherapy Unit, Department of Experimental & Clinical Biomedical Sciences, University of Florence, Firenze, Italy

Abstract

There is a growing interest in using stem cells for therapeutic and diagnostic application in the field of oncology. Stem cells have the intrinsic ability to ''home'' towards growing tumors and are hypo-immunogenic, and, thus they are very promising vehicles of gene therapy and immunotherapy of cancer. For hematological malignancies, intravenous injection of autologous and allogeneic bone marrow suspensions, including hematopoietic progenitors, is a consolidated strategy to support the delivery of otherwise lethal doses of radiation therapy or chemotherapy. In addition, it has been demonstrated that patients who develop graft-versus-host disease have lower incidence of relapse, showing that the donor-derived immune system contributes to the eradication of leukemia. This phenomenon is due to elimination of leukemic stem cells by alloreactivity of the transplanted stem cells. The tumor-specific homing of stem cells opens the possibility of using stem cells in early cancer diagnosis. Nowadays, it is well know that tumor is a "cancer stem cells disease." Tumor stroma is composed of a variety of cells, including proliferating tumor cells, cancer stem cells, tumor fibroblasts, endothelial cells, lymphocytes and other cells, while cancer stem cells are the main component involved in tumor maintenance and progression. The possibility to in vivo identify and track cancer stem cells is of pivotal importance for cancer diagnosis and therapy response assessment. This chapter focuses primarily on the capability of using non-invasive MR imaging to (1) monitor the transplantation of therapeutic cells to the tumor sites, where these cells subsequently differentiate and proliferate; and (2) non-invasively track individual cancer

* Corresponding author: Monica Mangoni, MD, PhD, Radiotherapy Unit, Department of Experimental and Clinical Biomedical Sciences, University of Florence, Largo Brambilla 3, 50134 Firenze, Italy (monica.mangoni@unifi.it).

cells, which is expected to provide more insight to the mechanisms of cancer development, dissemination, and responses to oncological therapies in the future.

Keywords: Oncology, cancer stem cells, chemotherapy/radiotherapy-induced damages, stem cells, non-invasive tracking

Introduction

Personalized diagnosis and treatment with allogenic or autologous cells are becoming a reality in modern medicine. In the field of oncology, there is a growing interest in using stem cells for diagnosis and therapy of various types of cancer. Stem cells have the intrinsic ability to "home" towards growing tumors and are hypo-immunogenic. Therefore, they can be used as either "Trojan Horses" to directly deliver therapeutic genes into tumors, or carriers of imaging-visible nanoparticles to allow cell tracking and cancer detection [1]. The ability to non-invasively track the delivery of various therapeutic cells to the tumor site, where the delivered cells subsequently differentiate and proliferate, should allow a better understanding of the mechanisms of cancer development and intervention. Moreover, the regenerative properties of stem cells offer interesting potential for prevention of chemotherapy- and radiotherapy-induced toxicities and tissue-damages.

In the last decades, numerous scientific evidences have supported the theory of cancer stem cells. The investigation on the behavior of cancer stem cells is of primary importance to provide more insights to carcinogenesis, as well as cancer progression and metastasis. Moreover, the possibility to detect and quantify cancer stem cells in vivo is expected to offer a reliable way for establishing prognostic stratification and assessing tumor responses to oncological therapies [2].

Research efforts have been dedicated to labeling stem cells with either reporter genes or various imaging contrast agents, which enables non-invasive cell tracking and quantifying the fate of administered cells in vivo using different imaging modalities (Figure 8.1), such as magnetic resonance imaging (MRI). An ideal imaging modality for tracking of therapeutic cells in cancer patients requires the imaging tags to be nontoxic, biocompatible, and highly specific [3]. In addition, the requirement for cell tracking techniques depends on the clinical scenario. In some cases, only short term tracking is needed, while in other cases long term survival and proliferation need to be monitored [3].

In this chapter, we first describe the potential application of stem cells in the field of oncology, and then overview the current status on MRI of stem cell application in cancer.

Application of Stem Cells in Oncology

Stem cell therapy represents an important field of interest in oncology. Main therapeutic applications of stem cells are in gene therapy, immunotherapy, and reduction of radio-/chemotherapy-induced damages. Moreover, it is nowadays accepted that cancer is a stem cells disease and that cancer stem cells have an increasing importance in the field of early tumor diagnosis and assessment of tumor prognosis.

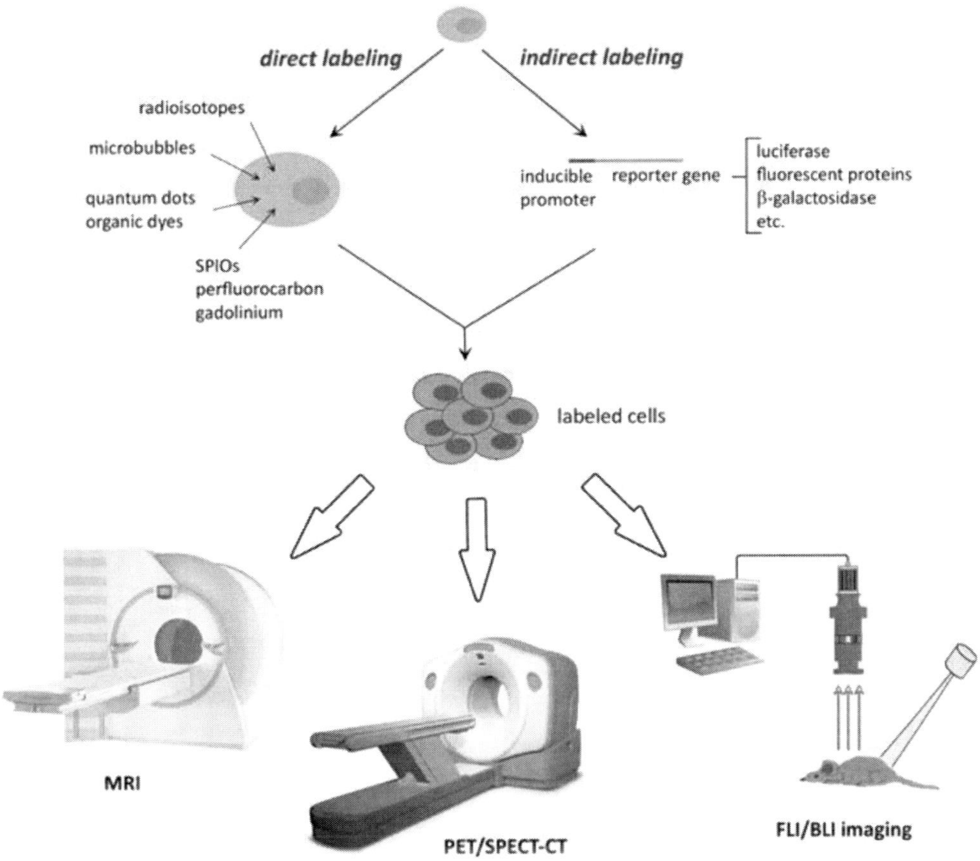

Figure 8.1. Schematic illustration of direct and indirect cell labeling modalities.
Direct labeling is based on incubation of cells with medium containing the imaging agents, which can be taken up by the cells with different mechanisms (i.e., transporter uptake, phagocytosis, macropinocytosis, passive diffusion etc.). In the indirect labeling, the cells are genetically modified by the introduction of a reporter gene. The transcription of the reporter gene under the control of a promoter and the subsequent translation of its mRNA in turn lead to the expression of different fluorescent or bioluminescent proteins. SPIONs: superparamagnetic iron oxide nanoparticles; MRI: magnetic resonance imaging; CT: computed tomography; PET: positron emission tomography; SPECT: single-photon emission computed tomography; FLI: fluorescence imaging; and BLI: bioluminescence imaging.

Gene Therapy

Gene therapy is one of the more exciting fields of research in the field of oncology. Using viral and non-viral vectors, therapeutic genetic materials can be specifically targeted to cancer cells (Figure 8.2), e.g., to compensate for mutations in tumor suppressor genes, to potentiate anticancer immune responses, or to initiate oncolysis [1, 4]. The ability of stem cells to elude immunological system clearance and to migrate towards pathological sites (such as wounds, ischemia, and cancer with micrometastases) offers an exciting paradigm for targeted cancer therapies [1]. Stem cells have the powerful advantage of being a vector or a cellular vehicle, which, along with their tumor homing ability, makes stem cells hold advantages for cancer gene therapy, superior to other vehicles such as proteins, antibodies, nanoparticles, and viruses. In particular, virus-mediated gene therapies have some limitation because of the difficulty in tracking cancer cells [5]. Prodrug cancer gene therapy represents an attractive therapeutic tool for the possibility of activating the prodrug directly within the tumor mass, thus avoiding systemic toxicity. Compared with conventional chemotherapy, suicide gene therapy using stem cells shows good safety and efficacy [6-8].

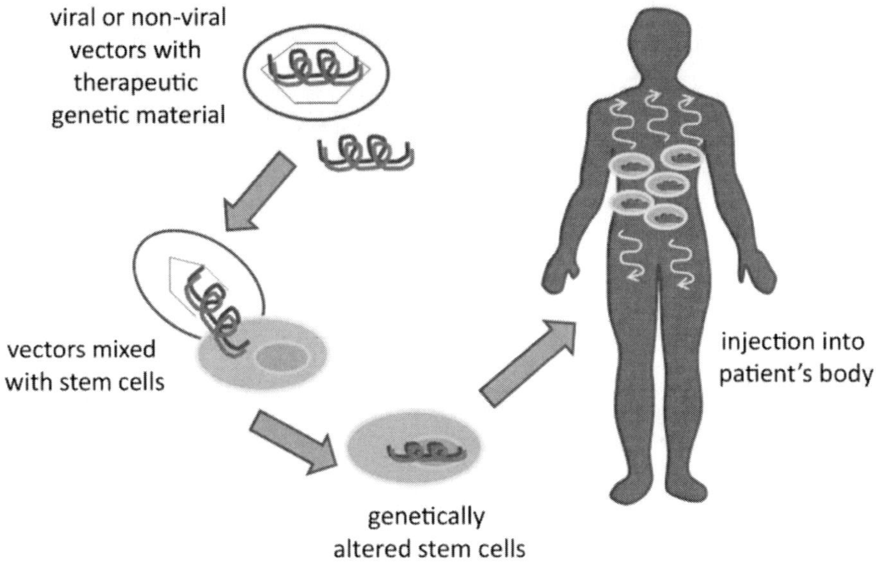

Figure 8.2. Gene therapy. A therapeutic gene is inserted in viral or non-viral vectors. The modified vectors are mixed with stem cells, so that the vectors are integrated into the cell's genome. The genetically altered stem cells are then introduced into the body of the patient, where they start producing the desired protein encoded by the inserted therapeutic gene.

Stem cells from different sources have been explored for biomedical applications, yielding embryonic, fetal multipotent, induced pluripotent, adult multipotent including neuronal, hematopoietic, and mesenchymal stem cells [1, 9]. Despite the tremendous interest in using different stem cells for gene therapy, the unpredictability of their in vivo biological properties, such as migration and the potential contribution to the neoplastic phenotype, poses a serious obstacle to their clinical use [1]. Indeed, there is the concern that the proangiogenic and immunomodulatory properties of different stem cells may potentiate growth and metastatic capacity of cancer cells. Thus, exhaustive investigative studies are essential before any clinical application [1].

Anticancer Immunotherapy

It is now accepted that tumor cells express neo-antigens, unique to the tumor (tumor-specific antigens; TSAs), or shared by other somatic cells (tumor-associated antigens; TAAs) [10, 11]. Unfortunately, tumors may lack immunogenicity, not for to the absence of TAAs per se but rather for their inability to activate the immune system [12]. The ultimate aim of cancer immunotherapy is to activate the immune system to recognize the tumor, and thereby generate a specific and durable-effected T-cell response (Figure 8.3).

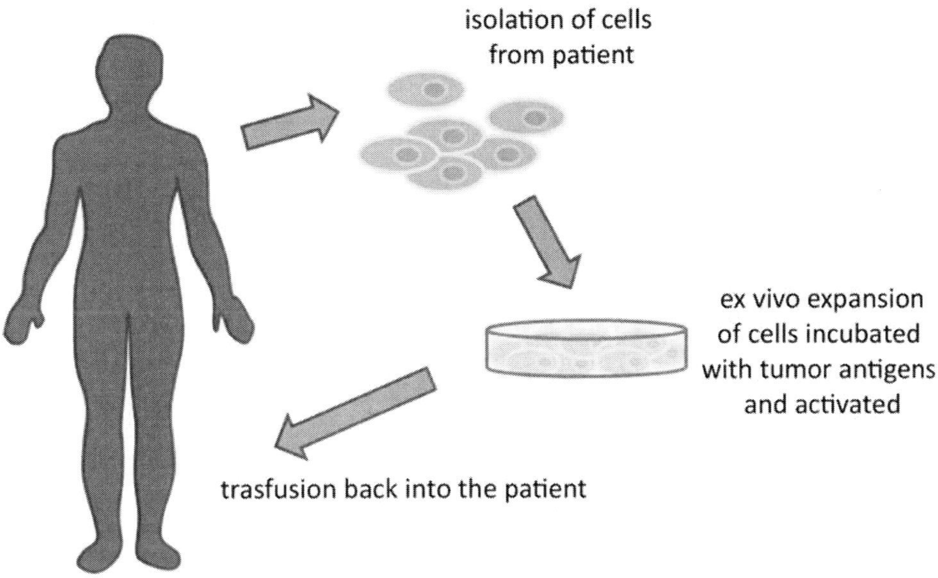

Figure 8.3. Anticancer immunotherapy. Anticancer immunotherapy involves the isolation of stem cells/induced pluripotent cells/immune cells from the patient. These cells are expanded and activated ex vivo by the incubation with tumor antigens. The activated cells are then reinfused back to the same patient to treat the disease.

In order to achieve this goal, adoptive transfer of TAA specific T cells has been explored. Adoptive T-cell transfer involves the isolation of T lymphocytes from the patient, ex vivo expansion of these T cells, and then reinfusion of them back to the same patient to treat the disease [13]. Natural killer (NK) cells have likewise been used for adoptive transfer, due to their innate ability to recognize tumor cells deficient in MHC class I. Alternatively, the ability of dendritic cells (DCs) to present TAAs to T cells has been harnessed to generate an immune response against tumor cells. Autologous monocyte-derived dendritic cells (moDCs) are cultured ex vivo and pulsed with soluble TAAs before re-administration to patients to induce a tumor-specific immune response [14].

Whereas adoptive T-cell transfer may generate a burst of T-cell immunity that is short-lived, DC-based vaccines have the potential to induce a sustained immune response, with the capacity for subsequent recall [15]. Interestingly, although the use of autologous cells is normally preferred, several studies have demonstrated that the use of allogeneic NK cells is significantly more effective [16, 17]. Given the difficulty of obtaining a sufficient number of cells to target tumors in vivo, the advent of induced pluripotency offers unrivaled opportunities. The proven ability to produce induced pluripotent stem (iPS) cells from individuals in a patient-specific manner, with the capacity for indefinite self-renewal and unrestricted differentiation potential, may facilitate the scale-up in the production of critical hematopoietic cell types, for many of which protocols have already been optimized [12].

Since their first description, embryonic stem (ES) cells have been regarded as the "gold standard" for pluripotency, displaying the capability for indefinite self-renewal and differentiation into any somatic cell type, irrespective of its embryonic germ-layer of origin [12] . However, their use has been controversial due to the ethical sensitivities surrounding their derivation from human blastocysts and the utilization of an allogeneic source of cells. In 2006, pluripotent stem cells were obtained from adult mouse fibroblasts by retroviral transduction with genes encoding Oct3/4, Sox2, c-Myc, and Klf4 [18]. These iPS cells are indistinguishable at the cellular level from conventional ES cells, have the capacity for indefinite self-renewal, unrestricted differentiation potential, and, following injection into mouse blastocysts, the ability to generate germline-competent chimeras. These findings were subsequently translated to human dermal fibroblasts [19, 20]. The production of iPS cells in an autologous fashion makes possible their use for immunotherapeutic intervention for numerous indications. For cancer immunotherapy, early research focused on the potential of pluripotency to provide a more homogenous source of DCs amenable to scale-up the significant donor-to-donor variability encountered in the use of moDCs. Moreover, NK cells were successfully differentiated from human iPS cells [21], obtaining a pure population.

Patients undergoing active anticancer immunotherapy based on TAA, can take advantage of an immunological conditioning prior and/or concomitant to immunization. Patients are treated with high dose chemotherapy followed by autologous or allogenic stem cells transplantation. Chemotherapeutic regimens that induce lymphopenia prior to adoptive T-cell therapy allow the efficient expansion of transferred T cells. Immunological conditioning has provided exiting results in melanoma patients [22, 23].

Hematopoietic Stem Cell Transplantation

In hematological malignancies, intravenous injection of autologous and allogeneic marrow suspensions, including hematological progenitors, was first used to support the delivery of otherwise lethal doses of radiation therapy or chemotherapy. The therapeutic potential of these progenitors was rapidly recognized and translated from hematological to solid malignancies [24].

The most common hematologic malignancy for which hematopoietic stem cell transplantation is used is acute myeloid leukemia [25]. The curative effect of hematopoietic stem cell transplantation results from both radiation and/or chemotherapy conditioning regimen and the graft-versus-leukemia effect of the donor immune system [26]. Chemotherapy used to treat hematologic malignancies is most effective in rapidly proliferating cells. Both normal and malignant stem cells, however, are quiescent and, in addition, they efficiently repair DNA, resist apoptosis and excrete toxic drugs. Thus, patients who achieved a complete response can relapse without post-remission therapy as a result of residual leukemic stem cells [27]. Lethal doses of radiation and chemotherapy can destroy leukemic cells along with normal marrow and the immune system of patients. In these cases, infusion of marrow from histocompatible donors can be used to rescue them [27]. It has been demonstrated that patients who developed graft-versus-host disease had lower incidence of relapse, showing that the donor-derived immune system contributed to the eradication of leukemia [26]. This phenomenon is due to elimination of leukemic stem cells by alloreactivity. Graft versus host and graft versus leukemia depend on the differential expression of the relevant minor histocompatibility antigens in each tissue [27].

Reduction of Radiation-Induced Normal Tissue Damages

Normal tissue damage after radiotherapy is a major problem in cancer treatment. Stem cell therapy provides a potential prevention or treatment of radiation-induced normal tissue damage and improves patients' quality of life [28]. Many factors play a role in the response of tissues to irradiation, but at the basis of the onset of radiation-induced damage in several tissues there are the influence of radiation in tissue homeostasis and the inability of stem cells to reconstitute functional cells. After the demonstration that bone marrow transplantation could rescue the hematopoietic system in animals that were exposed to lethal doses of total body irradiation, the first stem cell transplantations were developed. Currently, a wide variety of stem cell therapies are being investigated for their potential to treat a vast array of radiation-induced toxicities [28].

In the irradiated mouse salivary gland, it has been shown that stem cell therapy can be used to rescue an organ after radiation-induced damage. This has been the first time that bone marrow-derived stem cells have been successfully used for the repair of a solid organ [29]. To date, the only routinely applied clinical stem cell therapy is hematopoietic stem cell transplantation, which is used to restore blood production after treatment of patients suffering from leukemia, as well as from various other types of blood disorders [28]. The successes of stem cell therapy can be potentially translated to several radiotherapy settings, such as radiation-induced damage at skin, mammary gland, eye, inner ear, kidney, central nervous system, heart, muscle, and lung [28].

Cancer Diagnosis

Stem cells show preferential migration toward sites of inflammation, injury, and cancer. In several cancer animal models, the tropism of mesenchymal stem cells for the site of tumor has been demonstrated [1]. In particular, there are evidences in glioma [30, 31], pulmonary metastases [32-34], breast cancer metastases [35], ovarian carcinoma [36], and melanoma [37]. Stem cells and cancer stem cells homing to tumors in vivo are due to the release of growth factors and chemokines. Although this phenomenon is not completely understood, it is evident that some of the most important actors are stromal-derived growth factor (SDF)-1/CXC chemokine receptor-4 (CXCR4) [38, 39], monocyte chemotactic protein (MCP)-1/CC chemokine receptor-2 (CCR2) [35], hepatocyte growth factor (HGF)/c-met [40], and vascular endothelial growth factor (VEGF)/VEGF receptor [41], together with extracellular matrix (ECM) proteins. Stem cells appear to be attracted towards lesions where they engraft into the stroma and persist: in xenograft experiments, 40% of intratumoral fibroblasts in pancreatic lesions in mice were of bone marrow origin [42]. Although bone-marrow-derived cells are distributed throughout the tumor mass, this and subsequent studies have shown a greater concentration of them in the tumor periphery [1]. The tumor homing of stem cells opens the possibility of using them in early cancer diagnosis. Moreover, the possibility of non-invasive tracking of individual cancer cells is expected to give more information on cancer progression and metastasis in the future [43].

Cancer Stem Cells

Tumor stroma is composed of a variety of cells, including proliferating tumor cells, cancer stem cells, tumor fibroblasts, endothelial cells, lymphocytes, and other cells that infiltrate or are incorporated in the tumor mass. As already mentioned, it is now generally accepted that cancer is a stem cell disease [6]. The cancer stem cell theory holds that the cancer stem cell arises from either a stem cell with genetic or epigenetic mutations, resulting in the cancer phenotype, or from a transformed progenitor cell that also acquires the stem cell ability of self-renewal [2].

Cancer stem cells represent a rare population of cells, as low as 0.1% of cells within a human tumor, which gives rise to a hierarchy of progenitor and aberrantly differentiated cells and is therefore entirely responsible for the cellular heterogeneity of the tumor [44]. In addition, the observation that metastatic tumors tend to reproduce a cellular heterogeneity similar to that of the primary tumor has led to the hypothesis that cancer stem cells are the culprits of metastasis [2, 45].

A stem cell niche specific for cancer stem cells has not been identified; but if cancer stem cells derive from normal tissue stem cells, then it is very likely that signals that support and maintain the stem cell phenotype in normal tissue stem cells also support cancer stem cells. One important aspect of cancer stem cells is their relative resistance to chemotherapeutic agents and radiation. This resistance is based on their increased ability to scavenge free radicals formed in response to radiation and on their increased DNA repair activity. Furthermore, cancer stem cells are resistant to genotoxic chemotherapeutics via their increased drug pump activity and slowdown of the doubling time [2, 46-51].

The cancer stem cell model raises the concern that treatments targeting rapidly proliferating and/or non-stem-like cells are destined to fail. Therefore, the ability to identify and quantify cancer stem cells has therapeutic and prognostic value [2]. Cancer stem cells can be identified from clinical samples and cell lines on the basis of the expression of cell-surface markers, with substantial differences among different cancer cell lines. The possibility to track cancer stem cells will let to monitor the engraftment, propagation, and subsequent differentiation of cancer stem cells at a primary or metastatic site. The imaging and quantification of these cells will probably gain great importance in the future for the prognosis and the therapy response assessment of cancers. Considering their increased resistance to anticancer treatment and radiation, the possibility to get an imaging of the distribution of cancer stem cells and cancer stem cell niche could also largely influence radiotherapy treatment planning principles. Quantifying and mapping the distribution of cancer stem cells before the beginning of radiotherapy could lead to an adaptive radiotherapy, with modulation of the total dose on the basis of cancer stem cells early response [52, 53]. However, more knowledge on surface markers is still necessary for preclinical and clinical applications.

Circulating Tumor Cells

Circulating tumor cells (CTCs) are tumor-derived cells that can be found in the blood stream [54]. The detachment of cancer cells from a primary tumor into the blood system is due to a phenomenon called epithelial-mesenchymal transition (ETM). The CTC population is highly resilient, enabling the cells to colonize a foreign microenvironment. Detection of CTCs has been reported for most epithelial tumors and has been associated with an increased risk of local and regional recurrence, as well as the development of distant metastases. In CTCs, the presence of stem-cell properties is frequently observed, which contribute to the re-establishment of bulk tumor tissue at the metastatic site (for distance progression) or at the primary site (for tumor recurrence) [55]. Clinical trials indicated that CTCs are biomarkers that can be used for assessment or monitoring of prognosis. In metastatic breast, colon, prostate, as well as head and neck cancer patients, the presence of CTCs is related to poor prognosis [56-59]. Although the detection of CTCs has already shown to have a prognostic impact in many tumors, ongoing and future studies are aimed to explore whether CTCs can be used for individual therapies and immunotherapies [54]. Actually, CTCs are detected in blood samples as real time "liquid biopsies" on the basis of surface markers, but the possibility to detect them directly in vivo with tracking techniques is an exciting perspective for the future.

Non-Invasive Tracking of Stem Cells in Cancer

Stem cells can migrate to and proliferate within sites of inflammation and tumors as part of the tissue remodeling process, which has been exploited as a tumor-targeting strategy for cell-based cancer therapy [3]. However, once administered intravenously, the grafted stem cells migrate away from the initial delivery site toward tumor beds, which cannot be visualized in vivo [3]. Development of non-invasive cellular imaging techniques allows tracking of grafted cells and monitoring of their migration. There are several in vivo imaging techniques for tracking grafted cells, including optical imaging (bioluminescence imaging and fluorescence imaging), nuclear imaging (single photon emission computed tomography-SPECT and positron emission tomography-PET), computed tomography (CT), ultrasound imaging, and magnetic resonance imaging (MRI) [24]. The above mentioned imaging modalities are characterized by different sensitivities, tissue penetrations and spatial resolutions (Table 8.1).

Optical imaging systems are dependent on tissue depth and have not applications in humans [24, 60-62]. PET and SPECT have high sensitivity (>5 x10^3 cells) [63]; these techniques can be performed by direct labeling (that has the limitation of not being able to indicate cell viability) and by indirect or genetic labeling (that has the limitation of needing to introduce genetic material into the cells) [64]. Direct labeling of cells with radionuclide is basically an established method, which permits safe clinical application of cell tracking. However, the main shortcoming of nuclear imaging is the short half-life of clinically-applicable ligands, which restricts cell tracking to a few days at most [65]. CT has high spatial resolution, but needs high densities of metal-based contrast agents with risk of ionizing radiations [66].

Ultrasound imaging uses microbubbles as intravascular contrast agents, while microbubbles can be loaded with cells for the ultrasound-mediated delivery. The principal limit of the ultrasound imaging technique is the detection of cells that are engrafted within the vasculature, but not of components within the perivascular or interstitial compartments [67, 68].

Table 8.1. Comparison of different cellular imaging modalities

Imaging systems	Advantages	Limits
Bioluminescence imaging	High sensitivity Indicate cell viability	Dependent on tissue depth Not in humans
Fluorescence imaging	Not expensive Easy to use	Instability of fluorophores Overlap with autofluorescence (low specificity) Low resolution Not in humans
PET/SPECT	High sensitivity Small mass of radiotracer Genetic labeling: cell viability Low radiation exposure	Direct labeling: not indicates cell viability Genetic labeling: introduction of genetic material Lack of anatomical context
CT	High spatial resolution	Metal-based contrast agents (high density) Ionizing radiations
Ultrasound imaging	Non-invasive Ultrasound mediated cells delivery with microbubbles	No detection of cells within the perivascular or interstitial compartments Low resolution Restricted field of view
MRI	Excellent anatomic detection of cell location	Not yielding information about cell viability Magnetic labels can leak to nearby cells

MRI of Stem Cell Application in Oncology

MRI has been extensively attempted in stem cell imaging [69]. MRI provides accurate anatomical details and tomographic visualization of tumors with excellent soft tissue contrast. It can locate the cells of interest in the context of the surrounding milieu (edema or inflammation) [1, 70-72] without the use of ionizing radiations. In addition, MRI offers a greater tracking window in comparison to PET and SPECT that are limited by the decay of short-lived radioactive isotopes. The better contrast effect is obtained by superparamagnetic iron oxide nanoparticles (SPIOs) that not impair cell proliferative capacity, while gadolinium contrast agents have been shown to be toxic to stem cells. SPIOs are biocompatible and are eliminated through the body's normal iron metabolism. SPIOs have been studied for cancer therapy (hyperthermia), magnetic field-assisted targeting, and as contrast enhancers for MRI and targeted molecular imaging [1, 73, 74]. However, magnetic labels can leak into nearby cells, be up-taken by phagocytic cells, and rapidly cleared from the blood [75], thus resulting in measurement errors [24]. In addition, MRI of magnetic labels does not yield information about cell viability [76].

The ability to monitor SPIOs with MRI has been utilized to investigate the fate of labeled cells in tumors. Rodriguez et al. demonstrated that human and rodent prostate and breast cancer cell lines could be readily labeled by fluorescently tagged micron-sized superparamagnetic iron oxide particles (MPIOs) approximately 960 nanometers (nm). They further reported that the MPIOs were inert with respect to cellular division and tumor formation, and could pass along to daughter cells during mitosis. They also concluded that MPIO-labeled cancer cells and tumors were visible in vivo by MRI [43]. A recent study compared three labeling techniques for their abilities to track the migration of transplanted human mesenchymal stem cells (hMSC) in an orthotopic mouse xenograft model. The authors labeled the cells by three tags of fluorescence, luciferase or ferumoxide for comparison among fluorescent optical imaging, bioluminescence optical imaging, and MRI [77]. They confirmed that the labeled hMSC retained their migratory ability in vitro, similar to unlabeled hMSC, and that these cells could migrate to the tumor sites with their retention of tumor tropism. Although all three imaging modalities were able to conserve hMSC properties, only MRI provided both real time assessment and the high resolution imaging capability.

Loebinger et al. first evaluated the sensitivity of MRI by assessing the dose response of iron labeled cells in subcutaneous tumor xenografts [78]. hMSC were labeled in vitro with superparamagnetic iron oxide nanoparticles, with no effect on differentiation potential, proliferation, survival, or migration of the cells. In their initial experiments, the investigators double-labeled the MSC with fluorescent dye Dil and fluid MAG iron nanoparticles, and they then injected MDAMB231 human breast cancer cells (2×10^6) subcutaneously with increasing numbers of labeled MSC in nonobese diabetic/severe combined immunodeficient mice. The authors showed that as few as 1000 MSC carrying iron oxide nanoparticles could be detected by MRI in tumors 28 days after injection. Histopathological examination confirmed the presence of the iron nanoparticles only in the tumors injected with live labeled MSC. Subsequently, the investigators showed that intravenous injected iron-labeled MSC could be tracked in vivo to multiple lung metastases. Lung metastases were visualized as diffuse hyperintensities in all five lobes 38 days after tumor cell injection, using MRI without contrast agents. A few studies investigated the tumor tropism of SPIO nanoparticle-labeled cells in murine glioma models with MRI [3]. Wu et al. observed that systemically transplanted MSC migrated toward glioma with high specificity in a temporal-spatial pattern [31]. Seven days after transplantation, the labeled cells were distributed throughout the tumor, while after 14 days most of the MSC were found at the border between the tumor and the normal parenchyma.

Thu et al. demonstrated the tumor tropism of ferumoxide-protamine sulfate complex labeled neuronal stem cells to primary and invasive tumor foci in a murine glioma model [79]. These ferumoxide/protamine sulfate-labeled neuronal stem cells were found to retain their proliferative status, tumor tropism, and stem cell character, while allowing in vivo MRI tracking at 7 Tesla. Ferumoxide labeling of human mesenchymal stromal cells appeared feasible, did not alter migratory ability and allowed detection by MRI, so it was demonstrated to be a reliable technique for non-invasive tracking of transplanted therapeutic human mesenchymal stromal cells in the brain [77].

Tunici et al. [80] studied skin stem/progenitor cells derived from the dermis that in culture can generate mesodermal and neural progenies. To investigate their potential for the treatment of brain diseases, they first injected skin stem/progenitor cells into the brain of syngeneic mice. Brain histology indicated that most skin stem/progenitor cells remained undifferentiated. After labeling with magneto-dendrimers, murine and human skin stem/progenitor cells were detected by MRI even 5 months after brain injection. To evaluate the therapeutic potential of these cells on malignant gliomas, the authors transduced skin stem/progenitor cells by a lentiviral vector carrying the cDNA of the anti-glioma cytokine interleukin-4 (IL-4) and injected them into experimental gliomas. Cells were labeled with magneto-dendrimers (MD-100) before in vivo injection. After injection, animals appeared healthy and were followed up by MRI for 5 months, demonstrating the presence of an area of hypointensity, attributable to magneto-dendrimers. MRI demonstrated that IL-4-transducted skin stem/progenitor cells originally injected into the contralateral hemisphere were attracted into glioma. Moreover, IL-4-skin stem/progenitor cells significantly prolonged the survival of tumor-bearing mice.

Endothelial progenitor cells play a key role in the development and infiltration of gliomas and are promising vehicles for delivering anti-angiogenesis genes for tumor therapy.

Arbab et al. used ferumoxide-protamine sulfate complex labeling for human CD34+/AC133+ endothelial progenitor cells [81]. They documented the migration and incorporation of intravenously injected human endothelial progenitor cells into the neovasculature in a flank tumor model. Wang et al. [82] developed a non-invasive method to monitor the migration of endothelial progenitor cells to gliomas using 1.5-T MR scanning. They labeled endothelial progenitor cells isolated from cord blood with Resovist-PLL and they did not observed influence on the biological properties of these cells. After intravenous administration into glioma-bearing nude mice, the labeled endothelial progenitor cells specifically homed to gliomas and could be reliably tracked by 1.5-T MR as early as 1 day after transplantation, causing a signal loss on T2-weighted images. The investigators demonstrated that the transplanted cells may be able to differentiate into endothelial cells and become incorporated into glioma neovasculature. Moreover, this study showed that Resovist labeling of endothelial progenitor cells was feasible, efficient and safe for MRI tracking, and that 1.5-T MR could be a powerful method for in vivo monitoring of endothelial progenitor cells as an anti-angiogenic drug therapy vector target against glioma.

Trekker et al. synthesized polyethylene glycolated (PEG) magnetic nanoparticles and validated their suitability as MRI cell labeling agents in in vitro and in vivo experiments [83]. They evaluated the labeling of therapeutic potent MSC with small core and large core magnetic nanoparticles and observed that both magnetic nanoparticles were, in combination with a transfection agent, stably internalized into the MSC and didn't show any effect on cell metabolism. The labeled cells showed high contrast in MRI phantom studies. The in vivo final assessment with MRI and the subsequent histological validation of the distribution of the labeled cells were performed after intracranial injection in a glioma mouse model. Labeling only 1% of the injected cells allowed sufficient visualization of the labeled stem cells relative to the tumor lesion. The presented magnetic nanoparticles-based system enabled efficient and non-invasive imaging of the distribution of therapeutic cells after administration.

Recently, other authors reported the use of complexes between negatively charged fluorescent monodispersed SPIO nanoparticles and positively charged peptides to improve the MRI properties of labeled stem cells [84]. Stem cells labeled with this method exhibited a strong fluorescent signal and enhanced T2-weighted MRI both in vitro and in vivo in a flank tumor model [3].

Besides iron oxide nanoparticles, labeling cells with perfluorocarbon (PFC) nanoparticles for 19F MRI has also been explored [85]. It was found that CD34+CD133+CD31+ stem/progenitor cells readily internalized these PFC nanoparticles and remained functional in vivo. Furthermore, the PFC-labeled cells exhibited distinct 19F signals, which could be readily detected after both local and intravenous injection [3]. The therapeutic use of MSC in glioblastoma was recently investigated in a preclinical setting by Altaner et al. [86]. In this study of suicide gene therapy mediated by MSC, the authors evaluated the therapeutic efficacy of hMSC derived from bone marrow and from adipose tissue, engineered to express the suicide gene cytosine deaminase/uracil phosphoribosyltransferase to treat intracerebral rat C6 glioblastoma. They treated glioblastoma grown into the brain by resection and subsequently performed single or repeated intracerebral inoculations of therapeutic stem cells, followed by a continuous intra-cerebroventricular delivery of 5-fluorocytosine using an osmotic pump. Direct injections of therapeutic stem cells into the brain tissue surrounding the postoperative resection cavity led to a curative outcome in a significant number of treated animals. Moreover, the continuous supply of therapeutic stem cells into the brain with growing glioblastoma by osmotic pumps together with the continuous prodrug delivery also proved to be therapeutically efficient. Progress of C6 glioblastoma in rats during treatment mediated by therapeutic stem cells and delayed 5-fluorocytosine administration using osmotic pumps was followed by MRI.

The above mentioned optical imaging, MRI, SPECT, and PET are among the major imaging techniques used for cancer cell trafficking, similarly to immune cells and stem cells tracking [3]. SPIO nanoparticles have been also used to label and track tumor cells. Neumaier et al. [87] demonstrated that MRI at 1.5 T allowed the detection of ultrasmall superparamagnetic iron oxide nanoparticle conjugated antibody specifically bound to human tumor cells in vitro and in vivo, and that the magnetic resonance signal intensity correlated with the concentration of ultrasmall superparamagnetic iron oxide nanoparticle antibody used and with the antigen density at the cell surface. The experiments were performed using two different means of targeting: direct and indirect magnetic tumor targeting. Vuu et al., instead, used a dual-labeled gadolinium-rhodamine nanoparticle for labeling and tracking cells in vivo [88]. The authors inoculated labeled tumor cells subcutaneously into the flanks of C3H mice and were able to image these labeled tumor cells via MRI and optical imaging. Furthermore, the labeled tumor cells could be visualized via fluorescent microscopy after tissue biopsy.

Conclusion

Stem cell technology represents an important science of interest in the field of oncology. Main therapeutic applications of stem cells have been attempted in gene therapy, immunotherapy, and reduction of radio-/chemotherapy-induced damages. The tumor-specific homing of stem cells opens the possibility of using stem cells in targeted early cancer diagnosis and targeted therapies. Development of molecular-cellular imaging techniques has greatly promoted the advances of stem cell application in oncology. Among these imaging techniques, MRI offers several advantages of not only generating high resolution imaging of the tumors with excellent visualization of anatomic background, but also providing the opportunity to track, in vivo, the engrafted stem cells homing or trafficking to the tumor sites.

References

[1] Tang C, Russell PJ, Martiniello-Wilks R, Rasko JE, Khatri A. Concise review: Nanoparticles and cellular carriers-allies in cancer imaging and cellular gene therapy? *Stem Cells* 2010;28(9):1686-1702.

[2] Hart LS, El-Deiry WS. Invincible, but not invisible: imaging approaches toward in vivo detection of cancer stem cells. *J Clin Oncol* 2008;26(17):2901-2910.

[3] Hong H, Yang Y, Zhang Y, Cai W. Non-invasive cell tracking in cancer and cancer therapy. *Curr Top Med Chem* 2010;10(12):1237-1248.

[4] Majhen D, Ambriovic-Ristov A. Adenoviral vectors--how to use them in cancer gene therapy? *Virus Res* 2006;119(2):121-133.

[5] Pulkkanen KJ, Yla-Herttuala S. Gene therapy for malignant glioma: current clinical status. *Mol Ther* 2005;12(4):585-598.

[6] Cihova M, Altanerova V, Altaner C. Stem cell based cancer gene therapy. *Mol Pharm* 2011;8(5):1480-1487.

[7] Zarogoulidis P, Darwiche K, Sakkas A, Yarmus L, Huang H, Li Q, et al. Suicide Gene Therapy for Cancer - Current Strategies. *J Genet Syndr Gene Ther* 2013;4

[8] Kim JH, Lee HJ, Song YS. Stem cell based gene therapy in prostate cancer. *Biomed Res Int* 2014;2014:549136.

[9] Corsten MF, Shah K. Therapeutic stem-cells for cancer treatment: hopes and hurdles in tactical warfare. *Lancet Oncol* 2008;9(4):376-384.

[10] Burnet FM. The concept of immunological surveillance. *Prog Exp Tumor Res* 1970;13:1-27.

[11] Burnet M. Immunological Factors in the Process of Carcinogenesis. *Br Med Bull* 1964;20:154-158.

[12] Sachamitr P, Hackett S, Fairchild PJ. Induced pluripotent stem cells: challenges and opportunities for cancer immunotherapy. *Front Immunol* 2014;5:176.

[13] Palucka K, Banchereau J. Cancer immunotherapy via dendritic cells. *Nat Rev Cancer* 2012;12(4):265-277.

[14] Lesterhuis WJ, de Vries IJ, Adema GJ, Punt CJ. Dendritic cell-based vaccines in cancer immunotherapy: an update on clinical and immunological results. *Ann Oncol* 2004;15(Suppl 4):145-151.

[15] Park MY, Kim CH, Sohn HJ, Oh ST, Kim SG, Kim TG. The optimal interval for dendritic cell vaccination following adoptive T cell transfer is important for boosting potent anti-tumor immunity. *Vaccine* 2007;25(42):7322-7330.

[16] Ruggeri L, Mancusi A, Capanni M, Martelli MF, Velardi A. Exploitation of alloreactive NK cells in adoptive immunotherapy of cancer. *Curr Opin Immunol* 2005;17(2):211-217.

[17] Miller JS, Soignier Y, Panoskaltsis-Mortari A, McNearney SA, Yun GH, Fautsch SK, et al. Successful adoptive transfer and in vivo expansion of human haploidentical NK cells in patients with cancer. *Blood* 2005;105(8):3051-3057.

[18] Takahashi K, Yamanaka S. Induction of pluripotent stem cells from mouse embryonic and adult fibroblast cultures by defined factors. *Cell* 2006;126(4):663-676.

[19] Takahashi K, Tanabe K, Ohnuki M, Narita M, Ichisaka T, Tomoda K, et al. Induction of pluripotent stem cells from adult human fibroblasts by defined factors. C*ell* 2007;131(5):861-872.
[20] Nakagawa M, Koyanagi M, Tanabe K, Takahashi K, Ichisaka T, Aoi T, et al. Generation of induced pluripotent stem cells without Myc from mouse and human fibroblasts. *Nat Biotechnol* 2008;26(1):101-106.
[21] Knorr DA, Ni Z, Hermanson D, Hexum MK, Bendzick L, Cooper LJ, et al. Clinical-scale derivation of natural killer cells from human pluripotent stem cells for cancer therapy. *Stem Cells Transl Med* 2013;2(4):274-283.
[22] Muranski P, Boni A, Wrzesinski C, Citrin DE, Rosenberg SA, Childs R, et al. Increased intensity lymphodepletion and adoptive immunotherapy--how far can we go? *Nat Clin Pract Oncol* 2006;3(12):668-681.
[23] Wolf D, Heine A, Brossart P. Implementing combinatorial immunotherapeutic regimens against cancer: The concept of immunological conditioning. *Oncoimmunology* 2014;3(1):e27588.
[24] Mangoni M, Livi L, Biti G, Di Cataldo V, Capaccioli N, Castier Y, et al. Stem cell tracking: toward clinical application in oncology? *Tumori* 2012;98(5):535-542.
[25] Baldomero H, Gratwohl M, Gratwohl A, Tichelli A, Niederwieser D, Madrigal A, et al. The EBMT activity survey 2009: trends over the past 5 years. *Bone Marrow Transplant* 2011;46(4):485-501.
[26] Horowitz MM, Gale RP, Sondel PM, Goldman JM, Kersey J, Kolb HJ, et al. Graft-versus-leukemia reactions after bone marrow transplantation. *Blood* 1990;75(3):555-562.
[27] Hamilton BK, Copelan EA. Concise review: the role of hematopoietic stem cell transplantation in the treatment of acute myeloid leukemia. *Stem Cells* 2012;30(8):1581-1586.
[28] Coppes RP, van der Goot A, Lombaert IM. Stem cell therapy to reduce radiation-induced normal tissue damage. *Semin Radiat Oncol* 2009;19(2):112-121.
[29] Lombaert IM, Wierenga PK, Kok T, Kampinga HH, deHaan G, Coppes RP. Mobilization of bone marrow stem cells by granulocyte colony-stimulating factor ameliorates radiation-induced damage to salivary glands. *Clin Cancer Res* 2006;12(6):1804-1812.
[30] Nakamura K, Ito Y, Kawano Y, Kurozumi K, Kobune M, Tsuda H, et al. Antitumor effect of genetically engineered mesenchymal stem cells in a rat glioma model. *Gene Ther* 2004;11(14):1155-1164.
[31] Wu X, Hu J, Zhou L, Mao Y, Yang B, Gao L, et al. In vivo tracking of superparamagnetic iron oxide nanoparticle-labeled mesenchymal stem cell tropism to malignant gliomas using magnetic resonance imaging. Laboratory investigation. *J Neurosurg* 2008;108(2):320-329.
[32] Studeny M, Marini FC, Champlin RE, Zompetta C, Fidler IJ, Andreeff M. Bone marrow-derived mesenchymal stem cells as vehicles for interferon-beta delivery into tumors. Cancer Res 2002;62(13):3603-3608.
[33] Stoff-Khalili MA, Rivera AA, Mathis JM, Banerjee NS, Moon AS, Hess A, et al. Mesenchymal stem cells as a vehicle for targeted delivery of CRAds to lung metastases of breast carcinoma. Breast Cancer Res Treat 2007;105(2):157-167.

[34] Mohr A, Lyons M, Deedigan L, Harte T, Shaw G, Howard L, et al. Mesenchymal stem cells expressing TRAIL lead to tumour growth inhibition in an experimental lung cancer model. *J Cell Mol Med* 2008;12(6B):2628-2643.

[35] Dwyer RM, Potter-Beirne SM, Harrington KA, Lowery AJ, Hennessy E, Murphy JM, et al. Monocyte chemotactic protein-1 secreted by primary breast tumors stimulates migration of mesenchymal stem cells. *Clin Cancer Res* 2007;13(17):5020-5027.

[36] Komarova S, Kawakami Y, Stoff-Khalili MA, Curiel DT, Pereboeva L. Mesenchymal progenitor cells as cellular vehicles for delivery of oncolytic adenoviruses. *Mol Cancer Ther* 2006;5(3):755-766.

[37] Studeny M, Marini FC, Dembinski JL, Zompetta C, Cabreira-Hansen M, Bekele BN, et al. Mesenchymal stem cells: potential precursors for tumor stroma and targeted-delivery vehicles for anticancer agents. J Natl Cancer Inst 2004;96(21):1593-1603.

[38] Menon LG, Picinich S, Koneru R, Gao H, Lin SY, Koneru M, et al. Differential gene expression associated with migration of mesenchymal stem cells to conditioned medium from tumor cells or bone marrow cells. *Stem Cells* 2007;25(2):520-528.

[39] Gelmini S, Mangoni M, Serio M, Romagnani P, Lazzeri E. The critical role of SDF-1/CXCR4 axis in cancer and cancer stem cells metastasis. *J Endocrinol Invest* 2008;31(9):809-819.

[40] Forte G, Minieri M, Cossa P, Antenucci D, Sala M, Gnocchi V, et al. Hepatocyte growth factor effects on mesenchymal stem cells: proliferation, migration, and differentiation. *Stem Cells* 2006;24(1):23-33.

[41] Schichor C, Birnbaum T, Etminan N, Schnell O, Grau S, Miebach S, et al. Vascular endothelial growth factor A contributes to glioma-induced migration of human marrow stromal cells (hMSC). *Exp Neurol* 2006;199(2):301-310.

[42] Direkze NC, Hodivala-Dilke K, Jeffery R, Hunt T, Poulsom R, Oukrif D, et al. Bone marrow contribution to tumor-associated myofibroblasts and fibroblasts. *Cancer Res* 2004;64(23):8492-8495.

[43] Rodriguez O, Fricke S, Chien C, Dettin L, VanMeter J, Shapiro E, et al. Contrast-enhanced in vivo imaging of breast and prostate cancer cells by MRI. *Cell Cycle* 2006;5(1):113-119.

[44] Soltysova A, Altanerova V, Altaner C. Cancer stem cells. *Neoplasma* 2005;52(6):435-440.

[45] Brabletz T, Jung A, Spaderna S, Hlubek F, Kirchner T. Opinion: migrating cancer stem cells - an integrated concept of malignant tumour progression. *Nat Rev Cancer* 2005;5(9):744-749.

[46] Bao S, Wu Q, McLendon RE, Hao Y, Shi Q, Hjelmeland AB, et al. Glioma stem cells promote radioresistance by preferential activation of the DNA damage response. *Nature* 2006;444(7120):756-760.

[47] Sussman RT, Ricci MS, Hart LS, Sun SY, El-Deiry WS. Chemotherapy-resistant side-population of colon cancer cells has a higher sensitivity to TRAIL than the non-SP, a higher expression of c-Myc and TRAIL-receptor DR4. *Cancer Biol Ther* 2007;6(9):1490-1495.

[48] Tavaluc RT, Hart LS, Dicker DT, El-Deiry WS. Effects of low confluency, serum starvation and hypoxia on the side population of cancer cell lines. *Cell Cycle* 2007;6(20):2554-2562.

[49] Rich JN. Cancer stem cells in radiation resistance. Cancer Res 2007;67(19):8980-8984.

[50] Eramo A, Ricci-Vitiani L, Zeuner A, Pallini R, Lotti F, Sette G, et al. Chemotherapy resistance of glioblastoma stem cells. *Cell Death Differ* 2006;13(7):1238-1241.
[51] Tazzari PL, Cappellini A, Ricci F, Evangelisti C, Papa V, Grafone T, et al. Multidrug resistance-associated protein 1 expression is under the control of the phosphoinositide 3 kinase/Akt signal transduction network in human acute myelogenous leukemia blasts. *Leukemia* 2007;21(3):427-438.
[52] Duprez F, De Neve W, De Gersem W, Coghe M, Madani I. Adaptive dose painting by numbers for head-and-neck cancer. *Int J Radiat Oncol Biol Phys* 2011;80(4):1045-1055.
[53] Guckenberger M, Richter A, Wilbert J, Flentje M, Partridge M. Adaptive radiotherapy for locally advanced non-small-cell lung cancer does not underdose the microscopic disease and has the potential to increase tumor control. *Int J Radiat Oncol Biol Phys* 2011;81(4):e275-282.
[54] Gorges TM, Pantel K. Circulating tumor cells as therapy-related biomarkers in cancer patients. *Cancer Immunol Immunother* 2013;62(5):931-939.
[55] Tinhofer I, Saki M, Niehr F, Keilholz U, Budach V. Cancer stem cell characteristics of circulating tumor cells. *Int J Radiat Biol* 2014;90(8):622-627.
[56] Cristofanilli M, Budd GT, Ellis MJ, Stopeck A, Matera J, Miller MC, et al. Circulating tumor cells, disease progression, and survival in metastatic breast cancer. *N Engl J Med* 2004;351(8):781-791.
[57] de Bono JS, Scher HI, Montgomery RB, Parker C, Miller MC, Tissing H, et al. Circulating tumor cells predict survival benefit from treatment in metastatic castration-resistant prostate cancer. *Clin Cancer Res* 2008;14(19):6302-6309.
[58] Cohen SJ, Punt CJ, Iannotti N, Saidman BH, Sabbath KD, Gabrail NY, et al. Prognostic significance of circulating tumor cells in patients with metastatic colorectal cancer. *Ann Oncol* 2009;20(7):1223-1229.
[59] Grisanti S, Almici C, Consoli F, Buglione M, Verardi R, Bolzoni-Villaret A, et al. Circulating tumor cells in patients with recurrent or metastatic head and neck carcinoma: prognostic and predictive significance. *PLoS One* 2014;9(8):e103918.
[60] Massoud TF, Gambhir SS. Molecular imaging in living subjects: seeing fundamental biological processes in a new light. *Genes Dev* 2003;17(5):545-580.
[61] Li Z, Suzuki Y, Huang M, Cao F, Xie X, Connolly AJ, et al. Comparison of reporter gene and iron particle labeling for tracking fate of human embryonic stem cells and differentiated endothelial cells in living subjects. *Stem Cells* 2008;26(4):864-873.
[62] Arbab AS, Janic B, Haller J, Pawelczyk E, Liu W, Frank JA. In Vivo Cellular Imaging for Translational Medical Research. *Curr Med Imaging Rev* 2009;5(1):19-38.
[63] Love Z, Wang F, Dennis J, Awadallah A, Salem N, Lin Y, et al. Imaging of mesenchymal stem cell transplant by bioluminescence and PET. *J Nucl Med* 2007;48(12):2011-2020.
[64] Kraitchman DL, Bulte JW. In vivo imaging of stem cells and Beta cells using direct cell labeling and reporter gene methods. *Arterioscler Thromb Vasc Biol* 2009;29(7):1025-1030.
[65] McColgan P, Sharma P, Bentley P. Stem cell tracking in human trials: a meta-regression. *Stem Cell Rev* 2011;7(4):1031-1040.

[66] Torrente Y, Gavina M, Belicchi M, Fiori F, Komlev V, Bresolin N, et al. High-resolution X-ray microtomography for three-dimensional visualization of human stem cell muscle homing. *FEBS Lett* 2006;580(24):5759-5764.
[67] Xu YL, Gao YH, Liu Z, Tan KB, Hua X, Fang ZQ, et al. Myocardium-targeted transplantation of mesenchymal stem cells by diagnostic ultrasound-mediated microbubble destruction improves cardiac function in myocardial infarction of New Zealand rabbits. *Int J Cardiol* 2010;138(2):182-195.
[68] Kuliszewski MA, Fujii H, Liao C, Smith AH, Xie A, Lindner JR, et al. Molecular imaging of endothelial progenitor cell engraftment using contrast-enhanced ultrasound and targeted microbubbles. *Cardiovasc Res* 2009;83(4):653-662.
[69] Himmelreich U, Hoehn M. Stem cell labeling for magnetic resonance imaging. *Minim Invasive Ther Allied Technol* 2008;17(2):132-142.
[70] Kalish H, Arbab AS, Miller BR, Lewis BK, Zywicke HA, Bulte JW, et al. Combination of transfection agents and magnetic resonance contrast agents for cellular imaging: relationship between relaxivities, electrostatic forces, and chemical composition. *Magn Reson Med* 2003;50(2):275-282.
[71] Dodd CH, Hsu HC, Chu WJ, Yang P, Zhang HG, Mountz JD, Jr., et al. Normal T-cell response and in vivo magnetic resonance imaging of T cells loaded with HIV transactivator-peptide-derived superparamagnetic nanoparticles. *J Immunol Methods* 2001;256(1-2):89-105.
[72] Muja N, Bulte JW. Magnetic resonance imaging of cells in experimental disease models. P*rog Nucl Magn Reson Spectrosc* 2009;55(1):61-77.
[73] Shubayev VI, Pisanic TR, 2nd, Jin S. Magnetic nanoparticles for theragnostics. *Adv Drug Deliv Rev* 2009;61(6):467-477.
[74] Gao J, Gu H, Xu B. Multifunctional magnetic nanoparticles: design, synthesis, and biomedical applications. *Acc Chem Res* 2009;42(8):1097-1107.
[75] Neuberger T SpB, Hofmann H, Hofmann M, von Rechenberg B. Superparamagnetic nanoparticles for biomedical applications: Possibilities and limitations of a new drug delivery system. *Journal of Magnetism and Magnetic Materials* 2005;293(1):483-496.
[76] Kraitchman DL, Heldman AW, Atalar E, Amado LC, Martin BJ, Pittenger MF, et al. In vivo magnetic resonance imaging of mesenchymal stem cells in myocardial infarction. *Circulation* 2003;107(18):2290-2293.
[77] Menon LG, Pratt J, Yang HW, Black PM, Sorensen GA, Carroll RS. Imaging of human mesenchymal stromal cells: homing to human brain tumors. *J Neurooncol* 2012;107(2):257-267.
[78] Loebinger MR, Kyrtatos PG, Turmaine M, Price AN, Pankhurst Q, Lythgoe MF, et al. Magnetic resonance imaging of mesenchymal stem cells homing to pulmonary metastases using biocompatible magnetic nanoparticles. *Cancer Res* 2009;69(23):8862-8867.
[79] Thu MS, Najbauer J, Kendall SE, Harutyunyan I, Sangalang N, Gutova M, et al. Iron labeling and pre-clinical MRI visualization of therapeutic human neural stem cells in a murine glioma model. *PLoS One* 2009;4(9):e7218.
[80] Tunici P, Bulte JW, Bruzzone MG, Poliani PL, Cajola L, Grisoli M, et al. Brain engraftment and therapeutic potential of stem/progenitor cells derived from mouse skin. *J Gene Med* 2006;8(4):506-513.

[81] Arbab AS, Pandit SD, Anderson SA, Yocum GT, Bur M, Frenkel V, et al. Magnetic resonance imaging and confocal microscopy studies of magnetically labeled endothelial progenitor cells trafficking to sites of tumor angiogenesis. *Stem Cells* 2006;24(3):671-678.

[82] Wang S, Fang J, Zhang T, Wang B, Chen J, Li X, et al. Magnetic resonance imaging targeting of intracranial glioma xenografts by Resovist-labeled endothelial progenitor cells. *J Neurooncol* 2011;105(1):67-75.

[83] Trekker J, Leten C, Struys T, Lazenka VV, Argibay B, Micholt L, et al. Sensitive in vivo cell detection using size-optimized superparamagnetic nanoparticles. *Biomaterials* 2014;35(5):1627-1635.

[84] Lee JH, Smith MA, Liu W, Gold EM, Lewis B, Song HT, et al. Enhanced stem cell tracking via electrostatically assembled fluorescent SPION-peptide complexes. *Nanotechnology* 2009;20(35):355102.

[85] Partlow KC, Chen J, Brant JA, Neubauer AM, Meyerrose TE, Creer MH, et al. 19F magnetic resonance imaging for stem/progenitor cell tracking with multiple unique perfluorocarbon nanobeacons. *FASEB J* 2007;21(8):1647-1654.

[86] Altaner C, Altanerova V, Cihova M, Ondicova K, Rychly B, Baciak L, et al. Complete regression of glioblastoma by mesenchymal stem cells mediated prodrug gene therapy simulating clinical therapeutic scenario. *Int J Cancer* 2014;134(6):1458-1465.

[87] Neumaier CE, Baio G, Ferrini S, Corte G, Daga A. MR and iron magnetic nanoparticles. Imaging opportunities in preclinical and translational research. *Tumori* 2008;94(2):226-233.

[88] Vuu K, Xie J, McDonald MA, Bernardo M, Hunter F, Zhang Y, et al. Gadolinium-rhodamine nanoparticles for cell labeling and tracking via magnetic resonance and optical imaging. *Bioconjug Chem* 2005;16(4):995-999.

In: Magnetic Resonance Imaging of Stem Cell Applications ISBN: 978-1-63463-910-1
Editor: Xiaoming Yang

Chapter 9

Magnetic Resonance Imaging of Stem Cell Application in Heart

Morteza Mahmoudi and Phillip C. Yang [*]
Division of Cardiovascular Medicine, Department of Medicine
Stanford University School of Medicine, Stanford, California, US

Abstract

Stem cells therapy is recognized as one of the potential approaches for the treatment of end-stage cardiovascular diseases, especially for those which no effective therapeutic modalities exist. The regenerative potential of stem cells can be used to alleviate the manifestations of heart failure, coronary artery disease, peripheral vascular disease, and heart valve dysfunction. However, due to the special features of the heart as well as its unique morphology and contractility, the retention and viability of injected cells in the target region is a major issue. Progress in the field can be tremendously accelerated by tracking the number and engraftment (e.g., biodistribution, migration, survival, and differentiation) of stem cells post transplantation, preferably over a long period of time. However, in vivo tracking of single stem cell is still a considerable challenge. For this purpose, noninvasive real-time imaging techniques such as magnetic resonance imaging (MRI) of magnetic nanoparticle (NP)-labeled cells is being employed as one of the most promising approaches. Among various types of nanoparticles, superparamagnetic iron oxide nanoparticles (SPIONs) are recognized as the most suitable option for tracking of transplanted stem cells to the heart using MRI, mainly due to their unique physicochemical properties (e.g., superparamagnetism, broad safety margin, easiness of fabrication and further potential for surface engineering). Several methods such as surface conjugation, simple incubation, transfection, magnetoelectroporation, and magnetosonoporation can be used to label the stem cells with SPIONs. Then, the labeled stem cell can be delivered to the desired site of the myocardial infarction or ischemia, and

[*] Corresponding author: Phillip C. Yang, MD, Division of Cardiovascular Medicine, Department of Medicine, Stanford University School of Medicine, Stanford, California, USA (email: phillip@stanford.edu).
This work was supported by a National Institutes of Health grant (5 UM1 HL087318-08 Cardiovascular Cell Therapy Research Network).

then can be tracked by cellular MRI. In this chapter, we will review the applications of novel technology to track the transplanted stem cells with a special focus on cardiovascular diseases. The chapter will also cover the limitations and challenges of these strategies.

Keywords: Stem cell, magnetic resonance imaging, contrast agent, regenerative medicine

Introduction

The differentiation potential of progenitor and pluripotent stem cells gives them the capability to develop into mature cell types. Stem cells are likely to revolutionize medicine, especially in treatment of conditions for which no simple and effective treatment strategies exist at the moment. The regenerative potential of stem cells can be exploited to reconstruct injured or infarcted tissues of the heart. Several clinical trials are currently running or being planned to evaluate the applicability, efficacy, and safety of cell-based therapies in a variety of diseases [1].

While embryonic stem cells (ESCs), obtained from inner cell mass of blastocyst, and induced pluripotent stem cells (iPSCs), generated from genetic and epigenetic reprogramming of adult cells, can be differentiated into all mature cell types and are promising candidates for cell replacement therapies, their uncontrollable differentiation and proliferation, which can result in tumor formation, has limited their use [2]. Stem cells isolated from fetal organs, or so called "fetal stem cells (FSCs)", can produce multiple lineages upon differentiation. Not only do these cells have better homing and engraftment efficiencies than those of adult stem cells (ASCs), but also they show lower immunogenicity problems and raise less ethical concerns compared to ESCs. The only limiting factor for using FSCs is that due to their fetal origin, these cells are only available in little quantities. ASCs, undifferentiated cells from an adult organism, involve the least ethical issues. ASCs have clinical applications, since they can differentiate into lineage-specific cell types, and transplantation of autologous cells can eliminate the immunogenicity problem. For example, mesenchymal stem cells (MSC) are a class of adult progenitor cells that can be exploited as a promising cell source for cell therapy in myocardial infarction [3], peripheral arterial occlusive disease [4] or heart valve dysfunction [5].

The high rate of mortality and morbidity from cardiovascular diseases has led to the development of novel therapeutic strategies to mitigate heart failure by reversing myocardial damage. In the past decade, cardiovascular diseases have turned into one of the main targets of stem cell therapies [6, 7]. Most clinical studies and meta-analyses have indicated the safety of stem cell administration, and have suggested that they restore cardiac function [8-14].

Current stem cell delivery strategies, including intravenous, intracoronary, direct epicardial, and retrograde coronary sinus administration, suffer from low cell retention, and absence of targeted homing. While among the other mentioned methods, intravenous delivery of cells is the least invasive one, only less than 1% of the injected cells make their way to the infarcted heart and most cells are taken up by the lungs. However, intracoronary injection can be performed during angioplasty to deliver the cells to the target region. The problem with the latter methodology is that most cells (50-90%) are lost during extrusion and in the week post implantation, 90% of the remaining cells die. Only about 3% of the total numbers of delivered cells seem to engraft into the heart. In contrast, direct intramuscular injection of the cells into the myocardium result in a modest increase in the number of engrafted cells (up to 11%) [15]. Therefore, robust clinical application of cardiovascular cell therapy requires novel strategies to overcome several challenges. Specifically, the therapeutic approaches to the myocardial tissue must account for the independent contractile motion of the myocardium and the underlying electromechanical pathway. Moreover, the infarcted myocardium does not supply nutrients and oxygen for the newly-transplanted cells in the hostile ischemic environment [16]. Therefore, in vivo tracking of stem cells is essential to understand the stem cell engraftment kinetics after delivery to the desired target region and possibly elucidate our understanding of the mechanism to restore the regional myocardial viability and function.

Importance of Tracking Stem Cells and Methods

One important frontier in devising effective stem cell therapies is to detect cell survival, location, and differentiation. The therapeutic success of stem cell therapy will depend on understanding the biodistribution and migration/homing of stem cells post engraftment in the injured target tissue. In developing stem cell therapies, the importance of cell retention in the region of delivery and potential teratoma formation from the pluripotent stem cell require reliable method to monitor the cell engraftment dynamics and cell fate in a non-invasive and real time approach [17]. For example, in a study by Kraitchman et al. [18], superparamagnetic iron oxide nano-particle (SPION)-labeled MSCs were injected intramyocardially in a swine model of ischemic reperfusion injury. However, the injection was not completely successful, since only ~30% of the stem cells injected under X-ray fluoroscopic guidance could be visualized under MRI. Therefore, if unlabeled cells are used in clinical trials, one could expect recurrent failure in the delivery of stem cells, which could confound the interpretation of clinical trial results, i.e., one cannot decipher whether the failure of therapy is due to suboptimal cell delivery, cell engraftment, or cell type [19]. Although traditional histopathological methods might be used to address some of these issues, they do not provide any information *in* the living organism in real time. Several imaging techniques might be used to achieve in vivo imaging, such as MRI, X ray/computed tomography (CT), positron emission tomography (PET), single photon emission computer tomography (SPECT), optical imaging (bioluminescence imaging and fluorescence microscopy), and ultrasound imaging. These methods can also be of help to guide therapy to achieve maximum benefit. In a recent review, Azene et al. [19] have summarized approaches, advantages, and disadvantages of stem cell tracking strategies for cardiovascular applications and highlighted recent advancements in the field. Frangioni et al. [20] have reviewed the characteristics of an ideal imaging technology for stem cell tracking including: i) biocompatibility and safety; ii) no genetic modification or perturbation to the stem cells; iii) high spatial resolution, ideally single-cell detection at any given anatomic location; iv) quantification of cell number; v) no or minimal dilution during cell divisions; vi) no or minimal transfer of contrast agent to non-stem cells (e.g., macrophages) in the area; vii) noninvasive and provide longitudinal follow-up and finally; and viii) no requirement for injecting a contrast agent. Furthermore, it should be cheap and cause only minimal discomfort in patients.

MRI has several advantages over other imaging modalities. The primary characteristic is patient safety record. Second, MRI provides three-dimensional (3D) high resolution images, which is readily available and proven clinical utility. Third, MRI circumvents exposure to ionizing radiation. In addition, the maximum spatial resolution of the MRI systems is approximately 50 μm, which is higher than those of currently available CT, ultrasound imaging, PET and SPECT devices [21]. Finally, the exquisite native contrast and high spatial resolution provided by MRI allows additional detailed anatomical and morphological information on the effects of cell therapy on the surrounding tissue, which may be of clinical utility. The application of MRI in stem cell tracking is dependent on labeling the transplanted stem cells using a contrast agent. After the first observation made by the Weissleder group in the early 1990s, which showed that SPION docking in endosomal compartments after endocytosis can alter MRI susceptibility, several SPION-based contrast agents have been employed for stem cell tracking applications. Nanoparticles (NPs) are structures with at least one dimension below 100 nm.

The exceptional physicochemical properties of NPs compared to their identical bulk counterparts and their capability to accommodate functional moieties have made them unique candidates for applications in biological interfaces such as delivery, imaging and cell therapy applications in diseased hearts. Among different magnetic NPs that can be used as contrast media for cellular MRI, SPIONs demonstrate several favorable properties.

The detection of labeled stem cells using MRI depends on several factors, including the magnetic field strength, labeling efficiency, cell number, relaxivity of the SPION, spatial resolution and acquisition parameters [22]. Most MRI studies are performed at 1.5 T, which has limited signal, resulting in attenuated sensitivity and spatial resolution.

To improve the signal in cellular MRI, stronger magnetic fields must be used; however, the potential hazards of stronger magnetic fields are yet to be determined [23, 24] . One major shortcoming specifically affecting the imaging of stem cell therapies in cardiovascular disease is that implantable devices, such as pacemakers, stents and defibrillators, which may generate substantial artifact in MRI scanning. Since there is no single imaging modality for full-feature tracking of stem cell in vivo [17], multimodality imaging might also be used to obtain more reliable results in stem cell tracking experiments. For instance, Amado et al. [25] have used MRI and multi-detector CT (MDCT) to study MSC-treated pigs over a 2-month period after anterior myocardial infarction (MI). Using serially-obtained MRI and MDCT result, the study demonstrated restoration of contractile function. In other cardiac stem cell therapy studies, MRI has been also been coupled with PET [26, 27] and bioluminescence imaging to monitor multiple biological processes [16, 28]. The manganese-enhanced MRI (MEMRI) is another approach to track the stem cells [29]. MEMRI employs viability-specific cellular transport of Mn2+ via voltage-gated calcium channels. The intracellular accumulation of Mn2+ shortens the T1 relaxation time to generate positive signal. MEMRI combines the high spatial and temporal resolution of MRI with cell viability specific signal to enable dual assessment of peri-infarct viability and stem cell engraftment [29].

Superparamagnetic Iron Oxide Nanoparticles (SPIONs)

SPIONs are a special class of iron oxide NPs usually in the size range of below 30 nm in diameter and have extensive biomedical application as MRI contrast agents [30], drug/gene delivery systems [31], molecular/cellular tracking systems [21], magnetic separation technologies (e.g., rapid DNA sequencing) [32], magnetic hyperthermia cancer treatment [33], magnetotransfections [34], as well as ultrasensitive diagnostic assays [35]. Owing to their biocompatibility and strong effects on T2 relaxation, one can expect that SPIONs could be one of the best candidates for MRI method in stem cell tracking applications in the cardiovascular system. One of the most important advantages of SPIONs is that they can be synthesized in desirable shapes and sizes using a variety of techniques [21, 31, 36].

SPIONs have superparamagnetic properties (i.e., single magnetic domain NPs that their magnetization can be randomly flipped upon thermal excitations). In the absence of an external magnetic field, SPIONs have a magnetization of zero and are in the so called superparamagnetic state. When an external magnetic field is applied, the NPs are magnetized; however, they do not retain any magnetization in the absence of an external magnetic field. Two MRI relaxation time constants, T1 and T2, are affected by the local microenvironment. One of the microenvironmental parameters that effects the time constant T2* is a strong magnetic inhomogeneity in the target region. Since SPIONs have high magnetic susceptibilities, they alter one or both of these time constants. For example, SPIONs have the capability to shorten T2 and T2* relaxation. When these SPIONs are imaged with T2 or T2*-weighted pulse sequences, a hypointense signal is produced on the MRI. Thus, the magnetically labeled stem cells can be visualized after transplantation in the target organ.

Stem Cell Labeling Strategies

Most labeling strategies involve the conjugation of magnetic NPs to the cell surface or internalization of NPs into the cytosol [37]. While most of the studies have focused on internalization of SPION labels into cells, a few studies have conjugated SPION labels to the cell surface. For example, Chung et al. [38] developed a novel reporter gene for expressing hemagglutinin A and myc as well as luciferase antigens on the surface of ESCs (Figure 9.1). Subsequently, SPIONs attached to monoclonal antibody against these antigens, were used to label and track ESCs in vivo [38].

A number of methods such as simple incubation, transfection (magnetofection), magnetoelectroporation, and magnetosonoporation have been established to introduce SPIONs into the target stem cells. In most of these methods, the efficiency of magnetic labeling depends on the size of the SPIONs, cell membrane properties as well as the size of the cells of interest. Incubation of the cell suspension with SPIONs is the simplest strategy to label cells [39, 40]. However, for cells with inadequate self-uptake, other methods have been devised. For example, in viral capsid incorporation [41], a virus envelope, encapsulates the SPIONs and transports NPs inside cells upon infection. In the antibody-mediated uptake,

SPIONs are covalently attached to antibodies [42, 43], which can then target the complex to the desired cells.

Since the application of viral capsid elements and antibody attachment is tricky and should be optimized for each case, alternative methods such as polycation coating have been established to cover the negatively-charged SPIONs, and to facilitate their interaction with the anionic cell membrane, which eventually increases NP uptake [44-47]. For example, magnetodendrimers have been shown to be effectively internalized in human neural stem cells (NSCs) and MSCs after non-specific membrane adsorption [45].

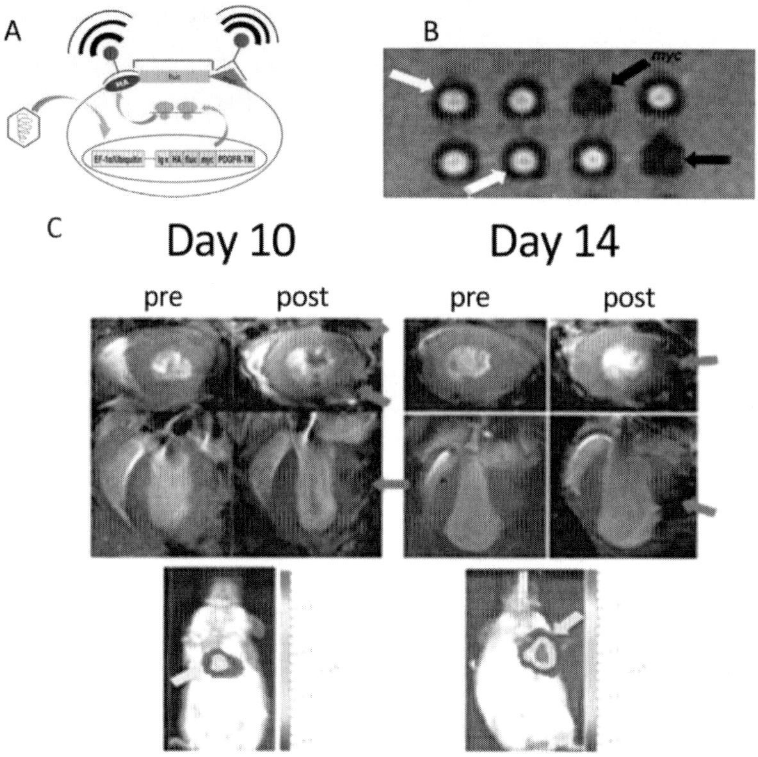

Figure 9.1. MRI of reporter gene. (A) HA-luc-myc is expressed on the cell membrane of human embryonic stem cells (hESC). HA and myc are the molecular targets for the microbeads to generate MRI signal, (B) in vitro MRI of red ginseng (RG)-hESCs (black) and hESCs (white arrows) after labeling with myc- and HA-microbeads, and (C) serial in vivo MRI of RG-hESCs in the mouse myocardium pre- and post-intravenous administration of microbeads on Days 10 and 14. In vivo RGMRI signal is validated by positive bioluminescence imaging (BLI). Reprinted, with permission, from [38].

Currently, polycationic transfection agents are popular in stem cell labeling and several of them are commercially available such as poly-L-lysine (PLL), protamine sulfate, and lipofectamine. When the labeling solution containing stable complexes of NP-transfection agent is added to the cell culture, the electrostatic interaction of the complexes with the cell membrane expedites the endocytosis or macropinocytosis of the contrast agent usually over a 24–48-h (sometimes shorter) labeling period [48, 49]. Using this method, Hinds et al. [48]

have labeled hematopoietic CD34+ cells and *mesenchymal stem cells* (MSCs) using micron-sized, iron oxide magnetic particles (Figure 9.2). This method allowed tracking of cells at a single cell resolution, while having no impact on biological activity, colony-forming ability and differentiation capacity of target stem cells. A big disadvantage of magnetofection is the relatively long incubation time needed for internalization of SPIONs. Such long incubation times are unacceptable for many of the bone marrow mononuclear stem cell trials [50].

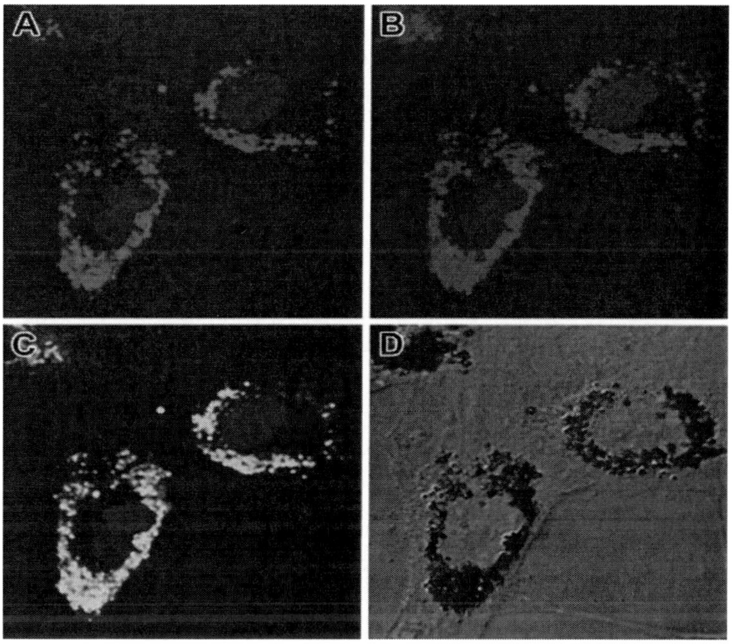

Figure 9.2. Confocal fluorescent microscopy image of porcine MSCs labeled with 10 μl/ml iron oxide fluorescent microparticles (× 100 magnification). (A) Green fluorescence from beads. (B) Red fluorescence from endosomal marker CM-DiI (3′,3′-dioactadecyl-5-5′-di(4-sulfophenyl) oxacarbocyanine, sodium salt). (C) Co-localization of the 2 colors confirms the endosomal uptake of microparticles. (D) Nomarski optics shows the outlines of the cells as well as the clustering of iron particles in perinuclear organelles. Reprinted, with permission, from [18].

Since some of these coating agents are not yet approved for clinical use, some research groups have tried to devise transfection agent-free systems for enhancing NP uptake. For example, Mailänder et al. [51] have tested the efficiency of labeling human MSCs and HeLa cells with two commercially available Resovist® and Feridex® SPION formulations without addition of transfection agents. Both tested cell lines internalized more Resovist® than the latter agent. The amount of intracellular iron reached in this protocol was comparable with the case in which SPIONs are added with transfection agents. The authors further confirmed that the higher uptake efficiency of Resovist® compared to Feridex® is somehow associated with the carboxyl groups present in the carboxydextran shell of Resovist® (while Feridex® shell is only composed of dextran). Similarly, in another study, human ESCs have been labeled with small iron oxide particles in an additive-free manner [52].

Electroporation is a quick delivery method, which is based on the temporary disruption of cell membrane [53, 54]. In this method, an externally applied electrical field induces transient porosity in the cell membrane, opening the way for internalization of exogenous substances.

However, unlike electroporation for DNA and protein delivery, in magnetoelectroporation of stem cells, lower voltage pulses are exploited to induce the stem cells to endocytose contrast agents; therefore, no channels or pores might be created in the process. A wide variety of stem or progenitor cells have been labeled using this technique without loss of viability or metabolic changes [54, 55]. The amount of NP uptake using magnetoelectroporation is associated with cell size, e.g., since MSCs are larger than neural stem cells, they can accommodate higher number of SPIONs in their cytoplasm [53]. Furthermore, the absence of transfection agents in the protocol facilitates approval of the labeling technique by regulatory agencies such as Food and Drug Administration (FDA). In a similar fashion, ultrasound generates transient non-specific disturbance in the cell membrane and facilitate NP internalization [56, 57].

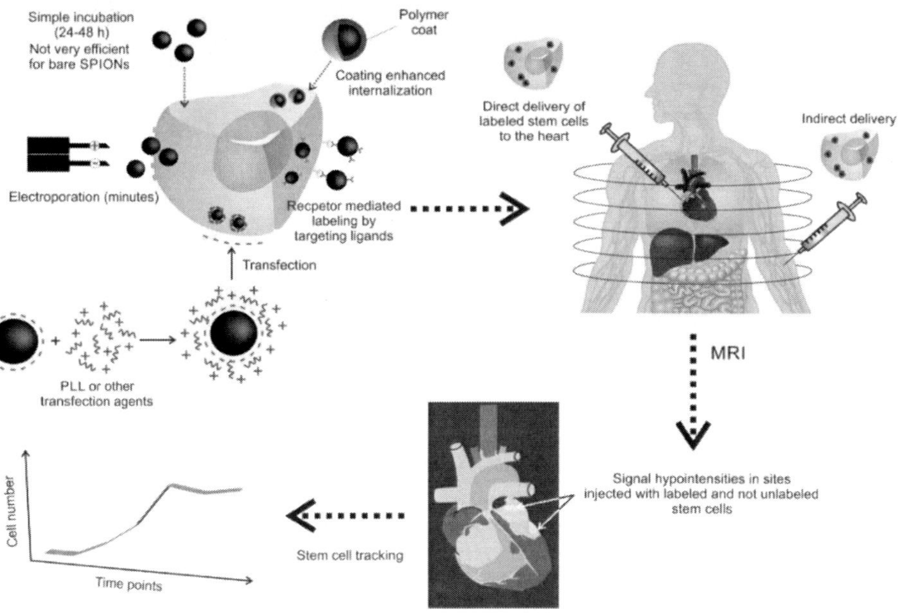

Figure 9.3. An overall scheme for labeling stem cells, delivering them to the heart, MR imaging and final image processing in stem cell tracking applications.

The advantage of the electroporation and ultrasound techniques, compared to the other ones, is that the stem cell labeling skips the incubation step. Not only does this shorten the length of the protocol, it also eliminates some concerns when working with sensitive cells such as the primary cells. However, the main issue with membrane-disrupting methods is that cell viability might be significantly reduced [58]. Furthermore, the parameters of the labeling experiment must be optimized for each cell type in a case by case manner. In every one of these methods, obviously, it is important to validate the efficiency of the labeling procedure for each cell type before clinical application. A washing step should also be included to remove any cell debris and to remove excess NPs, since they can produce unwanted reactions or false positive signals in vivo.

Several validation experiments must also be conducted to confirm the viability and fidelity of the labeled stem cells. An overall scheme for labeling stem cells and a typical stem cell tracking experiment using MRI has been depicted in Figure 9.3.

Application of SPIONs in Stem Cell Tracking: Animal Studies

Stem cell therapies hold great promise for treatment of several cardiovascular conditions including myocardial infarction (MI) [12], peripheral arterial occlusive disease [4] or heart valve dysfunction [5]. The retention and subsequent proliferation of stem cells in the target region have the potential to restore the activity of injured tissues. Cardiac imaging is already established in clinical settings, and is a valuable tool in studying the size of the infarcted area as well as performing interventional procedures. Similarly, the advent of non-invasive imaging for tracking stem cell therapies will provide unprecedented tools for treating cardiovascular disease.

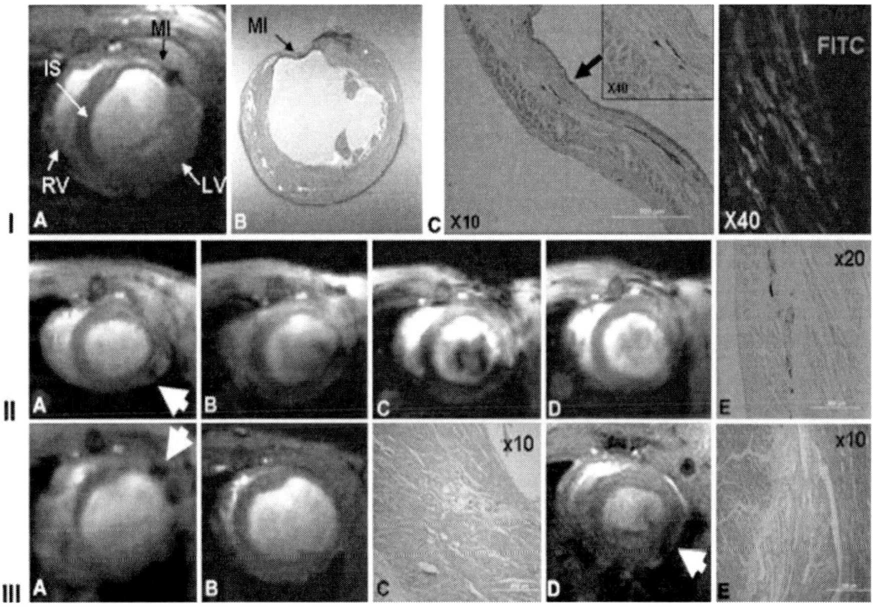

Figure 9.4. (IA) MR image of labeled cells in the myocardium 2 days after cell transplantation and (IB) ex vivo MR microscopy image of the same heart 6 weeks after cell transplantation. (IC) Prussian blue staining shows the presence of labeled cells, while fluorescence microscopy detects the FITC label. (IIA–D) MR images of the same animal at day 8, and week 3, 4 and 6 after administration of rat BMSCs. The hypointense region corresponding to the labeled rat BMSCs has been indicated with an arrow and the signal attenuation can be noted over time. (IIE) Prussian blue staining. (IIIA&B) MR images of the same rat 8 days (IIIA) and 6 weeks (IIIB) post-delivery of rat BMSCs and (IIIC) post-mortem Prussian blue staining. (IIID) MR images of a sham-operated rat 8 days post-delivery of rat BMSCs and (IIIE) Post-mortem Prussian blue staining. *LV, Left ventricle; IS, interventricular septum; RV, right ventricle. Reprinted, with permission, from [26].

Arai et al. [59] performed one of the first studies to assess the cardiac regenerative effects of mouse ESCs in a murine model of acute MI using a 1.5 T clinical MR scanner. The cell labeling was performed using Feridex and PLL. MRI results demonstrated a significant restoration of the injured myocardium 4 weeks after transplantation of mouse ESCs, manifested by improvements in the left ventricular (LV) ejection fraction (though not completely normalized) and conservation of LV mass. These findings were also verified by positive expression of viable green fluorescent protein (GFP)-expressing cells in the infarct area at weeks 1, 2, and 4. The results thus indicated that mouse ECSs can provide both early and long-term persistent improvements in myocardial function. The authors also made and optimized a small-animal coil in order to achieve an appropriate spatial resolution and signal to noise ratio at a 1.5 T MR scanner.

Multimodal imaging can help enhance reliability in stem cell tracking studies. For example, one study has used MRI and PET to track labeled bone marrow-derived stem cells (BMSCs) for cell therapy of rats [26]. In this study, BMSC labeling was performed with high efficiency of 98% using 15-20 nm dextran-coated NPs conjugated with tat-fluorescein isothiocyanate peptide. After injection in rat hearts, they were able to track live labeled stem cells for up to 6-weeks (Figure 9.4). However, Stucky et al. [60] had already reported a longer window of 16 weeks for detection of BMSCs labeled with relatively large 900 nm SPIONs. It is believed that the success/failure of these studies may depend on the infarction size and variations in tissue remodeling in different study designs [26, 60].

Suzuki et al. [61] combined positive contrast generated by an off-resonance sequence with bioluminescence detection of luciferase reporter gene to track the status of stem cells after in vivo transplantation in mouse hindlimb. The positive contrast imaging technique increased the signal-to-noise ratio (SNR) and contrast-to-noise ratio (CNR) in comparison with the results of a gradient recalled echo (GRE) sequence (Figure 9.5). There was a good correlation between the number of labeled ESCs and MRI signal immediately after transplantation with a statistically significant correlation of R2 = 0.74. Although bioluminescence imaging showed a significant enhancement of luciferase activity after 16 days, MRI failed to evaluate cell viability. The positive contrast generated by the off-resonance technique used in this study could yield reliable information on detection and quantification of the labeled cells following transplantation into the target organ.

Fast low angle positive contrast with steady-state free precession (FLAPS) [62] and positive contrast with alternating repetition time SSFP (PARTS) [63] are also among positive contrast MRI techniques. Although SPION-labeled cells can be effectively tracked by selective excitation and/or refocusing of off-resonant spins, spin-echo acquisitions and/or radiofrequency pulses generally used in these methods, leading to long scan times and high specific absorption rates, which limit the applicability of these techniques. PARTS technique provides fast, high resolution positive contrast MRI by coupling low tip angles for generating off-resonant signal with alternating repetition times and can provide reliable positive contrast with a wide choice of sequences and tissue parameters, while enhancing background suppression [63].

Inversion recovery with on-resonant water suppression (IRON) is yet another positive contrast imaging technique that can be used on the existing platforms without special pulse programming or image post-processing [64]. However, an anatomical reference image is needed to be matched with the susceptibility artifacts from the labeled cells. Dahnke et al. [65] have also devised a post-processing method for obtaining positive contrast images of SPION-labeled cells from the susceptibility gradient map of conventional gradient echo. Sweep imaging with Fourier transformation (SWIFT), is a newly developed technique for tracking of SPION-labeled stem cells in the rat heart [66].

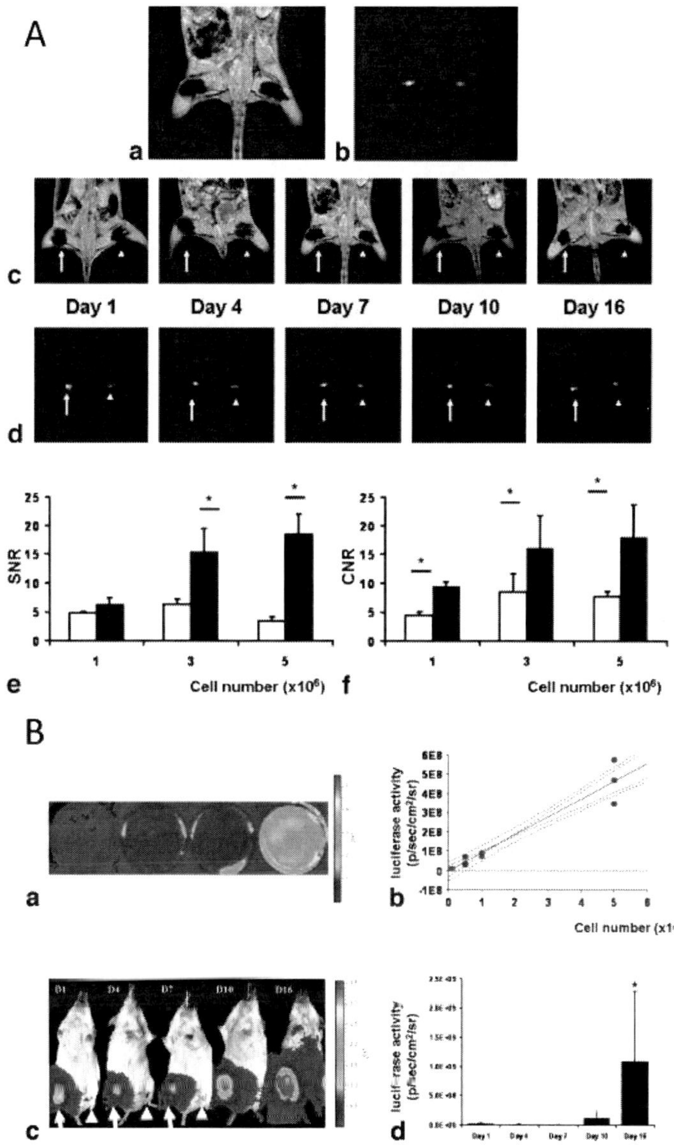

Figure 9.5. (A) In vivo a) GRE and b) off-resonance MR images. Serial in vivo MR images of labeled mouse ESCs during days 1–16 post-transplantation of stem cells; c) GRE and d) off-resonance (arrow: viable cells and arrowhead: nonviable cells). e) SNR and f) CNR of in vivo GRE (white bars) versus off-resonance (Black bars) *SNR, signal-to-noise ratio; CNR, contrast –to-noise ratio. (B) Serial in vivo bioluminescence imaging (BLI). a) In vitro BLI of mESC-luc+ showing direct relation between signal proportionate and the cell quantity (the wells contained 0.1, 0.5, 1, and 5 × 106luc-mESC); b) in vitro correlation between estimated number of luc-mESC and BLI activity; c) in vivo BLI shows a representative mice transplanted with luc-mESC reporter gene at 1, 4, 7, 10, and 16 days after cell transplantation (arrow: viable cells and arrowhead: nonviable cells); d) BLI signal of viable SPIO-luc-mESC increased significantly over time by day 16 (*P < 0.001). Reprinted, with permission, from [61].

SWIFT is well-suited for imaging iron oxide NPs with very short T2* relaxation time, because in this technique, there is only very little time between radiofrequency excitation and signal acquisition. Although SWIFT yields anatomical details on a magnitude image as well as a positive contrast image, this sequence cannot be implemented on currently available commercial MRI scanning machines.

Impact of Magnetic Labeling on Stem Cells

The whole process of preparing labeled stem cells can compromise the viability and function of stem cells. These changes might have an impact on differentiation capability of stem cells. Although SPIONs are generally considered to have a broad safety margin and acceptable biocompatibility, the studies performed with labeled stem cells should consider investigating the potential detrimental effects of cell labeling on phenotypic and genotypic changes. Overall, several criteria have been set for labeling procedures [67]: i) the labeling technique must be reproducible; ii) cells must retain their viability during the process; iii) cell phenotype must not undergo any changes as a result of labeling; iv) the differentiation capacity of stem cells after labeling should be the same as unlabeled cells and finally; and v) no toxins should be present in the final product.

Various studies have evaluated the cytotoxicity of SPIONs in different stem cell classes including human MSCs [23, 68], mouse ESCs [24, 59, 69] and NSCs [45, 70, 71]. These studies found no effects on cell viability, growth or differentiation. Most of the published studies on labeling stem cells with Feridex, an FDA approved SPION formulation in an off-label application, have not shown any unfavorable effects on stem cells at currently-used incubation times. In a study by Kedziorek et al. [72], gene expression profiling using microarrays and quantitative PCR (qPCR) only detected some early minor differential expression in a small group of genes, which largely got back to normal levels 1 week after labeling procedure. Taken together, the normal cellular functions of stem cells must be validated after labeling. For example, to confirm that SPION labeling has no effect on stemness of BMSCs, Balakumaran et al. [73] tested the capabilities of labeled BMSCs with regards to colony formation assay, CD146 expression, gene expression profiles, as well as bone and myelosupportive stroma formation in immuncompromised mice in vivo. SPION-labeling did not alter these assays. Furthermore, the in vivo self-renewal of the BMSCs in mice implanted with stem cells was verified by checking for PB+ adipocytes and PB+ pericytes from the donor origin. Therefore, this study confirmed that the differentiation potency of BMSCs was not reduced in presence of SPION labels. In the context of cardiogenic differentiation potential, one study demonstrated that SPION-labeled ESCs had equal cardiogenic potential as unlabeled cells [74].

However, different protocols can be tested on a specific cell line to identify the best labeling method. For example, Suzuki et al. [58] compared the biological effects of transfection with PLL, transfection with protamine sulfate and electroporation on mouse ESCs in vitro. The study involved testing for several criteria including cellular viability, apoptosis, proliferation, and cardiac differentiation of ferumoxides-labeled mouse ESCs. The viability and proliferation were the same across PPL and protamine sulfate methods; however, cell viability decreased immediately after electroporation. Overall, protamine sulfate was better than the other methods, in terms of SPION uptake and thus, demonstrated the largest MRI signal dephasing area. Among the tested methods, electroporation reduced the cardiac differentiation capacity of mouse ESCs the most, as assessed in both molecular and cellular levels. However, in one study [75], human MSCs were labeled with PLL-coated Feridex, and subsequently, five different assays were used to test the different inherent features of stem cells. MSCs showed the same viability and proliferation pattern and retained normal potential for adipogenic and osteogenic differentiation after labeling. However, chondrogenesis was inhibited significantly upon labeling. In another study, SPION labeling was shown to reduce the migration capacity and colony formation ability of human MSCs either in the absence or presence of a transfection agent [76].

Limitations of SPIONs

Since stem cells or progenitor cells are not terminally-differentiated cells and continue to proliferate after transplantation, the dilution of the iron oxide label among the daughter cells hinders long-term tracking as the MR signal becomes attenuated [77, 78]. This effect is even more prominent in the case of cells with fast turnover. Furthermore, the asymmetrical division of stem cells can result in an unequal distribution of labels within daughter cells [79]. Asymmetric division is a feature that empowers stem cells to use to maintain appropriate numbers of progeny, which is probably an inherent adaptation required for regeneration [80]. Thus, during asymmetric division of labeled stem cells, some daughter cells virtually become undetectable because of the quick dilution of the labels. This issue also complicates the quantification of the number of SPION-labeled cells. Since MRI is an indirect technique that works by measuring the overall concentration of SPIONs contained within cells (and not direct measurement of the actual number of cells), dilution and asymmetric division both affect the results of MRI [81].

Another disadvantage is that the signal from SPIONs ignores cell viability, i.e., MRI cannot differentiate between dead and live cells [82]. The persistence of SPIONs in the tissues and the engulfment of these particles by macrophages can also produce misleading MRI signals. For example, it has been reported that MRI overestimates ferumoxide-labeled stem cell survival after transplantation in the heart [83]. The engulfment of ferumoxide by macrophages was responsible for the false signal even 3 weeks after stem cell delivery to rats. Such an issue makes the long term tracking of stem cells very challenging. In this study, the authors injected labeled human and rat cardiac-derived stem cells expressing β-galactosidase intramyocardially to normal rats. Hypointensities were detected for 3 weeks by MRI. However, histological studies could not detect any stem cells. In a similar study, immunocompromised rats were injected with iron oxide-labeled human endothelial progenitor cells, which were also transfected with a sodium iodide symporter serving as PET reporter gene [27]. Twenty-four hours after intramyocardial injection, progenitor cells could be identified both using PET and MRI. Although hypointensities on MRI could be seen after 1 week, PET imaging or immunohistochemistry did not show the presence of any viable cells. However, staining for iron and Prussian blue indicated the co-localization of iron with macrophages (CD68+ cells). The progenitor cells most likely did not survive in the immunocompromised rats. Furthermore, the iron engulfed by macrophages may generate a false positive result at 1 week post-injection of labeled stem cells. In yet another study, the authors injected SPION-labeled MSCs directly into the hearts of immunocompetent Sprague-Dawley rats after ischemic injury [84]. Four weeks post-injection, no SPION was detected within MSCs, but they were present in cardiac macrophages. Interestingly, macrophages loaded with hemosiderin, an endogenous iron-storage complex of ferritin resulting from hemorrhage, are usually present in an infarcted myocardium and it may not be feasible to distinguish between the hypointense signals of hemosiderin and SPION-labeled cells [84, 85]. Overall, these complications can make the long-term tracking of NPs very challenging as shown in Figure 9.6.

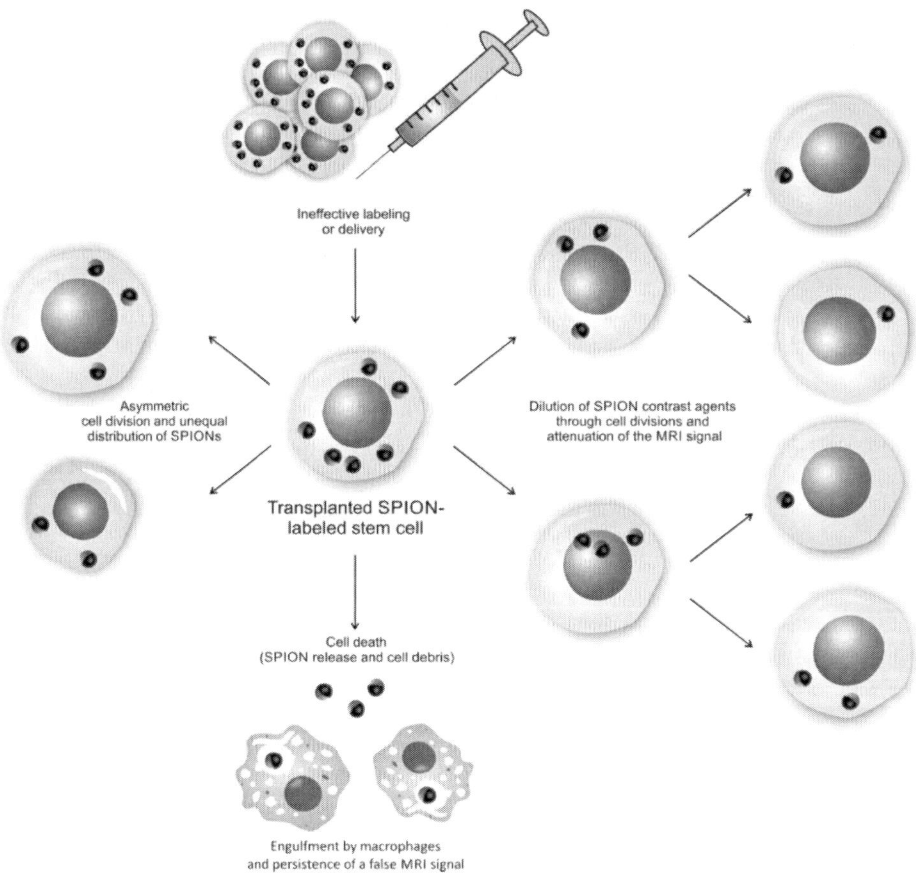

Figure 9.6. Challenges and problems with MRI tracking stem cells in vivo. First, ineffective labeling or delivery of labeled stem cells to the target region can spoil subsequent stem cell tracking. Second, in vivo proliferation of stem cells results in the dilution of SPION labels between the daughter cells, leads to attenuation of MRI signal and hampers long-term tracking. Third, through asymmetric division of labeled stem cells, some daughter cells become virtually undetectable because of the quick dilution of SPION labels. Finally, if transplanted cell die, SPIONs can be engulfed by cardiac macrophages in the area and thus, a false MRI signal might persists.

One strategy to circumvent this issue and prolong the imaging window is to decelerate the metabolic rate of SPIONs once within cells. This can be achieved by coating the SPION core with phospholipids. After internalization, the phospholipid layer will protect the SPIONs against endosomal degradation. Using this strategy, Soenen et al. [86] could acquire MRI signals for at least 1 month. As also discussed above, coating with enzyme and acid-resistant substances can help to prolong the tracking time.

To overcome the limitations of NPs as labeling agents, an innovative study has investigated the potential of ferritin, as a reporter gene, for tracking of stem cells in vivo using MRI [87]. In this study, a lentiviral vector was used to transfect swine cardiac stem/progenitor cells with human ferritin heavy chain (hFTH). After induction of MI in rats, hFTH-transduced cells were injected through myocardial route in the border zone. Iron-bearing tissues could only be detected in the hearts treated with hFTH-transduced cells and not in non-transduced cells. The signal could be detected for 1 week after infarction and persisted for more than 4 weeks. The treatment improved the left ventricular function and reduced the infarct size by 36% in treated animals. The presence of differentiated iron-bearing porcine cells was also validated using Prussian blue staining. Therefore, this methodology can be used to track stem cells in vivo without altering their function or differentiation capacity. Reporter genes such as GFP [59] and luciferase [16] have been used to assess the viability and tracking of stem cells post transplantation. Evidence suggests that reporter gene methodology is better than SPION labeling for monitoring cell viability, while SPION labeling of stem cells is a better approach for high-resolution detection of cell location by MRI [61, 88, 89]. For example, in a study by Chen et al. [88], firefly luciferase reporter gene and Feridex (SPION) were both used as cell markers to monitor cardiomyoblast survival after intramyocardial transplantation by bioluminescence imaging and MRI, respectively. The longitudinal cell viability monitoring gave different results in different methods. While cell survival half-life was 2.65 days for bioluminescene imaging, the half-life obtained from MRI was 16.8 days. These data confirms that bioluminescence imaging is more reliable for assessing the survival of stem cells post-transplantation.

One of the important issues compromising the efficacy of stem cell therapy in MI is the fact that the infarcted tissue may not be able to support the survival and proliferation of transplanted stem cells. Hung et al. [16] have used multimodality imaging of mouse ESCs dual labeled with luciferase and SPIONs, to monitor the cellular localization, viability and cardioreparative potential after injection of cells to different zones of MI (i.e., intra-infarct, peri-infarct, and normal (remote)). While MRI allowed for accurate tracking of cells, bioluminescence imaging analyzed cell viability by detecting luciferase activity. Furthermore, cardiac activity was monitored through MRI and pressure–volume loop analysis. The remotely-injected cells were shown to have significantly higher viability than the other two groups transplanted in the intra-infarct and peri-infarct regions. MRI and pressure–volume loop analysis demonstrated the restoration of cardiac functions. More importantly, the region of injection was found to be critical for successful stem cell therapy in cardiovascular disease and that the delivery of cells to the peri-infarct region was found to be the best option in regenerating the injured myocardium and restoring cardiac functions [38]. Furthermore, stem cell survival and engraftment are very critical issues that needs to be studied by a variety of methods [17]. Li and colleagues [90] isolated and characterized resident firefly luciferase and GFP-expressing cardiac stem cells (CSCs) from L2G85 transgenic mice. Subsequently, these CSCs were injected into the hearts of syngeneic FVB (Friend leukemia virus B strain) mice. CSCs demonstrated poor survival after 8 weeks, as shown by bioluminescence imaging. In addition, echocardiogram, invasive hemodynamic pressure-volume analysis, PET and MRI could not identify any significant difference in cardiac contractility and viability between treated and untreated animals. Monitoring for early and long-term viability of stem cells after transplantation is fundamental to the success of stem cell therapies in clinical trials.

Conclusion

The capability of stem cells to undergo differentiation and produce various mature cell types can be exploited to help regenerate defective tissues in the human body. Several clinical trials have already been planned with different categories of stem cells for proving their efficacy in treatment of various human conditions. In the realm of cardiovascular disease, stem cells might be used in the future to treat myocardial infarction, peripheral arterial occlusive disease or heart valve dysfunction. Therefore, researchers have been seeking in vivo imaging techniques to monitor the location, engraftment, and proliferation of stem cells after transplantation in the target organ. Among the multiple imaging techniques, MRI provides comprehensive analysis for stem cell tracking. Furthermore, the magnetic behavior and synthetic parameters of SPIONs allow some of the optimal properties as contrast agents to label stem cells for in vivo tracking. Great progress has been made in devising efficient labeling methods to achieve higher NP uptake while exerting no effects on cell viability, function and behavior. Despite great advances in the field, many challenges still remain to be overcome, including long-term tracking period and increased the stability of SPIONs within the cells to prevent dilution and loss of MRI contrast. Last but not least, preliminary studies must assess the safety of these cell therapies while clinical trials evaluate their efficacy.

References

[1] Wang J, Rao S, Chu J, Shen X, Levasseur DN, Theunissen TW, Orkin SW. A protein interaction network for pluripotency of embryonic stem cells. *Nature* 2006, 444:364-368.

[2] Takahashi K, Tanabe K, Ohnuki M, Narita M, Ichisaka T, Tomoda K, Yamanaka S. Induction of pluripotent stem cells from adult human fibroblasts by defined factors. *Cell* 2007;131(5):861-872.

[3] Amado LC, Saliaris AP, Schuleri KH, St John M, Xie JS, Cattaneo S, et al. Cardiac repair with intramyocardial injection of allogeneic mesenchymal stem cells after myocardial infarction. *Proc Natl Acad Sci U S A* 2005;102(32):11474-11479.

[4] Lawall H, Bramlage P, Amann B. Stem cell and progenitor cell therapy in peripheral artery disease. A critical appraisal. Thromb Haemost 2010;103(4):696-709.

[5] Loh Y, Oyama Y, Statkute L, Traynor A, Satkus J, Quigley K, et al. Autologous hematopoietic stem cell transplantation in systemic lupus erythematosus patients with cardiac dysfunction: feasibility and reversibility of ventricular and valvular dysfunction with transplant-induced remission. *Bone Marrow Transplant* 2007;40(1):47-53.

[6] Assmus B, Schachinger V, Teupe C, Britten M, Lehmann R, Dobert N, et al. Transplantation of Progenitor Cells and Regeneration Enhancement in Acute Myocardial Infarction (TOPCARE-AMI). *Circulation* 2002;106(24):3009-3017.

[7] Beltrami AP, Barlucchi L, Torella D, Baker M, Limana F, Chimenti S, et al. Adult cardiac stem cells are multipotent and support myocardial regeneration. *Cell* 2003;114(6):763-776.

[8] Schachinger V, Erbs S, Elsasser A, Haberbosch W, Hambrecht R, Holschermann H, et al. Intracoronary bone marrow-derived progenitor cells in acute myocardial infarction. *N Engl J Med* 2006;355(12):1210-1221.

[9] Leistner DM, Fischer-Rasokat U, Honold J, Seeger FH, Schachinger V, Lehmann R, et al. Transplantation of progenitor cells and regeneration enhancement in acute myocardial infarction (TOPCARE-AMI): final 5-year results suggest long-term safety and efficacy. *Clin Res Cardiol* 2011;100(10):925-934.

[10] Yang L, Soonpaa MH, Adler ED, Roepke TK, Kattman SJ, Kennedy M, Henckaerts E, Bonham K, Abbott GW, Linden RM, Field LJ, Keller GM. Human cardiovascular progenitor cells develop from a KDR+ embryonic-stem-cell-derived population. *Nature* 2008;453:524-528.

[11] Wollert KC, Meyer GP, Lotz J, Ringes-Lichtenberg S, Lippolt P, Breidenbach C, et al. Intracoronary autologous bone-marrow cell transfer after myocardial infarction: the BOOST randomised controlled clinical trial. *Lancet* 2004;364(9429):141-148.

[12] Lunde K, Solheim S, Aakhus S, Arnesen H, Abdelnoor M, Egeland T, et al. Intracoronary injection of mononuclear bone marrow cells in acute myocardial infarction. *N Engl J Med* 2006;355(12):1199-1209.

[13] Yamashita J, Itoh H, Hirashima M, Ogawa M, Nishikawa S, Yurugi T, Naito M, Nakao K, Nishikawa SI. Flk1-positive cells derived from embryonic stem cells serve as vascular progenitors. *Nature* 2000; 408: 92-96.

[14] Tse HF, Thambar S, Kwong YL, Rowlings P, Bellamy G, McCrohon J, et al. Prospective randomized trial of direct endomyocardial implantation of bone marrow cells for treatment of severe coronary artery diseases (PROTECT-CAD trial). *Eur Heart J* 2007;28(24):2998-3005.

[15] Barbash IM, Chouraqui P, Baron J, Feinberg MS, Etzion S, Tessone A, et al. Systemic delivery of bone marrow-derived mesenchymal stem cells to the infarcted myocardium: feasibility, cell migration, and body distribution. *Circulation* 2003;108(7):863-868.

[16] Hung TC, Suzuki Y, Urashima T, Caffarelli A, Hoyt G, Sheikh AY, et al. Multimodality evaluation of the viability of stem cells delivered into different zones of myocardial infarction. *Circ Cardiovasc Imaging* 2008;1(1):6-13.

[17] Yang PC. Is reliable in vivo detection of stem cell viability possible in a large animal model of myocardial injury? *Circulation* 2012;126(4):388-390.

[18] Kraitchman DL, Heldman AW, Atalar E, Amado LC, Martin BJ, Pittenger MF, et al. In vivo magnetic resonance imaging of mesenchymal stem cells in myocardial infarction. *Circulation* 2003;107(18):2290-2293.

[19] Azene N, Fu Y, Maurer J, Kraitchman DL. Tracking of stem cells in vivo for cardiovascular applications. *J Cardiovasc Magn Reson* 2014;16(1):7.

[20] Frangioni JV, Hajjar RJ. In vivo tracking of stem cells for clinical trials in cardiovascular disease. *Circulation* 2004;110(21):3378-3383.

[21] Mahmoudi M, Hosseinkhani H, Hosseinkhani M, Boutry S, Simchi A, Journeay WS, et al. Magnetic resonance imaging tracking of stem cells in vivo using iron oxide nanoparticles as a tool for the advancement of clinical regenerative medicine. *Chem Rev* 2011;111(2):253-280.

[22] Lewin M, Carlesso N, Tung CH, Tang XW, Cory D, Scadden DT Weissleder R. Tat peptide-derivatized magnetic nanoparticles allow in vivo tracking and recovery of progenitor cells. Nat. Biotechnol. 2000;18: 410-414.

[23] Hsiao JK, Tai MF, Chu HH, Chen ST, Li H, Lai DM, et al. Magnetic nanoparticle labeling of mesenchymal stem cells without transfection agent: cellular behavior and capability of detection with clinical 1.5 T magnetic resonance at the single cell level. *Magn Reson Med* 2007;58(4):717-724.

[24] Stroh A, Faber C, Neuberger T, Lorenz P, Sieland K, Jakob PM, et al. In vivo detection limits of magnetically labeled embryonic stem cells in the rat brain using high-field (17.6 T) magnetic resonance imaging. *Neuroimage* 2005;24(3):635-645.

[25] Amado LC, Schuleri KH, Saliaris AP, Boyle AJ, Helm R, Oskouei B, et al. Multimodality noninvasive imaging demonstrates in vivo cardiac regeneration after mesenchymal stem cell therapy. *J Am Coll Cardiol* 2006;48(10):2116-2124.

[26] Chapon C, Jackson JS, Aboagye EO, Herlihy AH, Jones WA, Bhakoo KK. An in vivo multimodal imaging study using MRI and PET of stem cell transplantation after myocardial infarction in rats. *Mol Imaging Biol* 2009;11(1):31-38.

[27] Higuchi T, Anton M, Dumler K, Seidl S, Pelisek J, Saraste A, et al. Combined reporter gene PET and iron oxide MRI for monitoring survival and localization of transplanted cells in the rat heart. *J Nucl Med* 2009;50(7):1088-1094.

[28] Hendry SL, 2nd, van der Bogt KE, Sheikh AY, Arai T, Dylla SJ, Drukker M, et al. Multimodal evaluation of in vivo magnetic resonance imaging of myocardial restoration by mouse embryonic stem cells. *J Thorac Cardiovasc Surg* 2008;136(4):1028-1037 e1021.

[29] Yamada M, Gurney PT, Chung J, Kundu P, Drukker M, Smith AK, et al. Manganese-guided cellular MRI of human embryonic stem cell and human bone marrow stromal cell viability. Ma*gn Reson Med* 2009;62(4):1047-1054.

[30] Wang YX. Superparamagnetic iron oxide based MRI contrast agents: Current status of clinical application. *Quant Imaging Med Surg* 2011;1(1):35-40.

[31] Laurent S, Saei AA, Behzadi S, Panahifar A, Mahmoudi M. Superparamagnetic iron oxide nanoparticles for delivery of therapeutic agents: opportunities and challenges. *Expert Opin Drug Deliv* 2014;1-22.

[32] Berensmeier S. Magnetic particles for the separation and purification of nucleic acids. *Appl Microbiol Biotechnol* 2006;73(3):495-504.

[33] Laurent S, Dutz S, Hafeli UO, Mahmoudi M. Magnetic fluid hyperthermia: focus on superparamagnetic iron oxide nanoparticles. *Adv Colloid Interface Sci* 2011;166(1-2):8-23.

[34] Saei AA BA, Majd MH, Asgari D, Omidi Y. Fe3O4 nanoparticles engineered for plasmid DNA delivery to Escherichia coli. *J Nanoparticle Res* 2014;16(8):11.

[35] Xu C, Sun S. Superparamagnetic nanoparticles as targeted probes for diagnostic and therapeutic applications. *Dalton Trans* 2009;29):5583-5591.

[36] Mahmoudi M, Sant S, Wang B, Laurent S, Sen T. Superparamagnetic iron oxide nanoparticles (SPIONs): development, surface modification and applications in chemotherapy. *Adv Drug Deliv Rev* 2011;63(1-2):24-46.

[37] Ferreira L, Karp JM, Nobre L, Langer R. New opportunities: the use of nanotechnologies to manipulate and track stem cells. *Cell Stem Cell* 2008;3(2):136-146.

[38] Chung J, Kee K, Barral JK, Dash R, Kosuge H, Wang X, et al. In vivo molecular MRI of cell survival and teratoma formation following embryonic stem cell transplantation into the injured murine myocardium. *Magn Reson Med* 2011;66(5):1374-1381.

[39] Yeh TC, Zhang W, Ildstad ST, Ho C. Intracellular labeling of T-cells with superparamagnetic contrast agents. *Magn Reson Med* 1993;30(5):617-625.

[40] Yeh TC, Zhang W, Ildstad ST, Ho C. In vivo dynamic MRI tracking of rat T-cells labeled with superparamagnetic iron-oxide particles. *Magn Reson Med* 1995;33(2):200-208.

[41] Hawrylak N, Ghosh P, Broadus J, Schlueter C, Greenough WT, Lauterbur PC. Nuclear magnetic resonance (NMR) imaging of iron oxide-labeled neural transplants. *Exp Neurol* 1993;121(2):181-192.

[42] Bulte JW, Hoekstra Y, Kamman RL, Magin RL, Webb AG, Briggs RW, et al. Specific MR imaging of human lymphocytes by monoclonal antibody-guided dextran-magnetite particles. *Magn Reson Med* 1992;25(1):148-157.

[43] Norman AB, Thomas SR, Pratt RG, Lu SY, Norgren RB. Magnetic resonance imaging of neural transplants in rat brain using a superparamagnetic contrast agent. *Brain Res* 1992;594(2):279-283.

[44] Arbab AS, Yocum GT, Kalish H, Jordan EK, Anderson SA, Khakoo AY, et al. Efficient magnetic cell labeling with protamine sulfate complexed to ferumoxides for cellular *MRI. Blood* 2004;104(4):1217-1223.

[45] Bulte JW, Douglas T, Witwer B, Zhang SC, Strable E, Lewis BK, et al. Magnetodendrimers allow endosomal magnetic labeling and in vivo tracking of stem cells. *Nat Biotechnol* 2001;19(12):1141-1147.

[46] Frank JA, Miller BR, Arbab AS, Zywicke HA, Jordan EK, Lewis BK, et al. Clinically applicable labeling of mammalian and stem cells by combining superparamagnetic iron oxides and transfection agents. *Radiology* 2003;228(2):480-487.

[47] Josephson L, Tung CH, Moore A, Weissleder R. High-efficiency intracellular magnetic labeling with novel superparamagnetic-Tat peptide conjugates. *Bioconjug Chem* 1999;10(2):186-191.

[48] Hinds KA, Hill JM, Shapiro EM, Laukkanen MO, Silva AC, Combs CA, et al. Highly efficient endosomal labeling of progenitor and stem cells with large magnetic particles allows magnetic resonance imaging of single cells. Blood 2003;102(3):867-872.

[49] Arbab AS, Wilson LB, Ashari P, Jordan EK, Lewis BK, Frank JA. A model of lysosomal metabolism of dextran coated superparamagnetic iron oxide (SPIO) nanoparticles: implications for cellular magnetic resonance imaging. *NMR Biomed* 2005;18(6):383-389.

[50] Kraitchman DL, Bulte JW. Imaging of stem cells using MRI. *Basic Res Cardiol* 2008;103(2):105-113.

[51] Mailänder V, Lorenz MR, Holzapfel V, Musyanovych A, Fuchs K, Wiesneth M, et al. Carboxylated superparamagnetic iron oxide particles label cells intracellularly without transfection agents. *Mol Imaging Biol* 2008;10(3):138-146.

[52] Tallheden T, Nannmark U, Lorentzon M, Rakotonirainy O, Soussi B, Waagstein F, et al. In vivo MR imaging of magnetically labeled human embryonic stem cells. Life Sci 2006;79(10):999-1006.

[53] Walczak P, Kedziorek DA, Gilad AA, Lin S, Bulte JW. Instant MR labeling of stem cells using magnetoelectroporation. *Magn Reson Med* 2005;54(4):769-774.

[54] Walczak P, Ruiz-Cabello J, Kedziorek DA, Gilad AA, Lin S, Barnett B, et al. Magnetoelectroporation: improved labeling of neural stem cells and leukocytes for

cellular magnetic resonance imaging using a single FDA-approved agent. *Nanomedicine* 2006;2(2):89-94.

[55] Tai JH, Foster P, Rosales A, Feng B, Hasilo C, Martinez V, et al. Imaging islets labeled with magnetic nanoparticles at 1.5 Tesla. *Diabetes* 2006;55(11):2931-2938.

[56] Qiu B, Xie D, Walczak P, Li X, Ruiz-Cabello J, Minoshima S, et al. Magnetosonoporation: instant magnetic labeling of stem cells. *Magn Reson Med* 2010;63(6):1437-1441.

[57] Xie D, Qiu B, Walczak P, Li X, Ruiz-Cabello J, Minoshima S, et al. Optimization of magnetosonoporation for stem cell labeling. *NMR Biomed* 2010;23(5):480-484.

[58] Suzuki Y, Zhang S, Kundu P, Yeung AC, Robbins RC, Yang PC. In vitro comparison of the biological effects of three transfection methods for magnetically labeling mouse embryonic stem cells with ferumoxides. *Magn Reson Med* 2007;57(6):1173-1179.

[59] Arai T, Kofidis T, Bulte JW, de Bruin J, Venook RD, Berry GJ, et al. Dual in vivo magnetic resonance evaluation of magnetically labeled mouse embryonic stem cells and cardiac function at 1.5 t. *Magn Reson Med* 2006;55(1):203-209.

[60] Stuckey DJ, Carr CA, Martin-Rendon E, Tyler DJ, Willmott C, Cassidy PJ, et al. Iron particles for noninvasive monitoring of bone marrow stromal cell engraftment into, and isolation of viable engrafted donor cells from, the heart. *Stem Cells* 2006;24(8):1968-1975.

[61] Suzuki Y, Cunningham CH, Noguchi K, Chen IY, Weissman IL, Yeung AC, et al. In vivo serial evaluation of superparamagnetic iron-oxide labeled stem cells by off-resonance positive contrast. *Magn Reson Med* 2008;60(6):1269-1275.

[62] Dharmakumar R, Koktzoglou I, Li D. Generating positive contrast from off-resonant spins with steady-state free precession magnetic resonance imaging: theory and proof-of-principle experiments. *Phys Med Biol* 2006;51(17):4201-4215.

[63] Cukur T, Yamada M, Overall WR, Yang P, Nishimura DG. Positive contrast with alternating repetition time SSFP (PARTS): a fast imaging technique for SPIO-labeled cells. *Magn Reson Med* 2010;63(2):427-437.

[64] Stuber M, Gilson WD, Schar M, Kedziorek DA, Hofmann LV, Shah S, et al. Positive contrast visualization of iron oxide-labeled stem cells using inversion-recovery with ON-resonant water suppression (IRON). *Magn Reson Med* 2007;58(5):1072-1077.

[65] Dahnke H, Liu W, Herzka D, Frank JA, Schaeffter T. Susceptibility gradient mapping (SGM): a new postprocessing method for positive contrast generation applied to superparamagnetic iron oxide particle (SPIO)-labeled cells. *Magn Reson Med* 2008;60(3):595-603.

[66] Zhou R, Idiyatullin D, Moeller S, Corum C, Zhang H, Qiao H, et al. SWIFT detection of SPIO-labeled stem cells grafted in the myocardium. *Magn Reson Med* 2010;63(5):1154-1161.

[67] Frank JA, Anderson SA, Kalsih H, Jordan EK, Lewis BK, Yocum GT, et al. Methods for magnetically labeling stem and other cells for detection by in vivo magnetic resonance imaging. *Cytotherapy* 2004;6(6):621-625.

[68] Lu CW, Hung Y, Hsiao JK, Yao M, Chung TH, Lin YS, et al. Bifunctional magnetic silica nanoparticles for highly efficient human stem cell labeling. *Nano Lett* 2007;7(1):149-154.

[69] Sykova E, Jendelova P. Magnetic resonance tracking of implanted adult and embryonic stem cells in injured brain and spinal cord. *Ann N Y Acad Sci* 2005;1049(146-160.

[70] Guzman R, Uchida N, Bliss TM, He D, Christopherson KK, Stellwagen D, et al. Long-term monitoring of transplanted human neural stem cells in developmental and pathological contexts with MRI. *Proc Natl Acad Sci U S A* 2007;104(24):10211-10216.

[71] Wang. FH, Lee. IH, Holmström. N, Yoshitake. T, Kim. DK, Muhammed. M, et al. Magnetic resonance tracking of nanoparticle labelled neural stem cells in a rat's spinal cord. *Nanotechnology* 2006;17(8):1911-1915.

[72] Kedziorek DA, Muja N, Walczak P, Ruiz-Cabello J, Gilad AA, Jie CC, et al. Gene expression profiling reveals early cellular responses to intracellular magnetic labeling with superparamagnetic iron oxide nanoparticles. *Magn Reson Med* 2010;63(4):1031-1043.

[73] Balakumaran A, Pawelczyk E, Ren J, Sworder B, Chaudhry A, Sabatino M, et al. Superparamagnetic iron oxide nanoparticles labeling of bone marrow stromal (mesenchymal) cells does not affect their "stemness". *PLoS One* 2010;5(7):e11462.

[74] Au KW, Liao SY, Lee YK, Lai WH, Ng KM, Chan YC, et al. Effects of iron oxide nanoparticles on cardiac differentiation of embryonic stem cells. *Biochem Biophys Res Commun* 2009;379(4):898-903.

[75] Kostura L, Kraitchman DL, Mackay AM, Pittenger MF, Bulte JW. Feridex labeling of mesenchymal stem cells inhibits chondrogenesis but not adipogenesis or osteogenesis. *NMR Biomed* 2004;17(7):513-517.

[76] Schafer R, Kehlbach R, Muller M, Bantleon R, Kluba T, Ayturan M, et al. Labeling of human mesenchymal stromal cells with superparamagnetic iron oxide leads to a decrease in migration capacity and colony formation ability. *Cytotherapy* 2009;11(1):68-78.

[77] Riviere C, Boudghene FP, Gazeau F, Roger J, Pons JN, Laissy JP, et al. Iron oxide nanoparticle-labeled rat smooth muscle cells: cardiac MR imaging for cell graft monitoring and quantitation. *Radiology* 2005;235(3):959-967.

[78] Sun R, Dittrich J, Le-Huu M, Mueller MM, Bedke J, Kartenbeck J, et al. Physical and biological characterization of superparamagnetic iron oxide- and ultrasmall superparamagnetic iron oxide-labeled cells: a comparison. *Invest Radiol* 2005;40(8):504-513.

[79] Walczak P, Kedziorek DA, Gilad AA, Barnett BP, Bulte JW. Applicability and limitations of MR tracking of neural stem cells with asymmetric cell division and rapid turnover: the case of the shiverer dysmyelinated mouse brain. *Magn Reson Med* 2007;58(2):261-269.

[80] Morrison SJ, Kimble J. Asymmetric and symmetric stem-cell divisions in development and cancer. *Nature* 2006;441(7097):1068-1074.

[81] Liu W, Frank JA. Detection and quantification of magnetically labeled cells by cellular MRI. *Eur J Radiol* 2009;70(2):258-264.

[82] Berman SC, Galpoththawela C, Gilad AA, Bulte JW, Walczak P. Long-term MR cell tracking of neural stem cells grafted in immunocompetent versus immunodeficient mice reveals distinct differences in contrast between live and dead cells. *Magn Reson Med* 2011;65(2):564-574.

[83] Terrovitis J, Stuber M, Youssef A, Preece S, Leppo M, Kizana E, et al. Magnetic resonance imaging overestimates ferumoxide-labeled stem cell survival after transplantation in the heart. *Circulation* 2008;117(12):1555-1562.

[84] Amsalem Y, Mardor Y, Feinberg MS, Landa N, Miller L, Daniels D, et al. Iron-oxide labeling and outcome of transplanted mesenchymal stem cells in the infarcted myocardium. *Circulation* 2007;116(11 Suppl):I38-45.

[85] van den Bos EJ, Baks T, Moelker AD, Kerver W, van Geuns RJ, van der Giessen WJ, et al. Magnetic resonance imaging of haemorrhage within reperfused myocardial infarcts: possible interference with iron oxide-labelled cell tracking? *Eur Heart J* 2006;27(13):1620-1626.

[86] Soenen SJ, Vercauteren D, Braeckmans K, Noppe W, De Smedt S, De Cuyper M. Stable long-term intracellular labelling with fluorescently tagged cationic magnetoliposomes. *Chembiochem* 2009;10(2):257-267.

[87] Campan M, Lionetti V, Aquaro GD, Forini F, Matteucci M, Vannucci L, et al. Ferritin as a reporter gene for in vivo tracking of stem cells by 1.5-T cardiac MRI in a rat model of myocardial infarction. *Am J Physiol Heart Circ Physiol* 2011;300(6):H2238-2250.

[88] Chen IY, Greve JM, Gheysens O, Willmann JK, Rodriguez-Porcel M, Chu P, et al. Comparison of optical bioluminescence reporter gene and superparamagnetic iron oxide MR contrast agent as cell markers for noninvasive imaging of cardiac cell transplantation. *Mol Imaging Biol* 2009;11(3):178-187.

[89] Li Z, Suzuki Y, Huang M, Cao F, Xie X, Connolly AJ, et al. Comparison of reporter gene and iron particle labeling for tracking fate of human embryonic stem cells and differentiated endothelial cells in living subjects. *Stem Cells* 2008;26(4):864-873.

[90] Li Z, Lee A, Huang M, Chun H, Chung J, Chu P, et al. Imaging survival and function of transplanted cardiac resident stem cells. *J Am Coll Cardiol* 2009;53(14):1229-1240.

In: Magnetic Resonance Imaging of Stem Cell Applications ISBN: 978-1-63463-910-1
Editor: Xiaoming Yang

Chapter 10

Creation of Animal Models for Magnetic Resonance Imaging of Stem cell Application in Vasculatures

***Feng Zhang*[1], *Yaoping Shi*[1,2] *and Xiaoming Yang*[1*]**
[1]Image-Guided Bio-Molecular Intervention Research, Department of Radiology University of Washington School of Medicine, Seattle, Washington, US
[2]Department of Radiology, Sir Run Run Shaw Hospital, Zhejiang University School of Medicine, Hangzhou, Zhejiang, China

Abstract

Laboratory animal model is one of the key components for basic research on magnetic resonance imaging (MRI) of atherosclerotic cardiovascular disease - the leading cause of death across the world. Successful development of animal models with arterial injuries or atherosclerotic lesions offers great opportunities for investigating the pathogenesis, prevention, and treatment of atherosclerosis. Stem cells-based cell therapy has been emerging as a promising therapeutic approach to manage atherosclerotic cardiovascular disease. Creating the reliable animal models with arterial injuries and atherosclerotic plaques, which mimic the pathophysiologic progress of human vascular diseases, can lay the groundwork for the basic research on in vivo MRI of stem cell-based therapies. In this chapter, we emphasize the techniques for creation of animal models with arterial injuries, and currently widely available approaches for establishing animal models with atherosclerotic plaques. We first address the techniques, histologic characteristics and the potential application of each specific animal model with arterial injury and atherosclerotic plaque, and then describe the advantage and inherent drawbacks of each animal model for cellular MRI.

* Corresponding author: Xiaoming Yang, MD, PhD, Image-Guided Bio-Molecular Intervention Research, Department of Radiology, Institute for Stem Cell and Regenerative Medicine, University of Washington School of Medicine, Seattle, Washington, USA (xmyang@uw.edu).
This work was supported by a National Institutes of Health grant (R01EB012467).

Keywords: MRI; animal models; artery injury; atherosclerosis; stem cell; vasculature

Introduction

Atherosclerotic cardiovascular disease remains the leading cause of mortality in the world [1-3]. The formation of atherosclerotic plaques is a progressive, chronic and inflammatory process, characterized by the accumulation of a lipid core, inflammatory cells, smooth muscle cells and extracellular matrix proteins in the arterial wall [3-5]. Plaques can evolve to an extent, which causes either flow-limited vessel stenosis leading to distal organ/tissue ischemia, or the exposed matrix and thrombogenic core triggering the cascade of arterial thrombosis due to the abrupt plaque rupture or its surface erosion. These pathophysiological events ultimately lead to severe clinical outcomes, acute coronary syndrome (ACS), myocardial infarction, or stroke [2, 4, 6].

Creation of appropriate animal models with atherosclerosis and arterial injury have played an important role in increasing our understanding of atherosclerotic cardiovascular disease, and helping us to develop the innovative diagnostic and therapeutic techniques to manage this illness [1]. In the past decades, great progresses have been made in unraveling some of the principles of atherosclerotic pathophysiology through experimental works on various animal models of atherosclerosis [7, 8]. However, it is unfortunate that there is no ideal animal model of atherosclerosis that completely resembles the pathophysiologic natures of human atherothrombotic disease so far [7]. Huge gaps remain in translation of findings in atherosclerotic research on animals to the clinical practice on humans. Bridging the gaps is the important element to achieve the full promise of scientific advances in atherosclerotic cardiovascular disease [8]. Being aware of the disadvantages and advantages of different atherosclerotic animal models is the essential step to select the proper animal models for the specific research purposes, such as cellular MRI for stem cell therapy of atherosclerotic cardiovascular disease.

Creation of Animal Models with Artery Injuries

Intimal thickening is an essential early stage in the development of vascular injury. Arterial injury results in proliferation and migration of smooth muscle cells (SMCs) and the development of intimal hyperplasia, a critical component of restenosis after angioplasty of human arteries and an important feature of atherosclerotic lesions. Several models of vascular injuries have been shown to produce neointima-like hyperplasia, which are used to evaluate the susceptibility of transgenic/knock-out rodents (such as mice and rats) to vascular lesion formation, as well as investigate the participating role of stem cells-derived smooth muscle progenitor cells and endothelial progenitor cells in the repair and remodeling of injured arteries.

Surgical Cuff-Induced Artery Injury

Placement of a cuff around an arterial segment in rodents via a surgical approach can result in a concentric intimal hyperplasia [9-11]. Although the mechanisms of intimal hyperplasia in such cuff-injury model have not been fully elucidated, recent reports have suggested that adventitial inflammatory cell infiltration may be involved. The technique for surgically placing a cuff around a peripheral artery to induce the arterial injury is straightforward. A target artery (such as a femoral artery or a carotid artery) of a mouse is isolated and exposed surgically from surrounding tissues. A polyethylene tube (e.g., PE-160; 5 mm in length, 1.14 mm at the inner diameter and 1.57 mm at the outer diameter; Becton Dickinson and Company, NJ, USA) is longitudinally opened and loosely placed around the artery, and then the skin incision closed. Two weeks after the cuff placement, an obstruction of the target artery can be achieved, which manifests primarily as extensive intimal hyperplasia of smooth muscle cells with pathology (Figure 10.1).

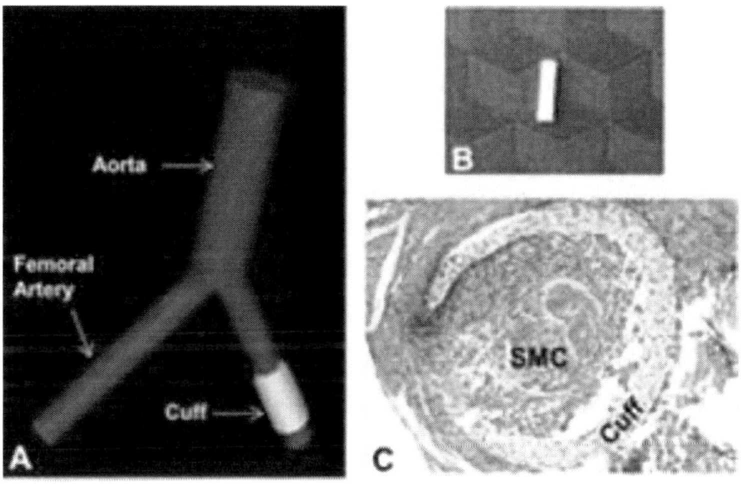

Figure 10.1. (A) Schematic description of the surgical procedure to place the cuff (B) around the target femoral artery. (C) Pathology with hematoxylin & Eosin (H&E) staining shows the extensive hyperplasia due to the proliferation of smooth muscle cells, which completely occludes the arterial lumen in this case.

Endovascular Intervention-Induced Artery Injury

Balloon Inflation-Induced Artery Injury

Balloon-based angioplasty is the mostly used method to induce the arterial injury, with its primary mechanism of causing endothelial denudation. However, due to the size limit of commercially available balloons, balloon angioplasty is usually used for creation of artery injuries in middle-to-large sized animals, such as rabbits and pigs. For example, when creating a rabbit model, a 4 French Fogarty balloon catheter is usually placed into the target artery, where the over-inflated balloon can damage the endothelium. The balloon is manually inflated for 20 to 30-second duration in order to have an overstretching of 30%, and then withdrawn for five separate occasions with an interval of 60 seconds between inflations [12].

Wire-Induced Artery Injury

Unlike those of middle- or large-sized animals, the rodent arteries are too small to be denudated via an endovascular balloon catheter. Thus, a wire-induced artery injury technique has been developed for creation of rodent models with artery injuries [13-15]. Briefly, an open surgical procedure is used to expose a muscular branch of the femoral artery, followed by a dilation of the arteries by topical application of one drop of 1% lidocaine hydrochloride. Transverse arteriotomy is then performed in the muscular arterial branch with Vannas style iris spring scissors to achieve an access to the target femoral artery segment. After extending the arteriotomy with microsurgery forceps, a straight spring wire (e.g., 0.38mm in diameter, No. C-SF-15-15, COOK, Bloomington, IN, USA) is carefully inserted into the femoral artery toward the iliac artery for more than 5-mm distance. The wire is left in the place for 1 minute to cause over-expansion and thereby sufficient denudation of the artery endothelium. Then, the wire is removed and the proximal portion of the accessed muscular branch artery is ligated by a thin (6-0) silk suture. Blood flow in the femoral artery is restored by releasing the sutures placed in the proximal and distal segments to the damaged femoral artery portion. The skin incision is closed with a 5-0 silk suture. The blood flow to the hindlimbs can be measured immediately after the surgery by laser Doppler perfusion imaging.

Histologically, the media is markedly thinned and the injured artery remains dilated from 1 day to 8 weeks. At 1 week, immunostaining for proliferating cell nuclear antigen (PCNA) identified proliferating cells in the media with initial neointimal hyperplasia on the luminal side of the internal elastic lamina. The neointimal hyperplasia continues to extend up to 3 or 4 weeks, and then the created lesions do not advance further. The lesion is concentric and very homogenous in the artery segment where the wire is inserted. An immunohistochemical study of smooth muscle actin confirmed that the neointimal hyperplasia was exclusively composed of smooth muscle cells. The luminal side of the intima is almost completely re-endothelialized at 4 weeks after the endothelial denudation, as determined by anti-CD31 staining [10].

Image-Guided Wire-Induced Artery Injury

Precise creation of controlled artery injuries on small animal models (such as mice and rats) facilities basic research in investigating the mechanism on stabilization of vulnerable plaques and repair of ruptured plaques, which is critical for developing novel techniques, such as imaging-interactive regenerative medicine and gene therapy. To this end, an ultrasound imaging-guided intima injury technique on rats was developed [16].

Under general anesthesia, the right carotid artery is surgically exposed, and proximal and distal Sentinel loops (Sherwood Medical, St Louis, Montana) are placed for temporary vascular control. Transverse arteriotomy is performed in the exposed artery with Vannas style iris spring scissors (Roboz Surgical Instrument Co., Gaithersburg, Maryland). Through the arteriotomy, a 0.014-inch conventional guidewire (Terumo Co., Tokyo, Japan) is advanced into the ascending aorta. Then, a custom-made, 2F micro-catheter is advanced into the ascending aorta over the guidewire. Through the micro-catheter, the conventional guidewire is exchanged for a custom-made, 0.014-inch angled-metal-device, which has a 7-mm long and 120°-angled tip. Under real-time ultrasound imaging (as described below), the micro-catheter/angled-metal-device system is advanced until the tips of the catheter and the angled-metal-device reach the aortic root. After walking the micro-catheter back to the innominate artery, the intima of the aorta is damaged by withdrawing the angle-metal-device over a distance of approximately 5 mm. To ensure the sufficient damage of the intima, for each animal the injury process is repeated 5-10 times by rotating the tip of the angled-metal-device at different directions (Figure 10.2).

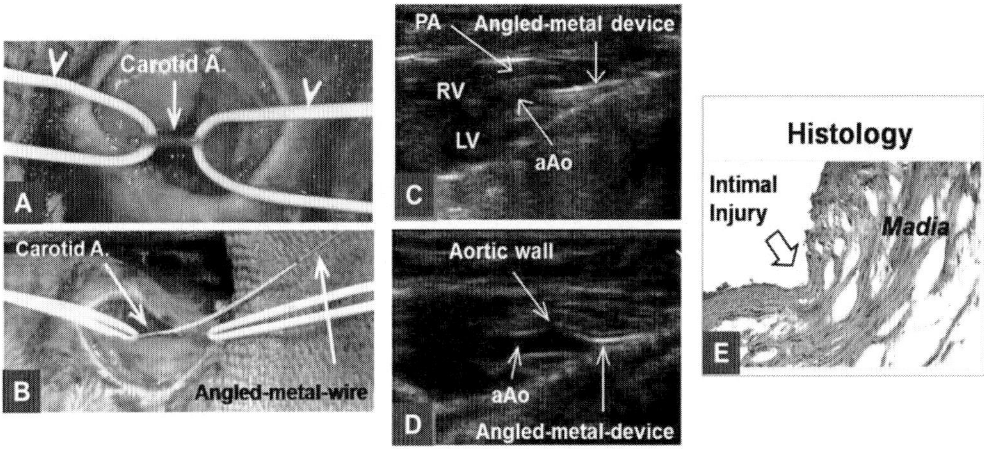

Fig. 10.2. Ultrasound-guided insertion of an angled-metal device into the ascending aorta of a rat. (A) Surgery for exposing the right carotid artery (arrow), with two Sentinel loops (arrowheads) placed for the temporary vascular control. (B) The angled-metal-wire is placed into the carotid artery. (C) At an oblique ultrasound projection, the great vessels and the entire heart can be clearly seen. PA=pulmonary artery, aAo=ascending aorta, RV=right ventricle, LV=left ventricle. (D) The location of the angled-metal-device and subsequent denudation of the aorta wall by the device can be visualized and monitored under real-time ultrasound imaging. (E) Histology immediately post-denudation shows an intimal injury of the aortic wall. Reprinted, with permission, from [16].

Analysis of histologic changes at the injured sites shows the discontinuation of intimal layers with no neointimal reaction after the acute sacrifice. The neointimal hyperplastic reactions became exuberant as the animal survival period increases. The intima at the injured sites appears to be re-endothelialized one week after the endovascular procedure, with several layers of infiltrative endothelial cells covering the injured intima.

Subsequently, the similar ultrasound-guided approach was successfully applied in creation of arterial intimal hyperplasia on near-human-sized animals, pigs [17]. These studies have proved the usefulness and benefits of imaging guidance in assisting the precise creation of controlled artery injuries for basic research on preclinical validation of novel MRI-guided stem cell therapies of vascular diseases.

Artery Injury Animal Models in Stem Cell Applications

One study reported a cuff-induced vascular injury model to investigate the role of bone marrow (BM) stem cell-derived smooth muscle cells (SMC) and endothelial cells (EC) in repair of injured arterial intima [9]. BM stem cells, collected from donor green fluorescent protein (GFP)-transgenic mice, were transplanted into the recipient mice with cuff-induced arterial injuries. The authors found that macrophages were major cells recruited to the adventitia of the vascular injury lesion along with SMCs and ECs. While investigating whether those cells were derived from the donor bone marrow, they found that most of the macrophages were GFP-positive, as some of SMCs and ECs were. Thus, by using the mouse model with artery injury, this study confirms that both BM-derived SMCs and ECs are recruited to the cuffed vascular remodeling lesions (Figure 10.3).

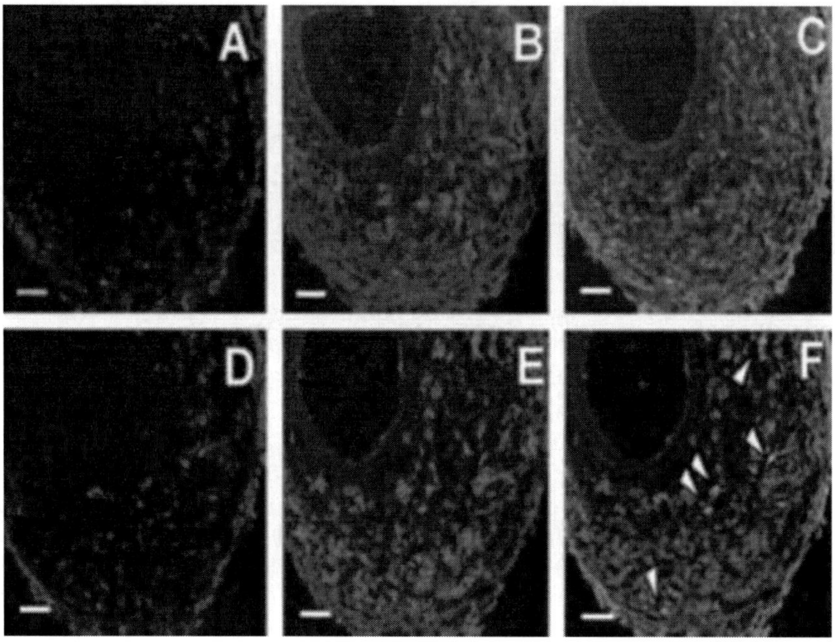

Figure 10.3. Extensive hyperplasia of smooth muscle cells in the thickened intima is visualized in the cuff-induced injury site of a mouse femoral artery. Bone marrow (BM) stem cells collected from a donor green fluorescent protein (GFP)-transgenic mouse are transplanted to the recipient mouse with cuff-induced arterial injury. Arterial tissues are subjected to immunostaining with anti-vWF antibody. A, B, and C are 1 week after cuff placement, and D, E, and F are 2 weeks after cuff placement. A&D indicate GFP signals and B&E indicate vWF signals. C is a merged image of A and B, and F is a merged image of D and E. F implied that some GFP^+ endothelial progenitor cells are derived from the bone marrow stem cells. Reprinted, with permission, from [9].

Some scientists also investigated the role of BM-derived progenitor cells in repair of intraluminally injured aorta of rats. BM cells are extracted from donor Sprague Dawley (SD) rats. Purified BM cells are then labeled with a superparamagnetic T2 MR contrast agent, Feridex (Berlex Laboratories, Wayne, NJ), at 37.5 ng/ml in QBSP-58 medium overnight. Feridex-labeled BM cells are then intravenously transplanted into recipient rats. Before BM transplantation, the recipient rats are irradiated with a sublethal dose of 450 rad (Gammacell 40; MDS Nordion, Ottawa, Ontario, Canada) to destroy the native bone marrow. Then, each recipient rat receives approximately 2×10^6 cells, suspended in 0.3–0.4mL 10-mM phosphate-buffered saline (PBS). Approximately three weeks post-cell transplantation, in vivo MRI is used to detect the Feridex/BM cells migrated to the injured ascending aorta of the recipient rats. Subsequent histology using Prussian blue staining of the ascending aorta specimens is performed to detect Feridex-positive cells. For the rat group with Feridex/BM cell transplantation, in vivo MR imaging detects signal voids of the injured ascending aorta walls, which is confirmed by the histologic correlation, manifested as (i) intimal hyperplasia and/or thickening of medium; and (ii) blue-colored iron-containing cells distributed through the neointima and media (Figure 10.4). Thus, the successful creation of animal models with artery injuries have greatly promoted the advance of basic researches on stem cell therapy, providing insight into the mechanisms on migration and homing to the injured arteries, as well as repair of injured arteries after transplantation of magnetically-labeled stem cells.

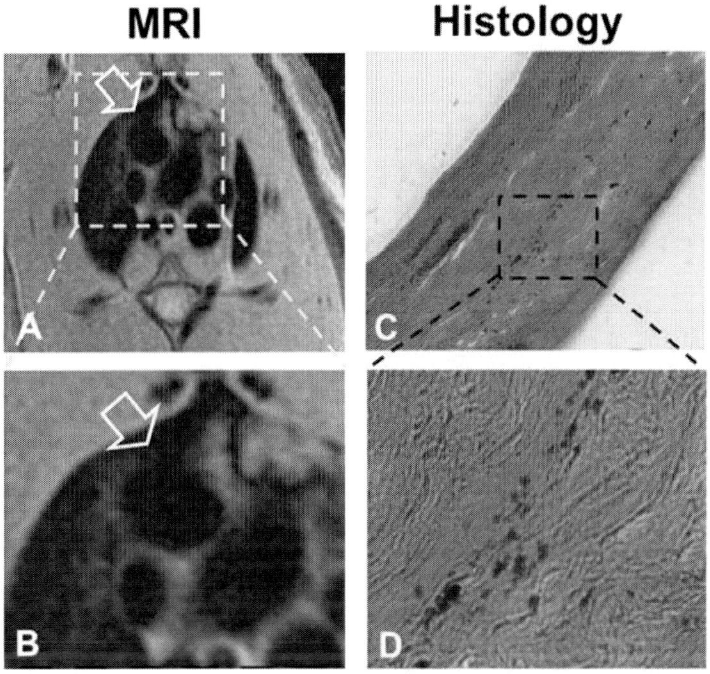

Figure 10.4. A&B (B=magnification of A): Axial MRI shows signal void (arrow) of the ascending aorta wall of the recipient rat due to T2-contrast agents within stem-progenitor cells migrated to injured site, which is confirmed by subsequent histology, presented as blue dots within the thickened aortic wall [C&D (D=magnification of C)].

Creation of Animal Models with Atherosclerosis

Pathogenesis of Atherosclerosis

Multiple systemic factors, such as hypercholesterolemia, diabetes, hypertension, and smoking, contribute to the formation and evolution of atherosclerosis [18]. The pathophysiologic mechanism behind the development of atherosclerotic plaques remains elusive. Hypercholesterolemia and hemodynamic alterations of arterial vessels are two important variables involving formation of atherosclerosis. Atherosclerosis occurs preferentially at particular atherosusceptible sites with disturbed blood flow characterized by low and oscillatory wall shear stress in branched or curved arteries. In contrast, straight arterial regions with a laminar flow are exposed to high and stable shear stress and are well protected from atherosclerosis [1, 3, 18].

Pathologic changes of the vessel wall in atherosclerotic disease mainly occur in the arterial intima and involve the infiltration of modified lipids, such as oxidized low density lipoprotein (LDL), macrophages, and smooth muscle cells [1, 2, 7]. Atherogenesis is initiated by endothelial dysfunction and structural alterations, including the integrity loss in a confluent luminal elastin layer, changes in endothelial permeability and the composition of the extracellular matrix beneath the endothelium, which facilitate the entry and subendothelial accumulation of LDLs [2, 8]. Elevated levels of circulating cholesterol transported by apolipoprotein B100 (ApoB100)-containing LDL further promote the atherosclerotic progress [2, 19]. ApoB100 binding to negatively charged extracellular matrix proteoglycans leads to retention of LDL particles in the intima, where they are susceptible to oxidative modification by reactive oxygen species or enzymes such as myeloperoxidase or lipoxygenases released from inflammatory cells. Oxidized lipids and LDL (oxLDL) trigger the expression of adhesion molecules, including vascular cell adhesion molecule-1 (VCAM-1) and E-selectin, as well as secretion of chemokines by endothelial cells, which, together with the deposition of platelet-derived chemokines, drive intimal immune cell infiltration. Endothelial activation facilitates recruitment of monocytes and other inflammatory cells, which are thought to play a central role in all stages of atherosclerosis. Inside the atherosclerotic intima, monocytes differentiate into macrophages and phagocytize modified LDL particles. This process leads to a transformation of macrophages into lipid-laden foam cells. At this stage of plaque development, lesions can be classified as fatty streaks, which can present in the arterial vessel wall at an early age [2, 4, 19]. Activated macrophages also express proinflammatory cytokines, matrix metalloproteinases, and tissue factors, contributing to the progression and potential destabilization of atherosclerotic lesions.

Formation of atherosclerotic lesions also involves the recruitment of smooth muscle cells (SMCs) from the tunica media - the middle layer of the artery wall - into the tunica intima [8, 20]. When vascular SMCs acquire the capability to migrate, they switch their phenotype from a contractile to a synthetic state, being able to synthesize more extracellular matrix (ECM) [12]. These proliferating smooth muscle cells constitute a substantial part of the neointima and produce ECM proteins, such as elastin and collagen, which form the fibrous cap that covers the plaque [8].

Hypoxia starts playing a central role as the plaque enlarges. Hypoxic conditions contribute to the apoptosis of inflammatory cells and the proliferation of new blood vessels into the atherosclerotic vessel wall, a process referred as neoangiogenesis [19, 21]. Inflammation exerts detrimental effects by degrading the fibrous cap, increasing apoptosis of the resident SMCs and increasing neovascularization in the plaque [21]. Free cholesterol originating from the membrane of red cells precipitates crystal formation, and contributes to the progression of one or multiple lipid-rich necrotic cores in the plaques [19, 21]. Unstable atherosclerotic plaques were shown to be associated with an increased density of neovessels, compared with stable plaques. If these fragile neovessels rupture, intraplaque hemorrhage due to the influx of red blood cells into the plaque is a consequence [4, 19]. The evolution of a stable, asymptomatic lesion to an unstable, ruptured plaque involves many processes, among which are inflammation, cellular breakdown, and expansion of a lipid-rich necrotic core. It is recognized that the death of macrophages and smooth-muscle foam cells, in addition to the aggregation of lipoproteins, contributes to the accumulation of extracellular free cholesterol within unstable plaques [4, 19, 22]. Plaques that rupture tend to have thin, collagen-poor fibrous caps with few SMCs but abundant macrophages [8]. The inflammatory cells may hasten plaque disruption by elaborating collagenolytic enzymes that can degrade collagen, and by generating mediators that provoke the death of SMCs, the source of arterial collagen. When the rupture of plaque occurs, blood gets to directly contact with exposed tissue factors and the plaque's matrix, while the coagulation cascade is triggered. If the newly formed thrombus occludes a downstream artery, an acute myocardial infarction or ischemic stroke can be the consequence [8]. Figure 10.5 shows the pathologic progression of a typical human coronary atherosclerosis [23].

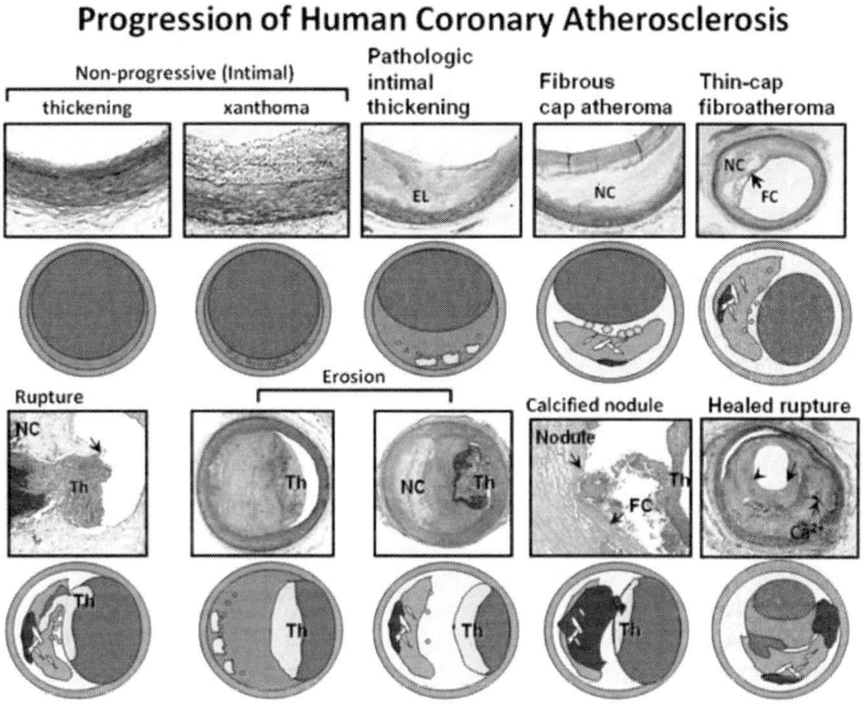

Figure 10.5. Typical pathologic progression of coronary atherosclerotic lesions, which is classified by American Heart Association (AHA). The two nonprogressive lesions are intimal thickening and intimal xanthomas (foam cell collections known as fatty streaks, AHA type II). Pathologic intimal thickening (PIT) (AHA type III transitional lesions) marks the first of the progressive plaques, which are the precursors to more advanced fibroatheroma (FA). Thin-cap fibroatheromas (TCFAs) are considered precursors to plaque rupture. Erosions can occur on a substrate of PIT or FA, whereas calcified nodules depict eruptive fragments of calcium that protrude into the lumen, causing a thrombotic event. Lastly, healed plaque ruptures are lesions with generally smaller necrotic cores and focal areas of calcification where the surface generally shows areas of healing rich in proteoglycans. Multiple healed plaque ruptures are thought responsible for progressive luminal narrowing. Ca2+ = calcium; EL = extracellular lipid; FC = fibrous cap; NC = necrotic core; Th = luminal thrombus. Reprinted, with permission, from [23].

Mouse Model of Atherosclerosis

Mice remain the favored species for basic research on atherosclerosis. The primary advantages of using mice for the study of atherogenesis and its complications include low cost, availability of genetic manipulation, high degree of genome similarity, easy handling in laboratories, ease of breeding, and small size that limits the quantities of new agents required for *in vivo* screening [2, 7, 24]. Genetic manipulation, which is capable of modifying some specific genes in mouse strains, can help us to elucidate the gene function and new pathways involved in the development of cardiovascular diseases [7].

Lipid metabolism of mice is quite different from that of humans. Wild-type mice are innately resistant to high-fat/high-cholesterol diet (HcD)-induced atherosclerosis because of their high levels of anti-atherosclerotic high-density lipoprotein cholesterol (HDL-C), as well as low levels of proatherogenic low-density lipoprotein cholesterol (LDL-C) and very-low-density lipoprotein cholesterol (VLDL-C) [6, 25]. Specific gene manipulation can alter mouse lipid metabolism to provide the feasibility of transforming the mouse from an atheroresistant phenotype to atherosusceptible phenotype [7, 24]. This is most readily accomplished by the genetic ablation of apolipoprotein-E (ApoE) or low-density lipoprotein cholesterol receptor (LDLR). Genetically-modified mice that lack ApoE or LDLR genes exhibit hyperlipidemia and atherosclerosis [26]. They differ in their dietary needs for developing atherosclerosis. The advantage of the $ApoE^{-/-}$ mouse model is that complex vascular lesions, comparable to those of human lesions, readily develop in animals fed the normal low-fat rodent chow, even when plasma cholesterol levels are between 300 to 500 mg/dL. The rate of atherogenesis can be notably accelerated by the feeding of a high-fat, high-cholesterol Western type diet (WTD) (typically 0.2% cholesterol with 21% milk fat), resulting in significant increases in plasma lipid levels (>1,000 mg/dL) [1]. While fed chow, foam cell lesions first appear at 8 to 10 weeks of age. After 15 weeks intermediate lesions are present, containing spindle shaped cells (mostly SMCs), and beyond 20 weeks, fibrous plaques are evident containing SMCs, extracellular matrix, and an overlying fibrous cap. This time course mainly refers to the aortic root, as lesions develop at different rates at each of the atherosclerosis prone sites [1] (Figure 10.6).

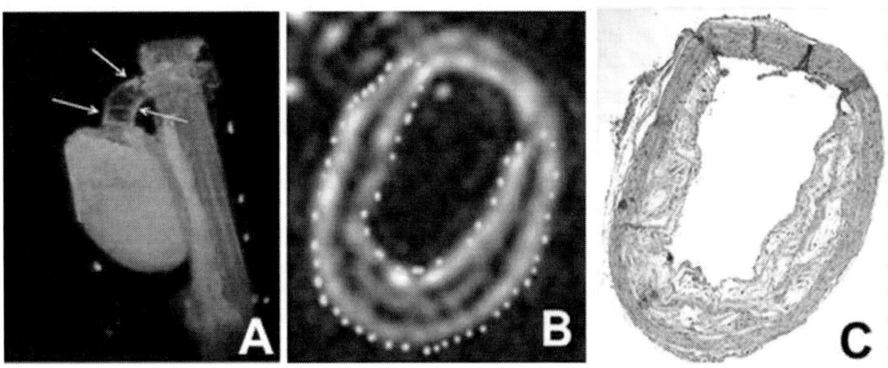

Figure10.6. Creation of ApoE-\- mouse model with aortic atherosclerotic plaques. (A) Ex-vivo three-dimensional (3D) 11.7T MRI of thoracic aorta (pseudo-colored) of an ApoE-/- mouse with atherosclerotic plaque formation (arrows). (B) Ex-vivo 11.7 T MRI of an atherosclerotic plaque in the mouse ascending aorta. The vessel wall is thickened with complicated, lipid-rich plaque (dashed line encircled). (C) Corresponding histology to the MRI, showing the atherosclerotic plaque featured as thickened vessel wall with the lipid core and thin fibrotic cap.

The atherosclerosis of $ApoE^{-/-}$ mouse models can be accelerated through an endovascular wire injury or placement of a perivascular shear modifier cuff around the target vessel segment [27]. The atherosclerotic plaques primarily occur at those atheroprone regions of arterial tree, such as lesser curvature of the aortic arch and root of innominate artery, because these regions are exposed to disturbed blood flow. In addition, these flow-disturbed areas in $ApoE^{-/-}$ and $LDLR^{-/-}$ mice develop measurable atherosclerotic lesions upon feeding atherogenic diets for at least 2–3 months [18].

Although mouse models of atherosclerosis have proven indispensable to studies of disease mechanisms, we should be very cautious to extrapolate the experimental finding to interpret human disease due to the inherent limitations of such mouse models [8]. Mice and humans differ in several parameters that may influence atherogenesis. In addition, their lesion distribution is not identical. Human atherosclerotic lesions predominate in the coronary arteries, carotids, and peripheral vessels, such as the iliac artery, which usually have a fibrous cap [20]. For mice, atherosclerotic lesions, however, more frequently occur in their aortic roots, aortic arches, and innominate arteries [1, 8]. The structure and hemodynamics of these smaller muscular arteries, and even the embryonic origin of their SMCs, differ markedly from the large elastic arteries. The proximal left anterior descending (LAD) coronary artery in humans, a frequent site of atherosclerotic lesion formation, characteristically contains a considerable population of intimal SMCs, even in early life — a major difference from mouse arteries [8]. Hypercholesterolemic $Apoe^{-/-}$ or $LDLR^{-/-}$ mice are frequently used to study mechanisms of disease initiation and progression, but are less suitable for investigations of advanced stages, such as plaque rupture or thrombosis, which continue to rely on histopathological and clinical studies [1, 2, 8].

Rabbit Model of Atherosclerosis

Rabbits are easy to handle and cost-effective. There are three breeds of rabbits that have been commonly used in biomedical research: New Zealand White, Dutch Belted, and Flemish Giant [7]. The New Zealand strain also appears in genetically altered strains, among which are the Watanabe, St Tomas, and Houston RT, presenting genetic abnormalities in lipid metabolism [1, 20]. These rabbits cannot develop spontaneous atherosclerotic plaques as they are vegetarian, but they are very sensitive to high cholesterol diet with the consequence of developing atherosclerotic lesions. The normal range of plasma cholesterol in New Zealand white rabbits is low (average 1.3 mmol/l), but it can increase by up to 2 to 8 times after the administration of a diet enriched with 0.1–2% cholesterol, within the first 20 days [20]. New Zealand rabbits with body weights between 2 and 5 kg are the most used ones in the laboratory. They can rapidly develop foam-cell-rich (fatty steaks) plaques after the administration of a rich atherosclerotic diet (0.5%–4% cholesterol content) during 8–16 weeks (Figure 10.7). The early lesions are characterized by the presence of foam cells originating from macrophages [1, 20]. Contrary to mice without the tendency of developing rupture-prone atherosclerotic plaques, rabbits have been used as a model to study plaque instability and rupture, besides their extended use in investigations of atherogenesis and myocardial infarction, as well as the efficacy of new antithrombotic and anti-atherosclerotic drugs. Moreover, transgenic rabbits have also been developed to obtain models of hereditary hyperlipidemia (WHHL-rabbit). Rabbits were fed 100g of cholesterol-supplemented chow per day for 28 to 29 months to promote the formation of aortic lesions. The cholesterol level in the diet was titrated between 0.125% and 0.25% (wt/wt) for the length of the lesion creation [28].

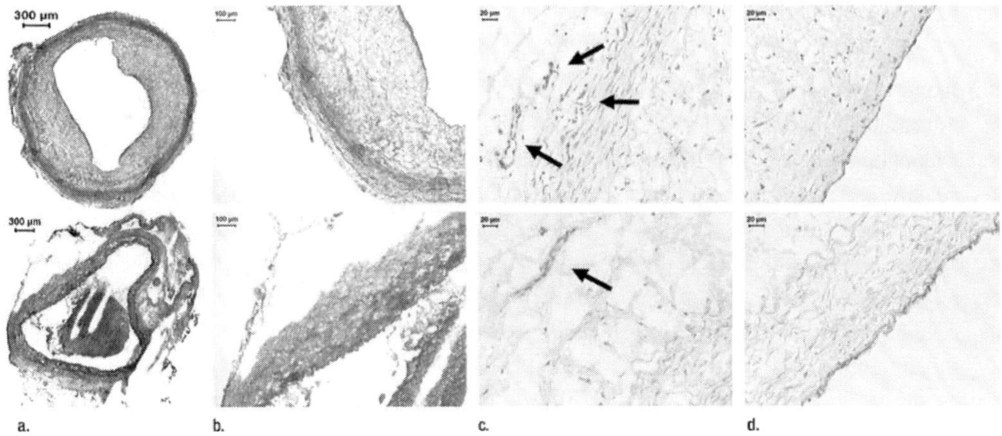

Figure 10.7. Examples of histologic findings in the aortic vessel wall of atherosclerotic (top row) and control (bottom row) rabbits. Atherosclerotic rabbits are fed with a 1.0% cholesterol–enriched diet for 2 weeks. (a) Hematoxylin-eosin–stained anatomic overview and (b) hematoxylin-eosin–stained detail of vessel walls show the thickened vessel wall and lipid-laden plaque in the aortic wall of atherosclerotic rabbits. Reprinted, with permission, from [22].

Combining cholesterol-rich feeding with arterial wall injury (e.g., balloon injury) can induce advanced lesions [7, 22]. Atherosclerosis in abdominal aorta of New Zealand white rabbits can be created by feeding the rabbits a cholesterol diet for two weeks before and six weeks after balloon injury of the abdominal aorta, followed by 4 weeks of normal chow diet [29].

In the rabbits, atherosclerotic lesions are distributed predominantly in the aortic arch and thoracic aorta, at the origins of intercostal arteries, and, to a lesser extent, in the abdominal aorta. In addition, atherosclerotic lesions of rabbits differ from human atheroma since lipid and macrophage content of rabbits is much higher due to their hypercholesterolemic index. Conversely, intermittent cycles of fat feeding with periods of normal diet has shown to induce plaques at more advanced stages that resemble human atheroma [7].

Swine Model of Atherosclerosis

Swine represent another useful animal model of atherosclerosis. In comparison to mice and rabbits, anatomy, physiology and habits of feeding and sleep of swine are very similar to those of humans [7, 25, 26]. Swine's hemodynamics, such as physiological cardiac function as well as mechanically induced myocardial infarction and the subsequent arrhythmogenic activity in reperfusion, is also analogous to humans [25, 30]. Three major coronary arteries of a swine can develop spontaneous atherosclerotic lesions [7, 25, 26]. Additional advantages of swine models are their large body sizes, which allow for imaging evaluation of atherosclerotic arteries, performing interventional procedures using commercially available devices, and harvesting sufficient arterial tissues for histologic analysis [26]. However, pig arteries are more friable and prone to vasospasm during manipulation, and thus require careful handling during interventional procedures [25, 30].

Atherosclerotic lesions in swine arteries generally occur at arterial bends, characterized by flow separation and low shear stress, which can be accelerated by feeding an atherogenic diet [1, 26]. Commercially available experimental miniature pigs (minipigs), such as Clawn, Gottingen, Chinese Bama and Yucatan minipigs, are smaller than domestic pigs, usually growing to a limited bodyweight less than 50 kilograms. Minipigs have much higher susceptibility than domestic pigs in term of developing atherosclerosis. Therefore, minipigs are thought to be appropriate experimental animals for research on atherosclerosis [26, 31, 32] (Figure 10.8).

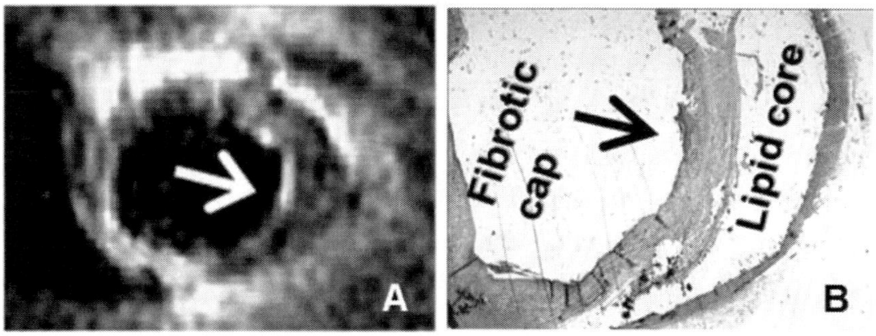

Figure 10.8. (A) A representative MRI of a Yucatan miniature pig with balloon-denudated intimal injuries of its aorta and iliac arteries, followed by a high-cholesterol diet for 18–24 months. 1.5 Tesla T1-weighted MRI shows the atherosclerotic plaque with a lipid core and a fibrotic cap (arrow). (B) Corresponding histology confirms a typical atherosclerotic plaque with the lipid core and fibrotic cap. Reprinted, with permission, from [32].

Atherogenic diet is one of the important environmental factors that may develop atherosclerosis. The shortest period when feeding minipigs a low percentage (2%) of cholesterol-containing diet in swine atherosclerosis models is three months. The superimposition of streptozotocin-induced diabetes onto the high-fat diet feeding of pigs has been used to induce complex atherosclerotic lesions in the first few centimeters of the coronary arteries without a major effect on plasma cholesterol levels. These lesions resemble human coronary lesions in complexity, with a thick fibrous cap, a necrotic lipid core, calcification, and hemorrhaging [1]. The locations of atherosclerotic lesions in these swine studies predominantly occur in coronary arteries and abdominal aortas [25, 26]. Nevertheless, it has been demonstrated that carotid arteries are generally spared of lesions in swine models. Carotid arteries in swine are quite straight at the neck and do not have major branches or curvatures that disturb the laminar blood flow pattern. Numerous studies suggest that disturbed flow patterns, particularly low or oscillatory wall shear stress, increase carotid artery susceptibility to atherosclerosis, whereas vessel regions exposed to high or laminar wall shear stress remain comparatively disease-free. A combination of hemodynamic instability with carotid arteries in hyperlipidemic swine can induce advanced atherosclerotic lesions [31].

Pig atherosclerosis, different from those of small animal models, generates usually quite slow. If allowed to develop over time, mild atherosclerotic lesions first appear in coronary arteries, and both atherosclerotic plaque distribution and composition (lipid, fibrinogen, smooth muscle cells, and macrophage content) follows a pattern comparable to those of humans. Humanlike pig lipoprotein metabolisms may help to explain, in part, the above mentioned similarities. Meanwhile, unlike other animal models, after gradual occlusion of the coronary vessels induced by both balloon injury and atherogenic diet, swine may develop the coronary restenosis syndrome as humans [25, 30].

The minipigs fed with high fat and cholesterol diet with sodium cholate (M-HFCD/SC) have an almost similar degree of atherosclerosis in the abdominal aorta, coronary arteries, aortic arch, pulmonary artery, and renal artery. The highest score for atherosclerosis is shown in the external and internal iliac arteries with M-HFCD/SC, which demonstrates thickening of the intima and arterial media. The thickest sections of the arteries display considerable foamy cell infiltration, extracellular lipid accumulation, and calcification. A fibrous cap is formed at the surface of the intima, at which collagen fiber proliferates while elastic fiber organization is widely damaged [25, 26].

Some authors demonstrated that aortic atherosclerotic lesions were significantly increased in the high cholesterol diet (HcD)-fed minipigs at all dietary cholesterol concentrations but unchanged in the NcD-fed controls. The atherosclerotic lesions developed first at the aortic arch and the entry of the spinal arteries and abdominal aorta, and progressed to involve the entire aorta as the cholesterol content in the HcD increased. The aortic atherosclerotic lesions were located in the intima with primary composition of infiltrated foam cells [26].

Some researchers had used a method, by combining extensive deep vascular injury with concomitant dietary hypercholesterolemia, to simulate and yield more advanced features in addition to intimal thickening. However, in such model, the high rate of acute thrombotic occlusion resulting from mechanical trauma remains a major drawback as the high expenses are encountered in working with such large laboratory animals [31]. This combination technique has been shown to induce intimal thickening in response to mechanical intimal-to-medial injury in virtually any sites within the vascular tree. However, several limitations are noted in this model. Atherosclerotic lesions usually lack advanced histologic features of "complicated atheroma," such as calcification, intraplaque hemorrhage, and necrotic cores, in contrast to lesions encountered in clinical practice [31].

Conclusion

A variety of animal models with arterial injury and atherosclerosis can be created for development of innovative diagnostic and therapeutic techniques to manage atherosclerotic cardiovascular disease, but none of them can replicate a human atherosclerotic plaque alike in the arteries.

Being aware of the biological and pathophysiological features of each arterial lesion on an animal model may be the pivotal step for selecting the appropriate animal model for specific research purposes. This chapter provides a comprehensive overview of the animal models with arterial intima injury or atherosclerosis, which is expected to be worthy of some help for the specialists in the scientific field of cardiovascular diseases, especially for selecting the suitable animal models for development of MRI-guided stem cell therapy.

References

[1] Getz GS, Reardon CA. Animal models of atherosclerosis. *Arterioscler Thromb Vasc Biol* 2012;32(5):1104-1115.

[2] Weber C, Noels H. Atherosclerosis: current pathogenesis and therapeutic options. *Nat Med* 2011;17(11):1410-1422.

[3] Chen YC, Bui AV, Diesch J, Manasseh R, Hausding C, Rivera J, et al. A novel mouse model of atherosclerotic plaque instability for drug testing and mechanistic/therapeutic discoveries using gene and microRNA expression profiling. *Circ Res* 2013;113(3):252-265.

[4] Kolodgie FD, Gold HK, Burke AP, Fowler DR, Kruth HS, Weber DK, et al. Intraplaque hemorrhage and progression of coronary atheroma. *N Engl J Med* 2003;349(24):2316-2325.

[5] Yao L, Heuser-Baker J, Herlea-Pana O, Iida R, Wang Q, Zou MH, et al. Bone marrow endothelial progenitors augment atherosclerotic plaque regression in a mouse model of plasma lipid lowering. *Stem Cells* 2012;30(12):2720-2731.

[6] Makowski MR, Forbes SC, Blume U, Warley A, Jansen CH, Schuster A, et al. In vivo assessment of intraplaque and endothelial fibrin in ApoE(-/-) mice by molecular MRI. *Atherosclerosis* 2012;222(1):43-49.

[7] Vilahur G, Padro T, Badimon L. Atherosclerosis and thrombosis: insights from large animal models. *J Biomed Biotechnol* 2011;2011(907575.

[8] Libby P, Ridker PM, Hansson GK. Progress and challenges in translating the biology of atherosclerosis. *Nature* 2011;473(7347):317-325.

[9] Xu Y, Arai H, Zhuge X, Sano H, Murayama T, Yoshimoto M, et al. Role of bone marrow derived progenitor cells in cuff-induced vascular injury in mice. *Arterioscler Thromb Vasc Biol* 2004;24(3):477-482.

[10] Revermann M, Schloss M, Barbosa-Sicard E, Mieth A, Liebner S, Morisseau C, et al. Soluble epoxide hydrolase deficiency attenuates neointima formation in the femoral cuff model of hyperlipidemic mice. *Arterioscler Thromb Vasc Biol* 2010;30(5):909-914.

[11] Gao F, Kar S, Zhang J, Qiu B, Walczak P, Larabi M, et al. MRI of intravenously injected bone marrow cells homing to the site of injured arteries. *NMR Biomed* 2007;20(7):673-681.

[12] Busnelli M, Froio A, Bacci ML, Giunti M, Cerrito MG, Giovannoni R, et al. Pathogenetic role of hypercholesterolemia in a novel preclinical model of vascular injury in pigs. *Atherosclerosis* 2009;207(2):384-390.

[13] Hosoda C, Hiroyama M, Sanbe A, Birumachi J, Kitamura T, Cotecchia S, et al. Blockade of both alpha1A- and alpha1B-adrenergic receptor subtype signaling is required to inhibit neointimal formation in the mouse femoral artery. *Am J Physiol Heart Circ Physiol* 2007;293(1):H514-519.

[14] Sata M, Saiura A, Kunisato A, Tojo A, Okada S, Tokuhisa T, et al. Hematopoietic stem cells differentiate into vascular cells that participate in the pathogenesis of atherosclerosis. *Nat Med* 2002;8(4):403-409.

[15] Sata M, Maejima Y, Adachi F, Fukino K, Saiura A, Sugiura S, et al. A mouse model of vascular injury that induces rapid onset of medial cell apoptosis followed by reproducible neointimal hyperplasia. *J Mol Cell Cardiol* 2000;32(11):2097-2104.

[16] Meng X, Zhang F, Valji K, Xie D, Gu H, Blair T, et al. Ultrasound guidance for the creation of a small animal model of aortic injury. *J Vasc Interv Radiol* 2011;22(8):1193-1197.

[17] Meng Y, Wang J, Sun J, Zhang F, Willis P, Li J, et al. 3.0-T MR imaging of intracoronary local delivery of motexafin gadolinium into coronary artery walls. *Radiology* 2013;268(2):556-562.

[18] Nam D, Ni CW, Rezvan A, Suo J, Budzyn K, Llanos A, et al. Partial carotid ligation is a model of acutely induced disturbed flow, leading to rapid endothelial dysfunction and atherosclerosis. *Am J Physiol Heart Circ Physiol* 2009;297(4):H1535-1543.

[19] Makowski MR, Botnar RM. MR imaging of the arterial vessel wall: molecular imaging from bench to bedside. *Radiology* 2013;269(1):34-51.

[20] Yanni AE. The laboratory rabbit: an animal model of atherosclerosis research. *Lab Anim* 2004;38(3):246-256.

[21] Wu X, Balu N, Li W, Chen Y, Shi X, Kummitha CM, et al. Molecular MRI of atherosclerotic plaque progression in an ApoE(-/-) mouse model with a CLT1 peptide targeted macrocyclic Gd(III) chelate. *Am J Nucl Med Mol Imaging* 2013;3(5):446-455.

[22] Lobbes MB, Miserus RJ, Heeneman S, Passos VL, Mutsaers PH, Debernardi N, et al. Atherosclerosis: contrast-enhanced MR imaging of vessel wall in rabbit model--comparison of gadofosveset and gadopentetate dimeglumine. *Radiology* 2009;250(3):682-691.

[23] Virmani R, Kolodgie FD, Burke AP, Farb A, Schwartz SM. Lessons from sudden coronary death: a comprehensive morphological classification scheme for atherosclerotic lesions. *Arterioscler Thromb Vasc Biol* 2000;20(5):1262-1275.

[24] Welch CL. Beyond genome-wide association studies: the usefulness of mouse genetics in understanding the complex etiology of atherosclerosis. *Arterioscler Thromb Vasc* Biol 2012;32(2):207-215.

[25] Kawaguchi H, Miyoshi N, Miura N, Fujiki M, Horiuchi M, Izumi Y, et al. Microminipig, a non-rodent experimental animal optimized for life science research:novel atherosclerosis model induced by high fat and cholesterol diet. *J Pharmacol Sci* 2011;115(2):115-121.

[26] Kawaguchi H, Yamada T, Miura N, Ayaori M, Uto-Kondo H, Ikegawa M, et al. Rapid Development of Atherosclerosis in the World's Smallest Microminipig Fed a High-Fat/High-Cholesterol Diet. J Atheroscler Thromb 2013;

[27] Liu Y, Pierce R, Luehmann HP, Sharp TL, Welch MJ. PET imaging of chemokine receptors in vascular injury-accelerated atherosclerosis. *J Nucl Med* 2013;54(7):1135-1141.

[28] Ronald JA, Chen JW, Chen Y, Hamilton AM, Rodriguez E, Reynolds F, et al. Enzyme-sensitive magnetic resonance imaging targeting myeloperoxidase identifies active inflammation in experimental rabbit atherosclerotic plaques. *Circulation* 2009;120(7):592-599.

[29] Phinikaridou A, Ruberg FL, Hallock KJ, Qiao Y, Hua N, Viereck J, et al. In vivo detection of vulnerable atherosclerotic plaque by MRI in a rabbit model. *Circ Cardiovasc Imaging* 2010;3(3):323-332.

[30] Miyoshi N, Horiuchi M, Inokuchi Y, Miyamoto Y, Miura N, Tokunaga S, et al. Novel microminipig model of atherosclerosis by high fat and high cholesterol diet, established in Japan. *In Vivo* 2010;24(5):671-680.

[31] Ishii A, Vinuela F, Murayama Y, Yuki I, Nien YL, Yeh DT, et al. Swine model of carotid artery atherosclerosis: experimental induction by surgical partial ligation and dietary hypercholesterolemia. *AJNR Am J Neuroradiol* 2006;27(9):1893-1899.

[32] Brushett C, Qiu B, Atalar E, Yang X. High-resolution MRI of deep-seated atherosclerotic arteries using motexafin gadolinium. *J Magn Reson Imaging* 2008;27(1):246-250.

In: Magnetic Resonance Imaging of Stem Cell Applications ISBN: 978-1-63463-910-1
Editor: Xiaoming Yang

Chapter 11

Magnetic Resonance Imaging of Stem Cell Application in Vasculatures*

Yanfeng Meng and Xiaoming Yang#*
Image-Guided Bio-Molecular Intervention Research, Department of Radiology,
Institute for Stem Cell and Regenerative Medicine,
University of Washington School of Medicine,
Seattle, Washington, US

Abstract

Regenerative medicine is one of the hottest scientific topics in modern medicine, aiming to treat the "roots" of different diseases. Recent progress in the field of cellular magnetic resonance imaging (MRI) has opened new avenues towards facilitating the regenerative medicine of vascular diseases. This chapter details the key components of cellular MRI in stem cell application in vasculatures, including the advanced techniques for magnetic labeling of stem cells, transplantation of these labeled cells, and MRI tracking of the cell migration/homing to the injured and atherosclerotic vessels for repair. In addition, the further efforts and potentials for translation of these new techniques from laboratory benches/small animals to preclinical suites/large animals, and ultimately to clinical practice in humans, will be addressed.

Keywords: MRI; atherosclerosis; stem cell; vasculature

Introduction

Atherosclerotic cardiovascular disease remains the leading cause of death worldwide [1]. One of the characteristic features of the disease is its diffuse involvement of arteries across

* This work is supported by a National Institutes of Health grant (R01EB012467).
# Corresponding author: Xiaoming Yang (xmyang@uw.edu).

the entire human body and the simultaneous presence of multiple atherosclerotic lesions or plaques. Surgical-based artery bypass grafting and percutaneous transarterial interventions are currently available methods for reducing the risk of myocardial infarction and stroke from atherosclerotic cardiovascular disease. However, these approaches have their drawbacks. Surgical grafting is an invasive approach, while percutaneous transarterial intervention only offers local treatment of limited numbers of atherosclerotic artery segments. Stem cell therapy is a frontier in modern medicine, and has three remarkable advantages in treatment of atherosclerosis and arterial injuries: (1) stem cells can automatically migrate into atherosclerotic or injured/ruptured lesion; (2) stem cells can differentiate to matured cells for repair; and (3) stem cells can transport nano-scaled agents or therapeutics for plaque-targeted imaging or therapy.

Recent studies have shown that stem cells can differentiate into smooth muscle cells (SMCs) and endothelial cells (ECs) of the vasculature [2, 3]. Furthermore, atherosclerotic lesion and injured artery can recruit circulating stem cells [4]. Clinical application of stem cell therapy requires methodologies that can monitor, in vivo, the migration to and tissue biodistribution of transplanted cells at the targets. Developments of cellular magnetic resonance imaging (MRI) technology have greatly facilitated the advances of stem cell applications in vascular diseases. These new MRI techniques enable labelling of the stem cells by MRI-detectable contrast agents, such as superparamagnetic iron-oxide (SPIO) agents [5-8]. Once they are magnetically labeled, stem cells can carry MR contrast agents specifically to the injured arteries or atherosclerotic lesions for specific cellular MRI of these targets.

MRI of Stem Cell-Based Repair of Injured Arteries

Arterial injury, which results in proliferation and migration of SMCs and thereafter neointimal hyperplasia, is a critical component of post-angioplasty/in-stent restenosis. The traditional method for assessing the successful migration of stem cells to the neointimal hyperplasia relies on staining of tissues obtained from invasive approaches, such as surgery, biopsy, or autopsy. For both basic science and clinical practice, it is essential to develop non-invasive imaging methods to monitor the trafficking of stem cells to the target vessels. Some authors reported their attempts on such development [9].

In their studies, the recipient mice were first irradiated with a sublethal dose to destroy their own bone marrows. Then, bone marrow-derived stem-progenitor cells from transgenic donor mice expressing β-galactosidase (LacZ) were labeled with Feridex, a SPIO nanoparticle contrast agent, which thereafter were systematically administered into the recipient mice. The unilateral femoral artery of each recipient mouse was mechanically injured by either a cuff-constricted approach or an endothelium-damaged approach [10, 11], while the contralateral femoral artery was not injured to serve as a control. In vivo visualization of the migrated Feridex/LacZ-labeled stem cells to the sites of injured arteries was performed using a 4.7 Tesla MR scanner, which detected large hypointense area at the site of the injured arteries, while no such signal change was detected in the controlled (uninjured) arteries (Figure 11.1). Subsequent histochemical staining confirmed

LacZ/Feridex-positive cells in the injured artery walls. This cellular MRI technique enables tracking of transplanted stem-progenitor cells in vivo.

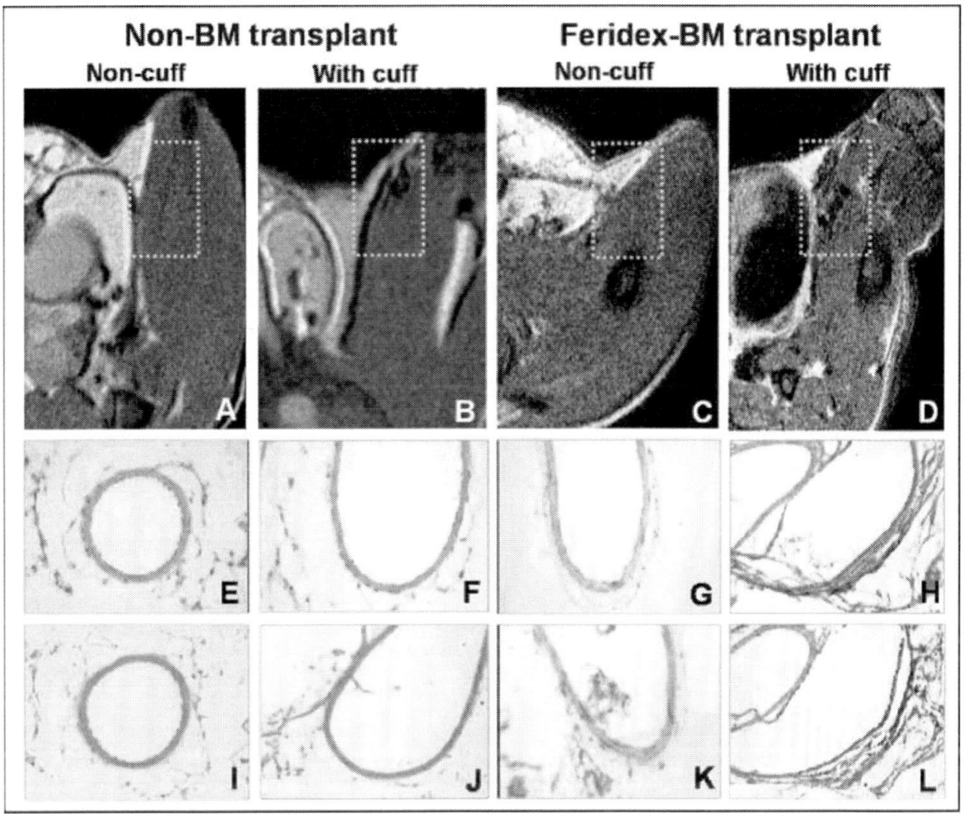

Figure 11.1. Upper panel: Cross sectional view of representative in vivo 4.7 T MR images of different arteries with various treatments (A–D). Images A and C are taken from the right legs of mice, which are vertically flipped for convenient comparison. Insets outline the femoral artery areas, showing larger hypointense areas at the site of the injured femoral artery in animal D with both Feridex-labeled stem cell transplantation and the cuff placement, whereas no such findings appear at the sites of the uninjured femoral arteries in animals A and C. In animal B, the cuff itself with circulated blood creates a small hypointense circle. Middle panel, Histochemical staining for iron with Prussian Blue (E–H). Lower panel: Histochemical staining for LacZ with X-gal (I–L). Numerous iron-positive cells (blue color on H) and LacZ-positive cells (blue color on L) are detected, which are not visualized in the control tissues (E–G and I–K). Original magnification 40X. Reprinted, with permission, from [9].

The MRI technique described above is based on allo-transplantation, which needs irradiation to destroy the immune system of the recipients for protection of the transplanted stem cells from immune rejection. This is not feasible in future clinical practice on humans. In order to avoid the immune rejection or immunosuppression and relief the side effect of allo-transplantation, scientists subsequently developed another new cellular imaging technique, MRI of auto-transplanted stem-progenitor cells [12]. The study of auto-transplantation of stem-progenitor cells was performed on near-human-sized animals, pigs. The unilateral iliofemoral artery was injured by pulling an overly-inflated Fogarty balloon or inflating a cutting balloon to injure the artery intima. One day after the endovascular intimal injury, Feridex and a fluorescent cell membrane dye, PKH26, were used to co-label bone marrow-derived stem-progenitor cells, which were harvested from the same pig with the iliofemoral artery injury. These Feridex/PKH26-labelled autologous cells were then intravenously administered back to the same pig. Three weeks after the cell transplantation, clinical 3 Tesla MRI was performed to detect the Feridex/PKH26-labeled cells migrated to the injured iliofemoral arteries. MRI detected hypointense area due to the successful migration of Feridex-labeled cells to the injured artery walls of auto-transplanted pigs, which were not seen in the control pigs transplanted with non-labeled stem-progenitor cells. Subsequent histology confirmed magnetic labeled cells migrated to the injured arteries, which matched the findings of MRI (Figure 11.2). These studies validate the feasibility of using cellular or clinical MRI to track the transplanted stem-progenitor cells that migrate to the injured arteries.

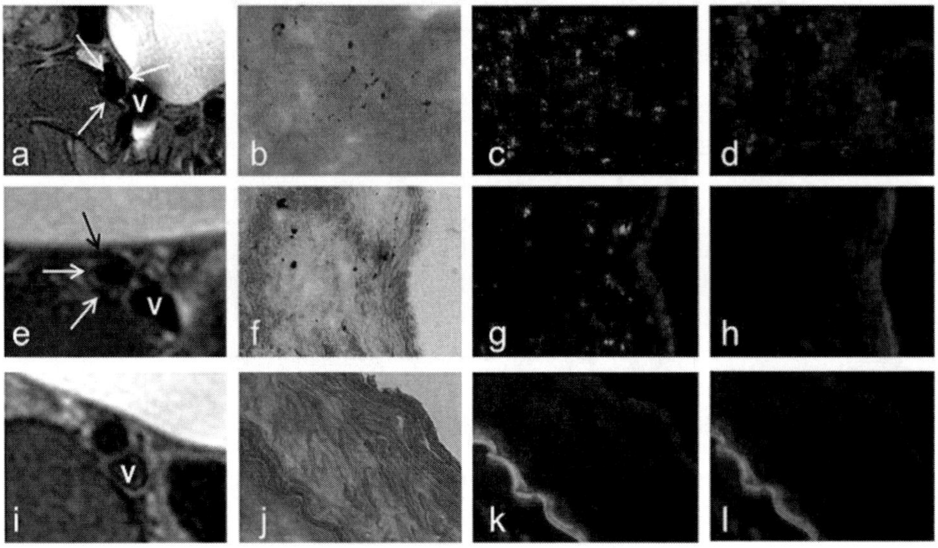

Figure 11.2. Representative MRI and corresponding histologic findings. (a–d) Animal group 1 with Feridex/PKH26-dual-labeled cell transplantation, showing MR signal void of the iliofemoral artery wall (arrows on a), where are confirmed by Prussian blue-positive cells (b), dextran-positive cells (c), and PKH26-positive cells (d), as blue and green as well as red spots or dots, respectively, in the artery wall. (e–h) Animal group 2 with Feridex-only-labeled cell transplantation, demonstrating MR signal void of the iliofemoral artery wall (arrows on e), which are confirmed by Prussian blue-positive cells (f), dextran-positive cells (g) and a negative PKH26 stain (h). (i–l) Animal group 3 (control group) with unlabeled cell transplantation or no cell transplantation, showing the intact artery wall on MRI (arrow on i), with a negative Prussian blue stain (j), a negative dextran stain (k), and a negative PKH26 stain (l). V = iliac vein. Reprinted, with permission, from [12].

MRI of Stem Cells Repair of Atherosclerotic Plaque

Atherosclerotic cardiovascular disease is a unique illness that produces diffuse and multiple lesions in nearly all arteries of the body. Different imaging techniques, such as digital subtraction angiography (DSA), computerized tomography (CT), ultrasound imaging, and MRI, have been used to localize and characterize atherosclerotic lesions. However, none of these imaging modalities are considered an ideal imaging tool for detecting atherosclerotic lesions in the early stage. Endovascular interventional procedures, such as angioplasty and stent placement, have been routinely used for the treatment of atherosclerotic arteries. These interventional techniques, however, function primarily as local therapies and thus do not enable the simultaneous treatment of diffuse and multiple atherosclerotic lesions around the entire body.

Stem cells can migrate to atherosclerotic arteries and differentiate into SMCs and ECs [2, 3, 11]. Intravenous transplanted stem cells circulate in the blood system, flow through the entire body, and can reach all atherosclerotic arteries. Thus, the characteristic of circulating stem cells with wide dissemination through the entire body may provide an approach for cell mediated therapy of multiple and diffuse atherosclerosis. Based on these principles, scientists developed a cellular MRI technique for tracking stem cell migration to the atherosclerotic plaques [13]. Atherosclerotic plaques were created on recipient $ApoE^{-/-}$ mice, which were fed with atherogenic diet to induce hyperlipidemia and subsequent atherosclerotic lesions. The recipient $ApoE^{-/-}$ mice received sublethal irradiation to destroy their own immune systems. Donor stem-progenitor cells were extracted from LacZ transgenic mice, labeled with Feridex, and then systemically transplanted into atherosclerotic recipient $ApoE^{-/-}$ mice [14].

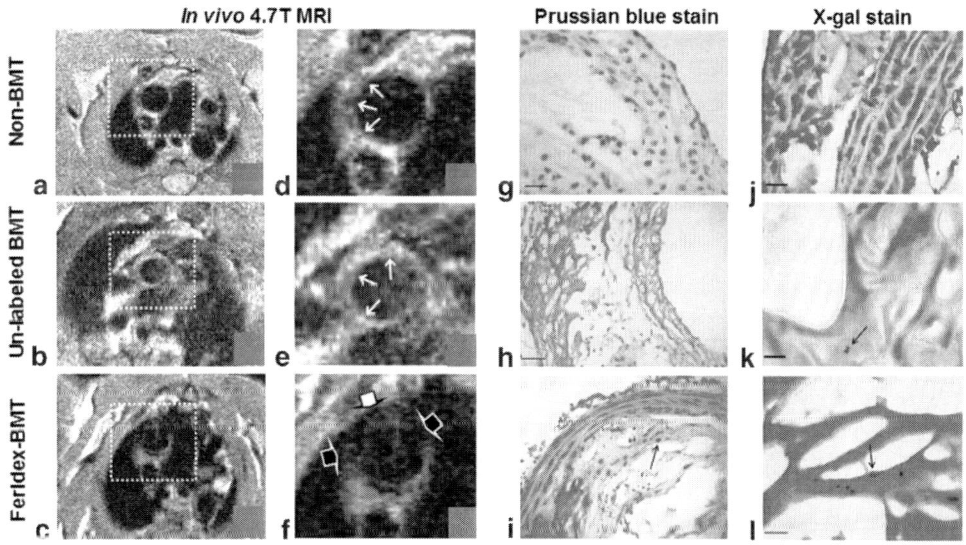

Figure 11.3. a–c: Cross-sectional view of representative in vivo 4.7T MR images of aortas from different $ApoE^{-/-}$ mice. Insets outline the ascending aorta, showing a large MR signal void of the aortic wall in animal (c) with Feridex-labeled stem cells, while the aortas of animals (a) and (b) appear as bright rings. d–f: Magnification of insets of (a– c). On images (d) and (e) (treated with no stem cell transplantation and unlabeled stem cell transplantation), the thickened aortic walls due to atherosclerotic plaques (arrows) are visualized and the aortic walls are basically shown as bright rings. On image (f) (treated with Feridex-labeled stem cells), larger signal voids (open arrows) of the aortic wall are seen. g–i: Histochemical staining for Feridex with Prussian blue (scale bar = 50 μm). j–l: Histochemical staining for LacZ with X-gal (scale bar = 20 μm). Numerous Feridex- and LacZ-positive cells (blue color, arrows) are detected in aortic tissues with stem cells (k, i, and l) that are not visualized in the control aortic tissues (g, j and h). Reprinted, with permission, from [13].

In vivo visualization of migrated Feridex/LacZ-cells to the atherosclerotic lesions of the aortas was performed on a 4.7 Tesla MR scanner, which showed atherosclerotic plaque can be detected, manifested as hypointense signals at the aortic walls due to Feridex-labeled stem cells migrated to the plaque. Subsequent histology confirmed the plaque formation, as well as stem cell accumulation in the plaque (Figure 11.3). These studies demonstrate the capability of using cellular or clinical MRI to monitor the transplantation of stem-progenitor cells that migrate to atherosclerotic lesions, which opens new avenues to develop new approaches for effective management of atherosclerotic cardiovascular disease.

MRI In Stem Cell-Mediated Gene Therapy of Atherosclerosis

Gene therapy is an exciting frontier in cardiovascular medicine [15-19]. The transfer of therapeutic gene into stem cells prior to their transplantation to the body may allow for the simultaneous treatment of diffuse and multiple atherosclerotic lesions through the stem cell mediated, plaque specific delivery of therapeutic genes. Interleukin 10 (IL-10) is proved to be able to reduce the atherosclerosis [20-22]. A recent study reported using cellular MRI to monitor stem cell-mediated IL-10 gene therapy of atherosclerosis [23].

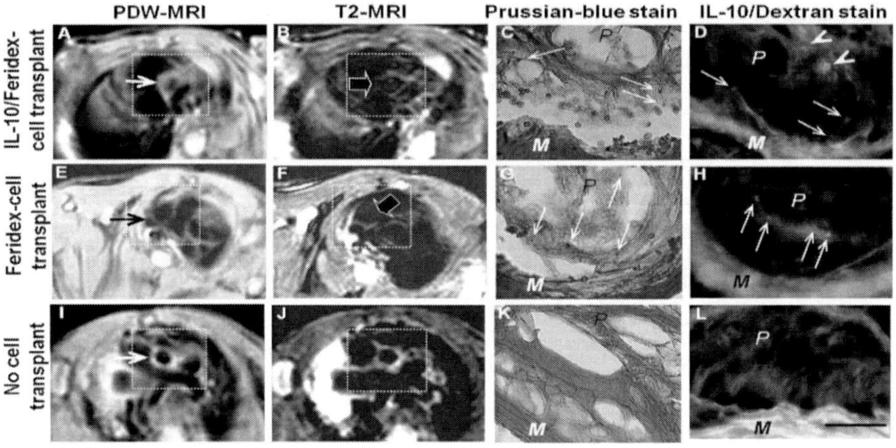

Figure 11.4. Representative MRI-histologic correlation of atherosclerotic ascending aorta (insets) of ApoE$^{-/-}$ mice. (A–D) ApoE$^{-/-}$ mice with IL-10/Feridex-stem cell transplantation. (E–H) ApoE$^{-/-}$ mice with Feridex-stem cell transplantation. (I–L) ApoE$^{-/-}$ mice with no cell transplantation as a control. (A, E, I) Proton-density-weighted (PDW) MRI shows thickening of the aortic walls due to formation of atherosclerotic lesions (arrows on A, E, I). (B, F, J) T2-weighted MRI shows signal voids (arrows on B and F) at the aortic walls with Feridex-labeled and/or IL-10-transduced stem cell transplantation, which are not seen in the aortic wall of the control group (J). (C, G, K) Prussian blue staining shows Feridex-positive stem cells migrated to the atherosclerotic aortic walls (arrows in C and G), which are not visualized in the aortic wall of the control group (K). (D, H, L) Immunofluorescent dual staining confirms simultaneous IL-10 gene expression (as red-colored spots, arrows on D), IL-10 overlap with dextran shells of Feridex particles (as orange-colored dots, arrowheads on D) and dextran shells of Feridex particles (as green-colored dots, arrows on H), which are not seen in the aortic wall of the control group (L). 400X. Bar: 100 mm. P = atherosclerotic plaque; M = medial. Blue color indicates nuclei. Reprinted, with permission, from [23].

In this study, authors transduced bone marrow-derived stem-progenitor cells with lentivirus-carrying IL-10 gene and then labeled the cells with Feridex. The transduced/labeled cells were systematically administered into recipient $ApoE^{-/-}$ mice with aortic atherosclerosis. MRI was performed to detect the migrated cells in atherosclerotic plaques, demonstrating Feridex-created signal voids around the atherosclerotic plaques of aorta. Subsequent histology confirmed Feridex labeled stem-progenitor cells really migrated into plaques, where there was presence of positive IL-10 expression from the transplanted cells by immunohistofluorescence examination (Figure 11.4). Most interestingly, the results also showed that the plaque size was significantly smaller than those with no gene transfer (Figure 11.5). Thus, it is feasible using cellular MRI to track IL-10/Feridex-stem cells migrating to atherosclerotic lesions, where IL-10 genes function to prevent or slow down the progression of atherosclerosis [23].

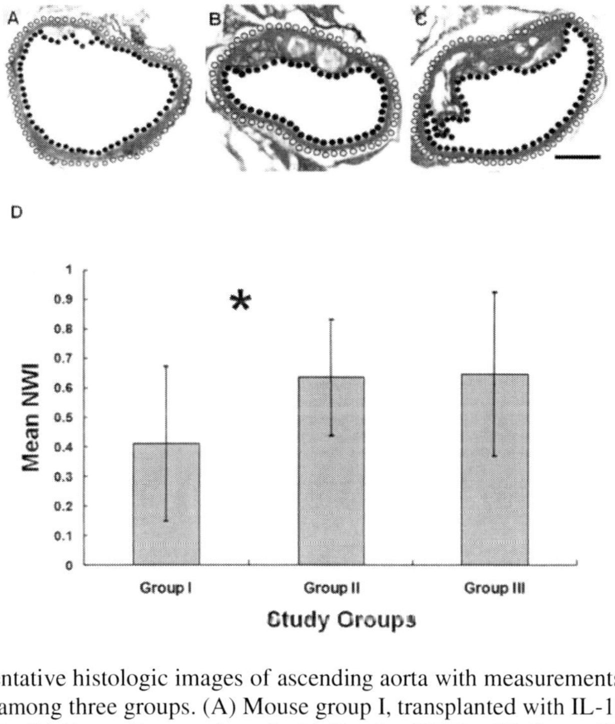

Figure 11.5. Representative histologic images of ascending aorta with measurements of normalized wall indexes (NWI) among three groups. (A) Mouse group I, transplanted with IL-10/Feridex-bone marrow cells (BMCs). (B) Group II, transplanted with Feridex-BMCs. (C) Group III with no cell transplantation. Yellow dotted line and black dotted lines outline the measured aortic wall area. Atherosclerotic plaques are clearly seen in groups II and III (B and C). 12.5 X. Bar: 200μm. (D) Comparison of NWIs among the three groups, demonstrating that the mean NWI of group I is significantly lower than those of the control group II and group III (* $P<0.05$), with no significant difference between two control groups II and III. Reprinted, with permission, from [23].

Conclusion

Cellular MRI is becoming a promising tool for non-invasive monitoring stem cell therapy of artery injury and atherosclerosis. Since auto-transplantation of stem cells can avoid immune rejection, the technique should be translatable to further clinical application. The tremendous efforts, as introduced in this chapter, have established groundwork to develop new techniques for effective management of multiple and diffuse distributed atherosclerotic cardiovascular disease, the number one killer worldwide, using MR-integrated stem cell therapy and stem cell-mediated gene therapy.

References

[1] Lloyd-Jones D, Adams RJ, Brown TM, Carnethon M, Dai S, De Simone G, et al. Heart disease and stroke statistics--2010 update: a report from the American Heart Association. *Circulation* 2010;121(7):e46-e215.

[2] Sata M, Saiura A, Kunisato A, Tojo A, Okada S, Tokuhisa T, et al. Hematopoietic stem cells differentiate into vascular cells that participate in the pathogenesis of atherosclerosis. *Nature medicine* 2002;8(4):403-409.

[3] Krause DS, Theise ND, Collector MI, Henegariu O, Hwang S, Gardner R, et al. Multi-organ, multi-lineage engraftment by a single bone marrow-derived stem cell. *Cell* 2001;105(3):369-377.

[4] Werner N, Nickenig G. Endothelial progenitor cells in health and atherosclerotic disease. *Annals of medicine* 2007;39(2):82-90.

[5] Shapiro EM, Sharer K, Skrtic S, Koretsky AP. In vivo detection of single cells by MRI. Magnetic resonance in medicine : official journal of the Society of Magnetic Resonance in Medicine / *Society of Magnetic Resonance in Medicine* 2006;55(2):242-249.

[6] Heyn C, Ronald JA, Mackenzie LT, MacDonald IC, Chambers AF, Rutt BK, et al. In vivo magnetic resonance imaging of single cells in mouse brain with optical validation. Magnetic resonance in medicine : official journal of the Society of Magnetic Resonance in Medicine / *Society of Magnetic Resonance in Medicine* 2006;55(1):23-29.

[7] Ruggiero A, Guenoun J, Smit H, Doeswijk GN, Klein S, Krestin GP, et al. In vivo MRI mapping of iron oxide-labeled stem cells transplanted in the heart. *Contrast media & molecular imaging.* 2013;8(6):487-494.

[8] Henning TD, Gawande R, Khurana A, Tavri S, Mandrussow L, Golovko D, et al. Magnetic resonance imaging of ferumoxide-labeled mesenchymal stem cells in cartilage defects: in vitro and in vivo investigations. *Molecular imaging* 2012;11(3):197-209.

[9] Gao F, Kar S, Zhang J, Qiu B, Walczak P, Larabi M, et al. MRI of intravenously injected bone marrow cells homing to the site of injured arteries. *NMR in biomedicine* 2007;20(7):673-681.

[10] Suzuki J, Iwai M, Nakagami H, Wu L, Chen R, Sugaya T, et al. Role of angiotensin II-regulated apoptosis through distinct AT1 and AT2 receptors in neointimal formation. *Circulation* 2002;106(7):847-853.

[11] Xu Y, Arai H, Zhuge X, Sano H, Murayama T, Yoshimoto M, et al. Role of bone marrow-derived progenitor cells in cuff-induced vascular injury in mice. *Arteriosclerosis, thrombosis, and vascular biology* 2004;24(3):477-482.

[12] Meng Y, Zhang F, Blair T, Gu H, Feng H, Wang J, et al. MRI of auto-transplantation of bone marrow-derived stem-progenitor cells for potential repair of injured arteries. *PloS one* 2012;7(2):e31137.

[13] Qiu B, Gao F, Walczak P, Zhang J, Kar S, Bulte JW, et al. In vivo MR imaging of bone marrow cells trafficking to atherosclerotic plaques. *Journal of magnetic resonance imaging : JMRI* 2007;26(2):339-343.
[14] Johnson J, Carson K, Williams H, Karanam S, Newby A, Angelini G, et al. Plaque rupture after short periods of fat feeding in the apolipoprotein E-knockout mouse: model characterization and effects of pravastatin treatment. *Circulation* 2005;111(11):1422-1430.
[15] Scimia MC, Gumpert AM, Koch WJ. Cardiovascular gene therapy for myocardial infarction. *Expert opinion on biological therapy* 2014;14(2):183-195.
[16] Wolfram JA, Donahue JK. Gene therapy to treat cardiovascular disease. *Journal of the American Heart Association* 2013;2(4):e000119.
[17] Yla-Herttuala S. Cardiovascular gene therapy with vascular endothelial growth factors. *Gene* 2013;525(2):217-219.
[18] Chen ZY, Lin Y, Yang F, Jiang L, Ge S. Gene therapy for cardiovascular disease mediated by ultrasound and microbubbles. *Cardiovascular ultrasound* 2013;11:11.
[19] Su CH, Wu YJ, Wang HH, Yeh HI. Nonviral gene therapy targeting cardiovascular system. *American journal of physiology Heart and circulatory physiology* 2012;303(6):H629-H638.
[20] Han X, Kitamoto S, Wang H, Boisvert WA. Interleukin-10 overexpression in macrophages suppresses atherosclerosis in hyperlipidemic mice. *FASEB journal: official publication of the Federation of American Societies for Experimental Biology.* 2010;24(8):2869-2880.
[21] Yoshioka T, Okada T, Maeda Y, Ikeda U, Shimpo M, Nomoto T, et al. Adeno-associated virus vector-mediated interleukin-10 gene transfer inhibits atherosclerosis in apolipoprotein E-deficient mice. *Gene therapy* 2004;11(24):1772-1779.
[22] Namiki M, Kawashima S, Yamashita T, Ozaki M, Sakoda T, Inoue N, et al. Intramuscular gene transfer of interleukin-10 cDNA reduces atherosclerosis in apolipoprotein E-knockout mice. *Atherosclerosis* 2004;172(1):21-29.
[23] Sun J, Li X, Feng H, Gu H, Blair T, Li J, et al. Magnetic resonance imaging of bone marrow cell-mediated interleukin-10 gene therapy of atherosclerosis. *PloS one* 2011;6(9):e24529.

In: Magnetic Resonance Imaging of Stem Cell Applications ISBN: 978-1-63463-910-1
Editor: Xiaoming Yang

Chapter 12

Magnetic Resonance Imaging in Clinical Application of Stem Cells: Current Status

Wayne L. Monsky*

Department of Radiology, University of Washington Medical Center, Seattle, Washington, US

Abstract

Stem cell therapy, with the potential to regenerate damaged tissue, is rapidly becoming a clinical reality. To be therapeutically efficacious, stem cells must successfully establish anatomic and physiologic function of the target organ. A sufficient number of the stem cells must accumulate and survive in the target organ. One key aspect of successful cell therapy is accurate injection into the target tissue. Without precise injection any therapy, no matter how sophisticated the approach, is guaranteed to fail. A number of imaging methods, including MRI, have been described for stem cell tracking and imaging of the stem cells at the target sites. Stem cell retention, migration and efficacy can be evaluated using cellular MRI. To date, it appears that only five clinical applications of MRI imaging of stem cell tracking and deposition as well as function have been described including; dendritic cell based cancer vaccines, traumatic brain injury, chronic spinal cord injury, multiple sclerosis/amyotrophic lateral sclerosis, and type 1 diabetes. The strengths and limitations of several techniques for these clinical applications have been described.

Keywords: Stem cell, MRI, tracking, clinical, in-vivo imaging

* Corresponding author: wmonsky@uw.edu

Introduction

An imaging technique for evaluation of stem cell therapy must have high spatial resolution and sufficiently high sensitivity and specificity to identify and map the fate of the stem cells. The ideal imaging method should permit noninvasive, longitudinal tracking of implanted cells, allowing long-term follow-up of tissue function and cellular survival, without affecting the cells or the target organ. Furthermore, it should enable a repeated and accurate assessment and should detect stem cell damage early enough to allow treatment. The contrast material, allowing imaging, must remain within viable cells and be rapidly cleared from tissue when stem cells die. A number of imaging approaches including Nuclear Medicine and MRI have been described. MRI is well suited for stem cell tracking, providing both whole-body and detailed images of the stem cells and targeted organ, with near microscopic anatomical resolution and excellent soft-tissue contrast. Super-paramagnetic iron oxide (SPIO) and ultra-small super-paramagnetic iron oxide (USPIO) have been used successfully to label stem cells for MRI. In this chapter, we will focus on MRI methods applied in the few clinical applications cited in the literature.

MRI Contrast Agents and Stem Cell Labeling

MRI contrast agents either alter the T1 and/or T2 relaxation time, making the local tissue hyper- or hypo-intense. The majority of the MR contrast agents used clinically is paramagnetic gadolinium-analogues ($Gd3+$-DTPA) or super-paramagnetic iron-oxide nanoparticles. Gadopentetate dimeglumine, the most widely used MRI contrast agent, is clinically safe because more than 99% of the dose is rapidly cleared and excreted by renal clearance. Its use for clinical MRI cell tracking is limited because stem cell labeling would result in long-term retention of gadopentetate dimeglumine in the body. Low pH in the lysosomes and endosomes of cells may lead to rapid dechelation. Free $Gd3+$ ions may result in nephrogenic systemic fibrosis [1]. Furthermore, intracellular gadopentetate dimeglumine has much reduced T1 relaxivity, and compartmentalization leads to local magnetic susceptibility effects that can produce ambiguous (e.g., positive vs negative) contrast enhancement [2]. Due to their biocompatibility and strong effect on T2 relaxation time, iron-oxide nanoparticles such as SPIO have been the MRI contrast agent of choice for cell labeling.

Superparamagnetic iron oxide (SPIO) particles are a different class of MRI contrast agent resulting in hypointense contrast enhancement [3]. One SPIO formulation, ferumoxides (Feridex, Bayer HealthCare), is FDA approved, as a liver contrast agent, which is taken up by Kupffer cells.

It has been used for clinical cell tracking. Ultra small superparamagnetic iron oxide (USPIO) are designed for longer blood half-life applications, such as lymph node imaging, and are much less efficient than SPIO in being taken up by cells after simple incubation. Prior to consideration of use of USPIO particles for stem cell tracking, USPIO particles had been used with success in clinical settings as an MRI contrast agent in patients with stroke [4] and for sentinel node identification in cancer patients [5].

Super-paramagnetic agents consist of an iron oxide core, typically 4-10 nm in diameter, containing several thousand iron atoms. A biocompatible polymer surrounds the core, providing stabilization. USPIOs are individual iron oxide surrounded by a polymer. These super-paramagnetic contrast agents provide predominantly a T2 effect, but smaller particles have shown to possess additional T1 properties [6]. A new class of USPIO known as cross-linked iron oxide (CLIO) can be conjugated to another agent by virtue of the dextran coat of the USPIO being cross-linked with an amine [7].

These contrast agents, used in clinical settings, were not designed for cellular internalization. Several strategies exist for SPIO labeling of cells. The easiest and safest method is spontaneous uptake of particles by phagocytic cells such as macrophages, microglia, and dendritic cells. For nonphagocytic cells, cationic (positively charged) transfection agents can be used to coat the anionic (negatively charged) ferumoxides particles using electrostatic interactions using poly-L-lysine [8, 9] or protamine sulfate [10] to allow for macropinocytosis and intra-cellular incorporation. Electroporation, electrical pulses, enable temporary membrane permeability without an additional compound [11, 12]. Strategies to optimize intracellular accumulation also include linking the nanoparticles to the highly cationic HIV-tat peptide [13] or a biological entity, such as an anti-transferrin receptor monoclonal antibody [14].

Pre-labeling of cells with SPIO has several limitations. Once cells die, the SPIO particles remain in and around dead cells. Misleading information is possible if macrophages or microglial cells phagocytize dying SPIO-labeled cells and actively move away from the site of cell implantation.

Furthermore, when cells divide rapidly after transplantation, SPIO is divided among daughter cell and the overall signal diminishes [15].

The limitation is based on the fact that the MRI signal depends on the presence of iron particles and not if the particles are actually still within the original labeled cells. Thus, the stem cells may not be viable or functional yet contrast related signal may still be present on MRI. This has been a major concern with this imaging method. Most pre-clinical studies have found that the labeled cells were still alive within the target tissue and not infiltrated by macrophages or monocytes [16-18]. Thus, phagocytic engulfment of injected cells seems uncommon.

An MR reporter gene that can serve as a beacon of cell survival and produce an even signal from cells regardless of the number of divisions, that is, a transfected gene product may avoid these limitations. However, this approach has not yet been well developed for clinical use. At the time this is written, only one clinical study has been performed with a reporter gene using PET scanning in a glioma patient who received autologous cytotoxic T cells transfected with the PET reporter gene herpes simplex virus thymidine kinase [19].

In most of the super paramagnetic cell tracking clinical studies the implanted cells were visible as hypointense areas on MRI in the entire follow-up period, between 16 and 26 months in longer studies. However, in most studies there was a gradual loss of the MRI intensity during the follow up period, which is to be expected as cell divisions and cell migration will dilute the contrast. How long super paramagnetic iron oxide labeled cells can actually be followed on MRI is still undetermined.

It is important to keep in mind that successful cell therapy depends on accurate injection into the target tissue. This was exemplified by the accidental misinjections in four of eight patients in the first clinical MRI cell tracking study [20].

This clinical study suggested the absolute necessity for monitoring in real time the actual anatomic accuracy of cell depositions. MRI-guided real-time cell injection with MRI labeled cells could allow this required precision during injection.

Clinical Applications

At the time this chapter is written, it appears there have been only five clinical studies in which stem cells were labeled and tracked using MRI.

Dendritic Cells for Melanoma Therapy

The first clinical application of this approach involved autologous dendritic cells labeled with a SPIO formulation (ferumoxides) or ^{111}In-oxine that were co-injected intra-nodally in the lymph nodes of 11 patients with advanced stage III melanoma, which has a poor prognosis and no other effective therapy [20] (Figure 12.1).

No secondary (transfection) agent was needed because immature dendritic cells are phagocytic by nature. Dendritic cells containing approximately 30 pg Fe/cell were used in 3-Tesla MRI performed with conventional pulse sequences [21]. A resolution of 0.5 × 0.5 × 3.5 mm was obtained with approximately 15,000 cells. The draining lymph node bed, into which the ferumoxides-labeled cells were injected, was resected after 2 weeks and histology of resected lymph nodes confirmed the presence of the original labeled cells. The SPIO-labeled cells were negative for the macrophage marker CD68, indicating that the SPIO positive cells were not macrophages. It was therefore suggested that the signal was not from phagocytosed, non-viable, stem cell.

The success of cellular therapies depends in part on accurate delivery of cells to target organs. In dendritic cell therapy, accurate delivery and subsequent migration of cells to regional lymph nodes is essential for effective stimulation of the immune system. De Vries et al. used in vivo cellular magnetic resonance tracking of magnetically labeled cells to detect very low numbers of dendritic cells in conjunction with detailed anatomical information. In contrast to scintigraphic imaging, MRI allows assessment of the accuracy of dendritic cell delivery and of inter- and intra-nodal cell migration patterns. MRI is superior to radionuclide imaging with regard to accurate detection of the number of nodes that contained injected dendritic cells because of its flexible three-dimensional (3D) multi-planar nature.

In general, the clinical benefit of cancer vaccine therapy varies widely. When cells are misinjected, there is no response because intrafollicular T cells must form rosettes with dendritic cells to become activated. Therefore, the need for a noninvasive technique that can be used to assess the accuracy of cell injections is clear. The study demonstrated feasibility to detect ferumoxides-labeled cells not only in the injected lymph node but also in nearby lymph nodes to which they migrate.

Neural Stem Cells for Brain Trauma

In a second clinical MRI study, two patients with traumatic brain injury received autologous neural stem cells, isolated after removal of brain tissue during emergency surgery, then labeled with ferumoxides [22]. Cells were stereotactically injected near the area of brain injury in one patient and 3T gradient-echo MR images obtained.

Over time, MRI detected dynamic changes in the hypointensity suggestive of movement of neural stem cells from the injection site to the border zone of the lesion. The signal intensity had disappeared completely 7 weeks after injection, as cells proliferated and daughter cells did not contain ferumoxide. No hypointensity was seen in the control subject, with brain trauma, who received unlabeled cells. Regeneration of damaged brain tissue with neural stem cells was suggested.

Following trauma, neural tissue from exposed brain was collected and cultured in a medium previously shown to select for neural stem cells. The day before implantation, cultured neural stem cells were incubated in Feridex, SPIO nanoparticles and Effectene (a lipofection reagent) in medium for 60 minutes, resulting in labeled stem cells. These cells were then implanted stereotactically around the region of brain damage. MRI with a 3.0-T system demonstrated marked signal dampening on T2-weighted MRI images, which were not seen before injection.

MRI demonstrated the injection sites as circular areas of dark tissue on the first day after implantation which faded thereafter. Cell accumulation and proliferation around the trauma site was seen at the periphery of the lesion and intensified during the second and third weeks, suggesting that the neural stem cells had migrated from the primary sites of injection to the border of the damaged tissue. However, no signal was seen after 7 weeks, due to cell proliferation and dilution of signal. MRI cell tracking was limited in the setting of traumatic injury, where hemorrhage is present since methemoglobin, exhibit significant hypointensity, making detection of further SPIO-induced loss of signal intensity difficult.

CD34(+) Bone Marrow Precursor Cells for Spinal Cord Injury

Callera et al. demonstrated the ability to deliver autologous bone marrow precursor cells, CD34(+), labeled with magnetic nanoparticles intrathecally via lumbar puncture technique (LP) in patients with chronic spinal cord injury (SCI), having sustained injury 2 or more years previously [23]. Sixteen patients with chronic SCI were divided into two groups. One group of 10 patients had 0.7 x 10 (range 0.45 to 1.22 x 10) labeled-CD34(+) cells injected into the spinal cord via LP. The control group of 6 patients received an LP spinal cord injection of magnetic beads without stem cells. CD34(+) cells were labeled with magnetic beads coated with a monoclonal antibody specific for the CD34 cell membrane antigen. Standard 1T, turbospin echo-T2 weighted sequence MRI was performed before as well as 20 and 35 days after transplantation.

Magnetically labeled CD34(+) cells were visible at the lesion site as hypointense signals in five patients at 20 and 35 days after transplantation of labeled-CD34(+) cells. However, these signals were not visible in any patient of the control group. Thus, the autologous bone marrow CD34(+) cells, labeled with magnetic nanoparticles, delivered via LP technique, migrated into the injured site in patients with chronic SCI. The labeled cells were not seen anywhere else in the central nervous system. The study focused on the capacity to perform MRI tracking and safety. However, clinical efficacy of the approach was not studied.

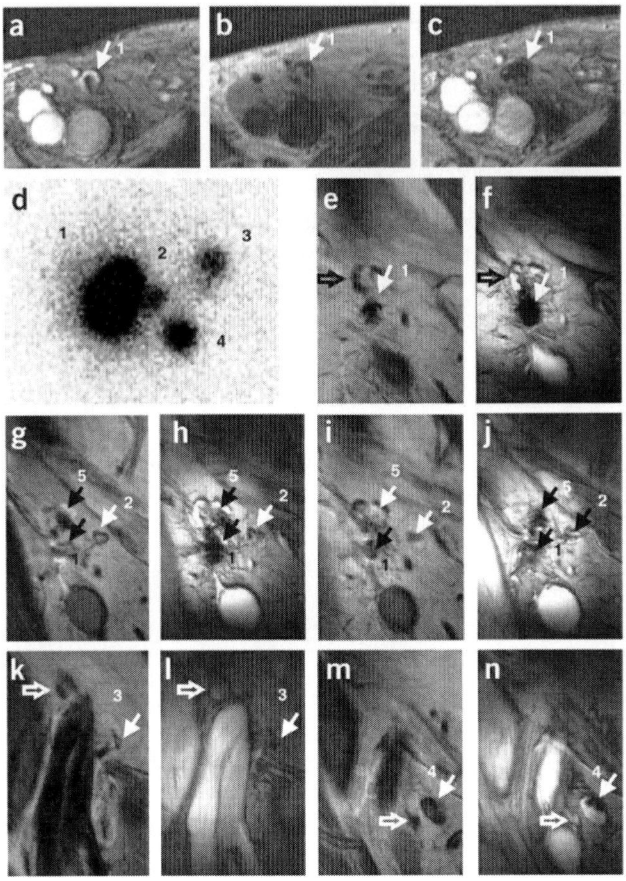

Figure 12.1. (a–c) Monitoring of the delivery of dendritic cells labeled with SPIO and ^{111}In by MRI before and after intranodal injection in a patient. (**a**) Gradient echo transversal magnetic resonance image before vaccination showing a right inguinal lymph node with a hyperintense signal area (1). (**b**) Spin echo (SE, technique much less sensitive for SPIO) transverse magnetic resonance image obtained from the same lymph node after vaccination. (**c**) Gradient echo transverse magnetic resonance images after vaccination in same position as **b** showing a decreased signal intensity of lymph node 1. (**d–n**) Monitoring of *in vivo* migration of SPIO and ^{111}In-labeled dendritic cells with MRI and scintigraphy after injection in a right inguinal lymph node in a patient. (**d**) *In vivo* scintigraphy 2 d after vaccination showing migration of the dendritic cells from the injection lymph node (1) to three following lymph nodes (2–4). (**e–n**) Five image pairs of a coronal gradient echo and SE image 2 d after vaccination showing migration of the dendritic cells from the injection lymph node 1 (**e** and **f**) to four following lymph nodes (**g–n**). Open arrows indicate lymph nodes that do not contain SPIO, on the SE images these nodes are dark-gray; on gradient echo images they are white. Closed arrows indicate lymph nodes that are positive for SPIO in the gradient echo magnetic resonance image. On gradient echo images SPIO-containing lymph nodes have a decreased signal intensity compared to SE images. The concentration of SPIO in lymph node 1 was very high, resulting even in a decreased signal intensity in the SE image. The lymph node that was identified by the scintigraphy as the injection lymph node (lymph node 1 in **d**) actually consisted of two distinct lymph nodes as evidenced by MRI (lymph nodes 1 and 5). Reprinted, with permission, from [20].

Islet cells for diabetes

The fourth clinical study using MRI for stem cell tracking was performed with human cadaveric islet cells, labeled with ferucarbotran and transplanted intraportally into the livers of four patients with type 1 diabetes [24]. Viability was first assessed by propidium iodide and fluorescein diacetate staining. In vivo function of both labeled and nonlabeled human islets was also assessed by transplanting the cells under the kidney capsule of athymic *nu/nu* (nude) diabetic mice.

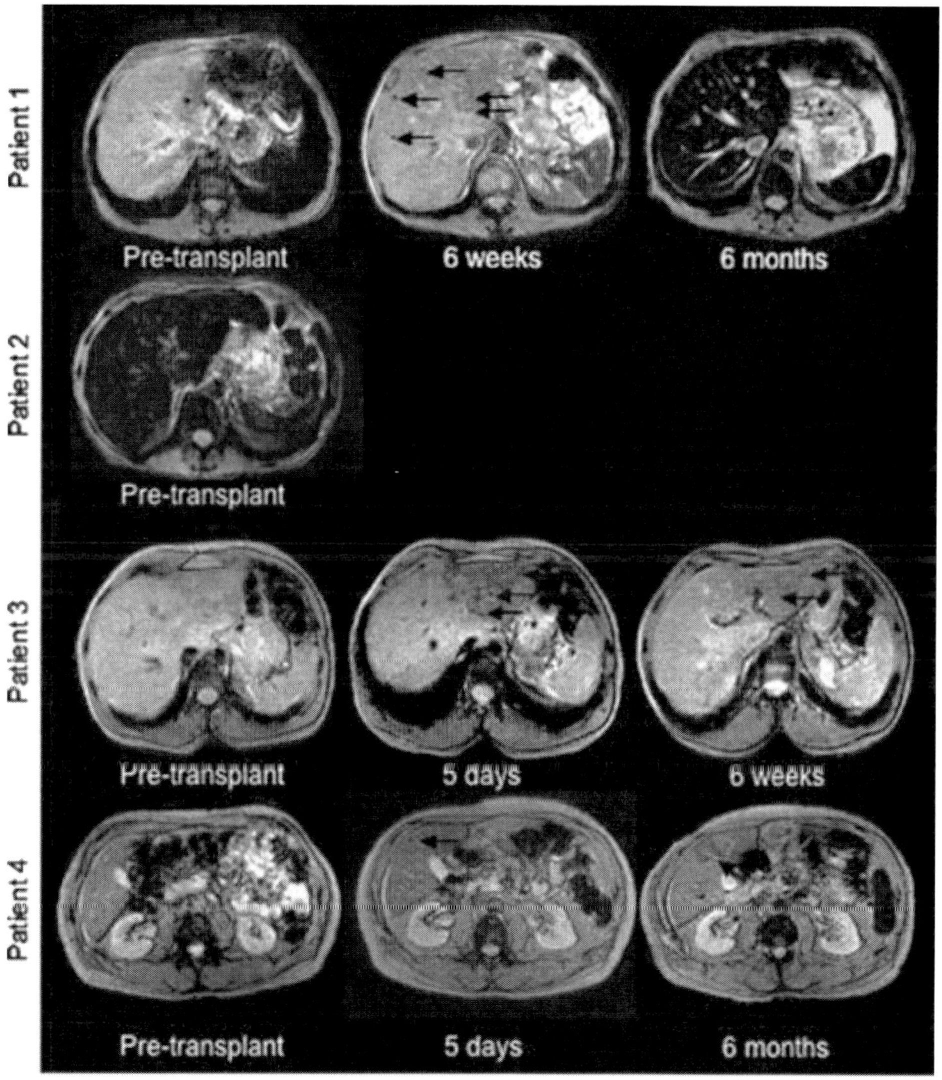

Figure 12.2. MRI images of patients 1–4 at various time points prior to and after transplant. The arrows indicate 'black spots' induced by iron-labeled islets. Reprinted, with permission, from [24].

T2*-weighted 1.5 T MRI was performed before and at 5 days, 6 weeks and 6 months after each transplant and whenever a significant metabolic event occurred. All patients became insulin-independent after transplantation, with normalized hemoglobin A1c (HbA1c) fewer than 6.5%. Insulin independence rates of approximately 10–15% were also demonstrated 5 years following transplantation. The liver exhibited normal signal intensity on pre-transplantation images, and iron-loaded islet cells were identified after transplantation as hypointense spots within the liver, in 3 of 4 patients, which were identified 6 months after transplantation (Figure 12.2). However the total number of hypointense spots, ranging from 3 to 138 in the first imaging after transplant, was much lower than the number of transplanted islet cells. There was no correlation between the number of injected islets and the number of spots. Therefore, MRI signal might represent clumps of cells. Furthermore, no clear correlation could be established between MRI signal and islet function.

The first patient had diffuse hypointense images on her baseline liver MRI, typical for spontaneous high iron content and transplant-related modifications could not be observed. In one patient, i.v. iron therapy prevented subsequent visualization of the spots because of diffuse hypointense liver background. Therefore, iron overload (spontaneous or induced) imposes a major obstacle to the technique.

Islet loss occurs in a two-step fashion. Early loss is linked to the low rate of engraftment. It is thought to be the result of damage during the isolation procedure or in the graft microenvironment within the liver, secondary to ischemia-reperfusion-like injury and to nonspecific inflammatory phenomena. Subsequent losses are usually more progressive, and are thought to involve allogeneic rejection, recurrence of autoimmunity, islet toxicity of the immunosuppressive drugs or 'exhaustion' of the islet graft.

Ideally, when imaging islet transplantation one should detect islet damage prior to a drop in serum C-peptide levels, an increase in fasting blood glucose levels, or the need to resume insulin. Animal studies have demonstrated that the iron contained in rejected cells is cleared from the liver, and MRI can detect a decrease in the number of spots at the time of rejection [25, 26]. However, this was not clearly seen in the clinical cases.

Mesenchymal Stem Cells for Multiple Sclerosis and Amyotropic Lateral Sclerosis

Previous efforts using various neuroprotective agents in progressive Multiple Sclerosis (MS) and Amyotropic Lateral Sclerosis (ALS) have not proven successful. Multipotential stem cells were hypothesized to be able to migrate locally into damaged central nervous system (CNS) areas where they could support local neurogenesis or myelogenesis through neurotrophic effects, stimulation of resident CNS stem cells, induction of in situ immunomodulation, or, theoretically, even transdifferentiation [27]. Mesenchymal stem cells (MSCs) are bone marrow–derived stem cells that normally generate osteocytes, adipocytes, and chondrocytes [28]. Mesenchymal stem cells have also been shown to possess immunomodulation properties, inducing suppression of various immune cell populations [29]. They can also give rise to neural-like, glial-like, and astrocytic-like cells in vitro [30]. In rats, mesenchymal stem cells migrated into the CNS, where they promoted brain-derived neurotrophic factor production and induced proliferation of a limited number of oligodendrocyte progenitors. Similar beneficial clinical effects of MSC transplantation were described in models of stroke and trauma [31].

Karussis et al. sought to evaluate the feasibility, safety, and immunological effects of intrathecal and intravenous administration of autologous MSCs in patients with multiple sclerosis and amyotrophic lateral sclerosis [27]. MSCs were injected, intrathecally (n = 34) and intravenously (n = 14), in 15 patients with multiple sclerosis and 19 patients with amyotrophic lateral sclerosis [27]. In nine cases, MSCs were magnetically labeled with the SPIO ferumoxides (Feridex) to track cell migration after local grafting [32]. Follow-up (≤25 months) included; MRI to exclude unexpected pathologies and to track the labeled stem cells, as well as evaluation of adverse events, neurological disability assessment by means of the Expanded Disability Status Scale (EDSS), and immunological tests to assess immunomodulatory effects.

Bone marrow aspiration yielded 200 mL of bone from each patient. Patients with MS received a mean of 63.2×10^6 cells; patients with ALS received 54.7×10^6. To label MSCs, ferumoxide was complexed with the cationic polymer poly-L-lysine, and the cells were incubated for 24 to 48 hours. MRI was performed within 4 to 48 hours after MSC infusion and again after 1 month and 3 to 6 months. All MRIs were performed at 1.5 T, with the exception of one performed at 3 T, using standard T1-, T2-, diffusion-, and postgadolinium T1–weighted sequences. During the 6-month follow-up no significant unexpected pathology was seen on MRI.

In those injected with labeled stem cells, hypointense signal, on T2-weighted images, indicated the presence of ferumoxides-positive cells. These cells were detected in the meninges of the spinal cord and nerve roots and in the spinal cord parenchyma [27]. In 1 patient, 3-T brain MRI, performed 18 hours after infusion, showed dependent layering of the intrathecally delivered cells in the occipital horns of the ventricles, suggesting dissemination of MSCs from the injection site to the occipital horns, meninges, spinal roots, and spinal cord parenchyma. No major adverse effects were reported during follow-up. The mean ALS Functional Rating Scale (ALSFRS) score remained stable during the first 6 months of observation, whereas the mean (SD) Expanded Disability Status Scale (EDSS) score improved from 6.7 (1.0) to 5.9 (1.6).

The intrathecal approach for cell-based therapies in neurological diseases, in which the areas of tissue damage are widespread throughout the neuroaxis, may increase the possibility of migration of the injected cells to the proximity of the CNS lesions. Circulating with the flow of the cerebrospinal fluid, stem cells may have a better chance of reaching the affected CNS areas. Intravenous injection may be equally effective because MSCs exert peripheral immune-modulating effects and may also migrate through the blood to the damaged areas of the CNS after receiving inflammatory signals [33]. However, the optimal route of stem cell delivery in patients with neurological diseases remains debatable. A possible drawback of the intravenous administration of MSCs is that most of the cells injected into the blood will home to the lungs, lymph nodes, and other reticuloendothelial system tissues, greatly reducing the number of cells available to migrate to the CNS. However, intrathecal delivery of cells may focus their immunomodulatory and trophic effects directly on the CNS. This could also be evaluated further with MRI.

Conclusion

Stem cell therapies offer great promise in a wide range of diseases. Magnetic resonance imaging of labeled stem cells allow non-invasive longitudinal tracking of the transplanted stem cells. The fate and longevity of the stem cells, injected distant to the target site, can be determined. Furthermore, MRI can be used for guidance during stem cell delivery. To date, only five clinical studies have been conducted utilizing MRI imaging of labeled stem cells. The studies suggest safety and efficacy of the approach. It is likely that stem cell therapy will become more common-place in clinical practice. An understanding of stem cell labeling techniques, imaging approaches and findings is important to the success of this therapeutic strategy.

References

[1] Thomsen HS. Nephrogenic systemic fibrosis: A serious late adverse reaction to gadodiamide. *Eur. Radiol.* 2006;16(12):2619-2621.

[2] Bulte JW. In vivo MRI cell tracking: clinical studies. *AJR Am. J. Roentgenol* 2009;193(2):314-325.

[3] Bulte JW, Kraitchman DL. Iron oxide MR contrast agents for molecular and cellular imaging. *NMR Biomed.* 2004;17(7):484-499.

[4] Nighoghossian N, Wiart M, Cakmak S, Berthezene Y, Derex L, Cho TH, et al. Inflammatory response after ischemic stroke: a USPIO-enhanced MRI study in patients. *Stroke* 2007;38(2):303-307.

[5] Dinniwell R, Chan P, Czarnota G, Haider MA, Jhaveri K, Jewett M, et al. Pelvic lymph node topography for radiotherapy treatment planning from ferumoxtran-10 contrast-enhanced magnetic resonance imaging. *Int. J. Radiat Oncol. Biol. Phys.* 2009;74(3):844-851.

[6] Sophie Laurent, Luce Vander Elst, Muller RN. Superparamagnetic Iron Oxide Nanoparticles for MRI, in: *The Chemistry of Contrast Agents in Medical Magnetic Resonance Imaging*. 2rd ed. André E Merbach, Lothar Helm, Tóth, Éva, 2013;427-444.

[7] Wunderbaldinger P, Josephson L, Weissleder R. Crosslinked iron oxides (CLIO): a new platform for the development of targeted MR contrast agents. *Acad Radiol.* 2002;9 Suppl 2(S304-306.

[8] Frank JA, Miller BR, Arbab AS, Zywicke HA, Jordan EK, Lewis BK, et al. Clinically applicable labeling of mammalian and stem cells by combining superparamagnetic iron oxides and transfection agents. *Radiology* 2003;228(2):480-487.

[9] Bulte JW, Arbab AS, Douglas T, Frank JA. Preparation of magnetically labeled cells for cell tracking by magnetic resonance imaging. *Methods Enzymol* 2004;386:275-299.

[10] Arbab AS, Yocum GT, Kalish H, Jordan EK, Anderson SA, Khakoo AY, et al. Efficient magnetic cell labeling with protamine sulfate complexed to ferumoxides for cellular MRI. *Blood* 2004;104(4):1217-1223.

[11] Walczak P, Kedziorek DA, Gilad AA, Lin S, Bulte JW. Instant MR labeling of stem cells using magnetoelectroporation. *Magn Reson Med.* 2005;54(4):769-774.

[12] Gilad AA, Walczak P, McMahon MT, Na HB, Lee JH, An K, et al. MR tracking of transplanted cells with "positive contrast" using manganese oxide nanoparticles. *Magn Reson Med.* 2008;60(1):1-7.

[13] Josephson L, Tung CH, Moore A, Weissleder R. High-efficiency intracellular magnetic labeling with novel superparamagnetic-Tat peptide conjugates. *Bioconjug Chem* 1999;10(2):186-191.

[14] Bulte JW, Zhang S, van Gelderen P, Herynek V, Jordan EK, Duncan ID, et al. Neurotransplantation of magnetically labeled oligodendrocyte progenitors: magnetic resonance tracking of cell migration and myelination. *Proc. Natl. Acad. Sci. USA* 1999;96(26):15256-15261.

[15] Walczak P, Kedziorek DA, Gilad AA, Barnett BP, Bulte JW. Applicability and limitations of MR tracking of neural stem cells with asymmetric cell division and rapid turnover: the case of the shiverer dysmyelinated mouse brain. *Magn. Reson. Med.* 2007;58(2):261-269.

[16] Stuckey DJ, Carr CA, Martin-Rendon E, Tyler DJ, Willmott C, Cassidy PJ, et al. Iron particles for noninvasive monitoring of bone marrow stromal cell engraftment into, and isolation of viable engrafted donor cells from, the heart. *Stem Cells* 2006;24(8):1968-1975.

[17] Yang K, Xiang P, Zhang C, Zou L, Wu X, Gao Y, et al. Magnetic resonance evaluation of transplanted mesenchymal stem cells after myocardial infarction in swine. *Can. J. Cardiol.* 2011;27(6):818-825.

[18] Ma GS, Qi CM, Liu NF, Shen CX, Chen Z, Liu XJ, et al. Efficiently tracking of stem cells in vivo using different kinds of superparamagnetic iron oxide in swine with myocardial infarction. *Chin. Med. J.* (Engl) 2011;124(8):1199-1204.

[19] Tjuvajev JG, Stockhammer G, Desai R, Uehara H, Watanabe K, Gansbacher B, et al. Imaging the expression of transfected genes in vivo. *Cancer Res.* 1995;55(24):6126-6132.

[20] de Vries IJ, Lesterhuis WJ, Barentsz JO, Verdijk P, van Krieken JH, Boerman OC, et al. Magnetic resonance tracking of dendritic cells in melanoma patients for monitoring of cellular therapy. *Nat. Biotechnol.* 2005;23(11):1407-1413.

[21] Verdijk P, Scheenen TW, Lesterhuis WJ, Gambarota G, Veltien AA, Walczak P, et al. Sensitivity of magnetic resonance imaging of dendritic cells for in vivo tracking of cellular cancer vaccines. *Int. J. Cancer* 2007;120(5):978-984.

[22] Zhu J, Zhou L, XingWu F. Tracking neural stem cells in patients with brain trauma. *N. Engl. J. Med.* 2006;355(22):2376-2378.

[23] Callera F, de Melo CM. Magnetic resonance tracking of magnetically labeled autologous bone marrow CD34+ cells transplanted into the spinal cord via lumbar puncture technique in patients with chronic spinal cord injury: CD34+ cells' migration into the injured site. *Stem Cells Dev.* 2007;16(3):461-466.

[24] Toso C, Vallee JP, Morel P, Ris F, Demuylder-Mischler S, Lepetit-Coiffe M, et al. Clinical magnetic resonance imaging of pancreatic islet grafts after iron nanoparticle labeling. *Am. J. Transplant* 2008;8(3):701-706.

[25] Kriz J, Jirak D, Girman P, Berkova Z, Zacharovova K, Honsova E, et al. Magnetic resonance imaging of pancreatic islets in tolerance and rejection. *Transplantation* 2005;80(11):1596-1603.

[26] Evgenov NV, Medarova Z, Pratt J, Pantazopoulos P, Leyting S, Bonner-Weir S, et al. In vivo imaging of immune rejection in transplanted pancreatic islets. *Diabetes* 2006;55(9):2419-2428.

[27] Karussis D, Karageorgiou C, Vaknin-Dembinsky A, Gowda-Kurkalli B, Gomori JM, Kassis I, et al. Safety and immunological effects of mesenchymal stem cell transplantation in patients with multiple sclerosis and amyotrophic lateral sclerosis. *Arch. Neurol.* 2010;67(10):1187-1194.

[28] Pittenger MF, Mackay AM, Beck SC, Jaiswal RK, Douglas R, Mosca JD, et al. Multilineage potential of adult human mesenchymal stem cells. *Science* 1999;284(5411):143-147.

[29] Tse WT, Pendleton JD, Beyer WM, Egalka MC, Guinan EC. Suppression of allogeneic T-cell proliferation by human marrow stromal cells: implications in transplantation. *Transplantation* 2003;75(3):389-397.

[30] Woodbury D, Schwarz EJ, Prockop DJ, Black IB. Adult rat and human bone marrow stromal cells differentiate into neurons. *J. Neurosci. Res.* 2000;61(4):364-370.

[31] Chen J, Li Y, Wang L, Lu M, Zhang X, Chopp M. Therapeutic benefit of intracerebral transplantation of bone marrow stromal cells after cerebral ischemia in rats. *J. Neurol. Sci.* 2001;189(1-2):49-57.

[32] Cunningham CH, Arai T, Yang PC, McConnell MV, Pauly JM, Conolly SM. Positive contrast magnetic resonance imaging of cells labeled with magnetic nanoparticles. *Magn. Reson. Med.* 2005;53(5):999-1005.

[33] Long CM, Bulte JW. In vivo tracking of cellular therapeutics using magnetic resonance imaging. *Expert Opin. Biol. Ther.* 2009;9(3):293-306.

Index

A

acid, 13, 17, 151
acidic, 53
acute myelogenous leukemia, 133
acute myeloid leukemia, 13, 17, 122, 131
acute promyelocytic leukemia, 17
ADC, 112
adhesion, 108, 113, 166
adipose tissue, 129
adsorption, 141
adult stem cells, 5, 83, 86, 138
advancement(s), 81, 139, 153
adventitia, 163
adverse conditions, 4
adverse effects, 195
adverse event, 195
age, 4, 166, 168
aggregation, 23, 107, 166
albumin, 107
ALS, 10, 194, 195
American Heart Association, 167, 184, 185
amine, 66, 189
mino acid(s), 66
amplitude, 28, 30
amyotrophic lateral sclerosis, 96, 187, 195, 198
anatomy, 34, 81, 170
angiogenesis, 128, 135
angiography, 72, 181
angioplasty, 138, 160, 161, 178, 181
angiotensin II, 184
antibody, 53, 60, 106, 108, 129, 141, 164
antigen, 35, 40, 42, 103, 108, 129, 162, 191
anus, 35
aorta, 42, 162, 163, 164, 165, 168, 170, 171, 172, 181, 182, 183
apoptosis, 36, 92, 122, 148, 166, 174, 184
aromatic rings, 46
arterial vessels, 165
artery(s), 84, 86, 96, 111, 152, 159, 160, 161, 162, 163, 164, 165, 166, 168, 169, 170, 171, 172, 173, 174, 175, 177, 178, 179, 180, 181, 183, 184
arthritis, 23, 40
ascending colon, 35
aspartic acid, 91
aspirate, 5
aspiration, 195
assessment, 14, 38, 55, 58, 59, 71, 79, 86, 92, 117, 118, 124, 125, 127, 128, 140, 173, 188, 190, 195
asymptomatic, 166
atherogenesis, 167, 168, 169
atherosclerosis, 54, 68, 72, 78, 159, 160, 165, 166, 167, 168, 169, 170, 171, 172, 173, 174, 175, 177, 178, 181, 182, 183, 184, 185
atherosclerotic plaque, 23, 40, 159, 160, 165, 166, 168, 169, 171, 172, 173, 174, 181, 182, 183, 185
atoms, 46, 48, 189
autoimmune disease(s), 15, 84
autoimmune hepatitis, 106
autoimmunity, 193
autopsy, 106, 178
axons, 24

B

back pain, 84
bacteria, 64, 65, 77
balloon angioplasty, 161
bandwidth, 30, 31
barium, 20
barriers, 53, 81, 82, 85
benefits, x, 34, 42, 83, 90, 163
biocompatibility, 93, 107, 108, 139, 141, 148, 188

biodistribution, ix, 47, 89, 90, 95, 96, 99, 137, 139, 178
biological activity, 142
biological processes, 94, 107, 133, 140
bioluminescence, 20, 58, 90, 91, 106, 119, 125, 127, 133, 139, 140, 142, 146, 147, 151, 158
biomarkers, 125, 133
biomedical applications, 120, 134
biomedical imaging, ix
biopsy, 90, 106, 129, 178
biotechnology, 114
bleeding, 84
blood, ix, 4, 5, 13, 15, 27, 29, 34, 37, 49, 69, 72, 78, 83, 84, 93, 98, 101, 107, 123, 125, 126, 128, 162, 165, 166, 169, 171, 179, 181, 188, 193, 195
blood flow, 162, 165, 169, 171
blood plasma, 49
blood stream, 107, 125
blood supply, ix
blood vessels, 37, 83, 166
bloodstream, 5
body size, 170
body weight, 169
bone, ix, 3, 4, 5, 6, 7, 8, 9, 15, 16, 23, 27, 42, 82, 83, 84, 85, 86, 97, 100, 102, 103, 109, 110, 112, 114, 117, 123, 129, 131, 132, 142, 146, 148, 153, 154, 156, 157, 163, 164, 173, 178, 180, 183, 184, 185, 191, 194, 195, 197, 198
bone cells, 9
bone marrow, ix, 3, 4, 5, 6, 15, 16, 23, 27, 42, 82, 83, 84, 85, 97, 100, 102, 103, 109, 110, 112, 114, 117, 123, 129, 131, 132, 142, 146, 153, 154, 156, 157, 163, 164, 173, 178, 180, 183, 184, 185, 191, 194, 197, 198
bone marrow aspiration, 4
bone marrow transplant, 4, 5, 123, 131
bowel, 35, 112
brain, 4, 8, 23, 24, 27, 28, 36, 39, 43, 44, 52, 59, 65, 66, 68, 72, 73, 78, 90, 95, 96, 97, 99, 102, 103, 127, 129, 154, 155, 157, 184, 191, 195, 197
brain damage, 23, 191
brain tumor, 95, 103
brainstorming, xi
breakdown, 166
breast cancer, 13, 64, 123, 127, 133
breast carcinoma, 131
breeding, 167
building blocks, ix
burn, 7
bypass graft, 178

C

Ca^{2+}, 167
CAD, 153
calcification, 167, 171, 172
calcium, 92, 140, 167
calibration, 28
cancer, x, 3, 4, 10, 11, 12, 13, 14, 15, 17, 35, 54, 63, 64, 117, 118, 119, 120, 121, 122, 123, 124, 125, 126, 127, 129, 130, 131, 132, 133, 141, 157, 187, 188, 190, 197
cancer cells, 13, 14, 35, 64, 117, 119, 120, 124, 125, 127
cancer progression, 118, 124
cancer stem cells, 4, 11, 12, 13, 14, 117, 118, 123, 124, 132
cancer therapy, 13, 125, 126, 130, 131
candidates, 138, 140, 141
capsule, 83, 193
carboxyl, 143
carcinogenesis, 118
carcinoma, 123, 133
cardiac activity, 151
cardiomyocytes, ix, 5, 6, 10, 25
cardiovascular disease(s), 101, 137, 138, 140, 145, 151, 152, 153, 159, 160, 168, 172, 177, 180, 182, 184, 185
cardiovascular system, 141, 185
caregivers, 4
carotid arteries, 171
cartilage, 7, 8, 184
castration, 133
catheter, 82, 83, 161, 162
cDNA, 128, 185
cell biology, 11, 13, 53, 89
cell culture, 8, 9, 10, 49, 92, 142
cell cycle, 12
cell death, 60, 92, 95, 97, 110
cell differentiation, 10, 37, 52, 94, 107
cell division, 20, 21, 22, 36, 38, 43, 62, 73, 94, 97, 139, 157, 189, 197
cell fate, 139
cell labeling, x, 14, 21, 23, 45, 46, 48, 49, 50, 51, 52, 53, 54, 55, 57, 58, 59, 60, 61, 62, 70, 73, 75, 97, 107, 108, 119, 128, 133, 134, 135, 142, 144, 145, 148, 155, 156, 188, 196, 197
cell line(s), 4, 60, 66, 83, 86, 124, 127, 132, 143, 148
cell membranes, 21, 48, 49, 50
cell metabolism, 128
cell size, 143
cell surface, 5, 59, 60, 73, 129, 141
cellular regulation, 79

central nervous system (CNS), 7, 23, 89, 90, 96, 99, 123, 192, 194, 195
cerebral arteries, 96
cerebrospinal fluid, 95, 98, 195
challenges, ix, 13, 17, 19, 20, 38, 69, 82, 89, 105, 130, 138, 139, 152, 154, 173
chelates, 20, 21, 93
chemical(s), x, xi, 10, 35, 39, 47, 48, 54, 58, 59, 62, 64, 71, 73, 75, 76, 77, 93, 94, 103, 134
chemical properties, 35, 39
chemical structures, 47
chemokine receptor, 123, 174
chemokines, 123, 166
chemotherapeutic agent, 86, 124
chemotherapy, 12, 13, 17, 86, 117, 118, 120, 122, 129, 154
China, v, xiv, xv, xvi, 97, 105
cholesterol, 166, 168, 169, 170, 171, 172, 174, 175
chromosome, 13
circulation, 6, 83, 86
cirrhosis, 106
classes, 92, 148
classification, 174
cleavage, 64
clinical application, xi, 3, 9, 11, 15, 16, 34, 39, 46, 51, 52, 53, 62, 92, 95, 97, 120, 124, 125, 131, 138, 139, 144, 154, 183, 187, 188, 190
clinical diagnosis, 14
clinical trials, ix, x, 6, 11, 14, 26, 89, 90, 99, 105, 138, 139, 152, 153
cloning, ix, 9, 60, 61
clustering, 32, 143
clusters, 50, 59
coatings, 107
cobalt, 38, 44
collaboration, 14
collagen, 37, 166, 172
colon, 125, 132
colon cancer, 132
colorectal cancer, 133
complications, 6, 84, 150, 167
compounds, 16, 48, 50, 64, 93, 97
computed tomography (CT), 20, 58, 59, 90, 91, 106, 119, 125, 126, 139, 140, 181
conservation, 43, 146
contamination, 48, 52
contralateral hemisphere, 95, 128
control group, 51, 84, 98, 109, 180, 182, 183, 191
contusion, 96
coronary arteries, 169, 170, 171, 172
coronary artery disease, 137, 153
cortex, 23
cost, 8, 51, 84, 106, 167, 169
creatine, 66, 72
cryopreservation, 8
CSCs, 151
CSF, 103
CT scan, 59
culture, 5, 8, 10, 11, 16, 50, 75, 127
culture conditions, 5
culture medium, 50
cure, 4, 10
current limit, x
CXC, 123
cycles, 51, 170
cyclophosphamide, 6
cytokines, 83, 166
cytoplasm, 48, 60, 144
cytosine, 129
cytotoxicity, 76, 100, 148

D

damages, 118, 129
data collection, 29
decay, 29, 30, 70, 79, 126
decomposition, 29
defects, 6, 184
deficiency, ix, 7, 173
degradation, 37, 79, 151
dendritic cell, 35, 97, 121, 130, 187, 189, 190, 192, 197
deposition, 37, 44, 85, 107, 166, 187
deposits, 27, 62
depth, 20, 58, 59, 125, 126
dermis, 127
descending colon, 35
destruction, 4, 6, 8, 81, 134
detectable, 22, 27, 35, 57, 60, 62, 66, 71, 97, 101, 111, 178
deviation, 107
diabetes, ix, 4, 11, 81, 165, 171, 193
diet, 72, 168, 169, 170, 171, 172, 174, 175, 181
diffusion, 26, 32, 36, 71, 91, 112, 119, 195
dilation, 162
direct chemical labels, x
direct measure, 149
discomfort, 139
discrimination, 42
discs, 84, 86
disease model, 10, 23, 134
disease progression, 133
diseases, ix, 3, 4, 6, 10, 11, 13, 81, 82, 89, 96, 99, 105, 106, 111, 127, 138, 177, 195, 196
dispersion, 36, 97, 98

distribution, 14, 24, 28, 95, 96, 98, 111, 124, 128, 149, 153, 169, 171
DNA, 10, 55, 74, 92, 122, 124, 132, 141, 143
DNA damage, 132
DNA repair, 124
DNA sequencing, 141
dogs, 25, 72
donors, 5, 10, 122
dopamine, 91
dopaminergic, ix, 83
dosage, 106
drug delivery, 54, 134
drug discovery, 10
drug testing, 173
drug therapy, 128
drugs, ix, 94, 122, 169
DWI, 114
dyes, 106

E

EAE, 16, 40, 95, 99, 102
echocardiogram, 151
ECM, 123, 166
ectoderm, 8
edema, 126
EDSS, 195
elastin, 165, 166
electron, 21, 35, 75
electron microscopy, 21
electroporation, 50, 78, 92, 143, 144, 148
emboli, 82, 83, 111
embolization, 82, 83, 111
embryonic stem cells (ESCs), ix, 8, 9, 10, 16, 23, 27, 74, 78, 102, 107, 114, 133, 138, 141, 142, 143, 145, 146, 147, 148, 151, 152, 153, 154, 155, 156, 157, 158
emergency, 97, 191
emission, 47, 58, 90, 91, 106, 119, 125, 139
emulsions, 35, 92
enamel, 4, 7
encephalomyelitis, 23, 40
encoding, 30, 60, 66, 77, 122
endoderm, 8
endothelial cells (ECs), 5, 74, 86, 117, 124, 128, 133, 158, 163, 166, 178, 181
endothelial dysfunction, 165, 174
endothelium, 161, 162, 166, 178
energy, 13, 47
engineering, xi, 14, 90, 137
environment, 8, 9, 10, 14, 59, 83, 139
environmental factors, 171
enzyme(s), 13, 20, 60, 61, 63, 64, 76, 91, 93, 108, 151, 166
epithelia, 12
epithelial cells, 4, 16
epithelium, 16
equilibrium, 69, 78
erosion, 160
ethical issues, 138
ethics, 15
etiology, 174
eukaryotic, 64, 74
eukaryotic cell, 64
Europe, 9, 10
europium, 54
evidence, 3, 6, 11, 13, 22, 23, 63, 89, 98
evolution, 165, 166
examinations, 106
exchange rate, 66
excitation, 30, 146, 148
exocytosis, 44
experimental autoimmune encephalomyelitis, 24, 28, 95
expertise, xi
exposure, 6, 52, 126, 139
extracellular matrix, 123, 160, 166, 168
extrusion, 138

F

fabrication, 137
false positive, 144, 150
family physician, 112
far right, 35
fasting, 193
fat, 9, 32, 34, 168, 170, 171, 185
FDA approval, 48
ferrite, 38
ferritin, 27, 58, 61, 62, 66, 67, 68, 69, 70, 74, 75, 77, 78, 79, 94, 107, 150, 151
fertility, 81, 82
fertilization, 3, 8, 9
fetus, 8
FFT, 32
fiber, 172
fibrin, 173
fibrinogen, 171
fibroblasts, 5, 9, 10, 16, 30, 92, 117, 122, 123, 124, 131, 132, 152
fibrosis, 82, 109, 110, 114, 188, 196
fibrous cap, 166, 167, 168, 169, 171, 172
fidelity, 144
filters, 33, 34
Finland, v

flank, 128
fluid, 127, 154
fluorescence, 20, 22, 27, 38, 46, 47, 53, 54, 58, 90, 91, 106, 113, 119, 125, 127, 139, 143, 145
fluorine, 19, 34, 54, 60, 93, 97, 102
fluorophores, 20, 94, 106, 126
Food and Drug Administration (FDA), 9, 40, 48, 49, 73, 96, 100, 107, 144, 148, 156, 188
formation, 9, 65, 74, 76, 77, 107, 114, 127, 138, 139, 148, 149, 155, 157, 160, 165, 166, 168, 169, 173, 182, 184
fragments, 97, 167
free radicals, 124
functional imaging, 20
functionalization, 35
funding, 8, 14
fusion, 13

G

gadolinium, 20, 21, 38, 46, 54, 59, 60, 64, 71, 76, 93, 95, 113, 126, 129, 174, 175, 188
gene expression, 24, 66, 67, 74, 75, 76, 77, 78, 103, 106, 113, 132, 148, 182
gene promoter, 60
gene regulation, 77
gene therapy, 54, 83, 117, 118, 120, 129, 130, 135, 162, 182, 184, 185
gene transfer, 183, 185
general anesthesia, 162
genes, 9, 10, 13, 58, 60, 62, 65, 89, 90, 94, 97, 118, 119, 122, 128, 148, 151, 168, 182, 183, 197
genetic alteration, 12
genetic disease, ix
genetic factors, 6
genetic mutations, 10
genetic predisposition, 6
genetics, 174
genome, 61, 62, 74, 92, 94, 120, 167, 174
genomics, 82
germ cells, 8, 14
Germany, 46
ginseng, 142
gland, 4, 65, 123
glia, 102
glial cells, 9, 101
glioblastoma, 13, 17, 129, 133, 135
glioma, 32, 42, 52, 66, 74, 92, 96, 123, 127, 128, 130, 131, 132, 134, 135, 189
globus, 84
glomerulus, 23
glucose, 91, 193
gold nanoparticles, 20, 91
growth, 4, 10, 12, 13, 17, 107, 120, 123, 132, 148, 185
growth factor, 123, 132, 185
Guangdong, xiv, xv, xvi, 105
Guangzhou, xiv, xv, xvi, 105
guanine, 91
guidance, 81, 85, 139, 163, 174, 196

H

hair follicle, 4
half-life, 20, 23, 90, 125, 151, 188
harvesting, 4, 11, 170
head and neck cancer, 125
healing, 4, 167
health, xi, 8, 184
health care, xi
heart failure, ix, 4, 11, 137, 138
heart rate, 69
heart transplantation, 22
hematopoietic stem cells, 3, 4
hematopoietic system, 4, 123
hemisphere, 95, 96
hemochromatosis, 28
hemodynamic instability, 171
hemoglobin, 193
hemorrhage, 27, 37, 38, 44, 60, 62, 90, 108, 150, 166, 172, 173, 191
hepatic failure, 113
hepatic injury, 112, 114
hepatitis, 106
hepatocytes, 5, 22, 23, 62, 67, 68, 75, 107, 113
herpes, 66, 91, 189
herpes simplex, 66, 91, 189
heterogeneity, 124
high fat, 172, 174, 175
histocompatibility antigens, 123
histology, 23, 69, 106, 128, 164, 165, 168, 171, 180, 182, 183, 190
HIV, 27, 108, 134, 189
HLA, 5, 10, 16
homeostasis, 77, 78
host, ix, 8, 14, 57, 59, 70, 117, 122
human body, 4, 7, 8, 10, 93, 97, 152, 178
human brain, 134
human cell populations, ix
human condition, 152
human leukocyte antigen, 10
human skin, 128
Hunter, 100, 135
hybrid, 38, 74
hydrocarbons, 93
hydrogels, 71, 101

hydrogen, 59
hydrolysis, 64
hydrophilicity, 107
hydroxyl, 70, 107, 114
hypercholesterolemia, 165, 172, 173, 175
hyperemia, 83
hyperlipidemia, 168, 169, 181
hyperplasia, 160, 161, 162, 163, 164, 174, 178
hypertension, 165
hyperthermia, 126, 141, 154
hypoxia, 110, 132

I

IBD, 35
identical twins, 4
identification, 33, 89, 188
imaging modalities, x, 14, 19, 20, 58, 59, 89, 118, 125, 126, 127, 139, 181
imaging systems, 38, 91, 125
imbalances, 31
immune response, 119, 121
immune system, 6, 117, 121, 122, 179, 181, 190
immunity, 121, 130
immunization, 122
immunocompromised, 149
immunodeficiency, 8
immunofluorescence, 50
immunogenicity, 58, 62, 120, 138
immunoglobulin, 6
immunohistochemistry, 97, 149
immunomodulation, 6, 194
immunomodulatory, 120, 195, 196
immunosuppression, 8, 15, 67, 86, 179
immunosuppressive drugs, 193
immunotherapy, 117, 118, 121, 122, 129, 130, 131
improvements, 82, 146
in vitro, 3, 4, 5, 6, 7, 8, 9, 10, 11, 13, 15, 39, 42, 52, 66, 68, 75, 76, 92, 95, 101, 112, 127, 128, 129, 142, 147, 148, 184, 195
incidence, 117, 122
incubation time, 21, 92, 142, 148
independence, 193
indirect genetic labels, x
indium, 91
individuals, 121
induced pluripotent stem cells, ix, 9, 16, 74, 131, 138
induction, 75, 92, 151, 175, 194
industries, 14
infarction, 6, 26, 37, 84, 146, 151
infection, 141
inflammation, ix, 35, 38, 40, 59, 64, 66, 90, 102, 123, 125, 126, 166, 174
inflammatory cells, 160, 166
infrastructure, 14
inguinal, 192
inhibition, 107, 132
inhibitor, 13, 17
inhomogeneity, 29, 31, 32, 36, 43, 141
initiation, 169
injections, 24, 84, 97, 108, 129, 190
injury(s), ix, xi, 10, 12, 23, 27, 37, 71, 83, 96, 97, 98, 106, 114, 123, 139, 150, 153, 159, 160, 161, 162, 163, 164, 168, 170, 171, 172, 173, 174, 178, 180, 183, 184, 191, 193
inner ear, 123
innominate, 162, 168, 169
insertion, 163
insulin, 193
integration, 10, 16, 61, 82, 89, 99, 107
integrity, 165
intercellular adhesion molecule, 86
interface, 27, 31
interference, 73, 158
interferon, 131
internalization, 21, 26, 92, 108, 141, 142, 143, 150, 189
internalizing, 92
intervention, 85, 118, 122, 178
intestine, 8
intima, 162, 163, 164, 165, 166, 172, 179
intramuscular injection, 83, 138
intravenously, 24, 41, 84, 109, 125, 128, 164, 173, 180, 184, 195
inversion, 31, 43, 156
iodine, 20, 91
ionizing radiation, xi, 20, 106, 107, 125, 126, 140
ions, 63, 75, 188
iPSCs, ix, 138
iris, 162
irradiation, 59, 123, 179, 181
ischemia, ix, 40, 71, 83, 85, 98, 99, 103, 111, 119, 137, 160, 193, 198
Islam, 39
isolation, 121, 156, 193, 197
isomers, 76
Italy, xiii, xiv, xv, 117

J

Japan, 10, 16, 162, 175
Jordan, 39, 40, 42, 43, 53, 54, 72, 73, 74, 99, 100, 101, 102, 155, 156, 196, 197

K

kidney(s), 23, 42, 82, 111, 114, 123, 193
kinetics, 139
knees, 23

L

labeling procedure, 144, 148
laminar, 165, 171
lanthanide, 54, 75
L-arginine, 66
lateral sclerosis, 195
layering, 195
LDL, 165, 168
lead, 13, 36, 90, 92, 97, 106, 107, 119, 124, 132, 160, 188
left hemisphere, 52
left ventricle, 25, 163
legs, 179
lesions, 24, 25, 28, 96, 97, 100, 111, 123, 159, 160, 162, 163, 166, 167, 168, 169, 170, 171, 172, 174, 178, 180, 181, 182, 183, 195
leukemia, 4, 13, 27, 117, 122, 123, 131, 151
leukocytes, 73, 156
liberation, 36
light, 15, 21, 67, 106, 133
lipid metabolism, 168, 169
lipid peroxidation, 107, 114
lipids, 165
lipoproteins, 166
liposomes, 20, 59, 100
liver, ix, x, 23, 27, 28, 39, 42, 78, 79, 82, 92, 100, 105, 106, 107, 109, 110, 111, 112, 113, 114, 115, 188, 193
liver cirrhosis, 82, 106, 113
liver disease, 105, 106, 111, 112
liver failure, 106, 112
liver transplant, 106
liver transplantation, 106
localization, 10, 54, 70, 143, 149, 151, 154
logistics, 14
longevity, 196
longitudinal study, 95
long-term retention, 188
low-density lipoprotein, 168
luciferase, 20, 91, 113, 127, 141, 146, 151
luciferin, 91
lumbar puncture, 97, 191, 197
lumen, 161, 167
lung cancer, 132, 133
lung metastases, 127, 131
Luo, 114
lymph, 6, 23, 35, 40, 92, 188, 190, 192, 195, 196
lymph node, 23, 35, 92, 188, 190, 192, 195, 196
lymphocytes, 6, 27, 117, 124, 155
lymphoma, 4, 11
lysine, 22, 23, 48, 49, 66, 94, 108, 142, 189, 195
lysis, 36
lysosome, 107

M

macromolecules, 66, 92
macrophages, 21, 23, 36, 57, 59, 70, 78, 92, 93, 108, 139, 149, 150, 163, 165, 166, 169, 185, 189, 190
macular degeneration, 4, 9, 10, 11, 15
magnetic field(s), 21, 23, 26, 28, 30, 32, 42, 43, 65, 109, 126, 140, 141
magnetic moment, 21, 26
magnetic particles, 39, 73, 97, 100, 142, 155
magnetic properties, 21
magnetic resonance image, 192
magnetic resonance spectroscopy, 64, 66, 99
magnetic structure, 65
magnetization, 32, 47, 69, 76, 141
malignancy, 8, 122
malignant cells, 13
mammalian cells, 16, 40, 41, 42, 65, 77, 100
mammals, ixmanagement, 182, 184
manganese, 59, 60, 62, 71, 72, 75, 93, 101, 113, 140, 197
manipulation, 13, 15, 167, 168, 170
mapping, 32, 42, 72, 77, 124, 156, 184
marrow, 5, 14, 27, 40, 84, 86, 97, 109, 122, 123, 131, 132, 153, 163, 164, 173, 178, 195, 198
Maryland, xiii, xv, 89, 162
mass, 8, 9, 12, 26, 52, 63, 120, 123, 124, 126, 138, 146
materials, 106, 119
matrix metalloproteinase, 166
MCP, 123
measurement(s), x, 26, 69, 70, 77, 79, 112, 126, 183
media, 20, 38, 140, 162, 164, 166, 172, 184
medical, ix, xi, 3, 54, 85, 114
medicine, ix, xi, 16, 38, 45, 57, 106, 112, 113, 118, 138, 177, 178, 182, 184
medulla, 23, 35
melanin, 63, 64, 75, 76, 77
melanoma, 63, 75, 76, 122, 123, 190, 197
membrane permeability, 189
membranes, 8, 48, 59, 61
meninges, 195
mesenchymal stem cells, 5, 6, 21, 23, 28, 41, 42, 44, 49, 50, 74, 75, 84, 85, 86, 99, 103, 106, 107, 112,

113, 114, 120, 123, 127, 131, 132, 134, 135, 138, 142, 152, 153, 154, 157, 158, 184, 195, 197, 198
mesoderm, 8
metabolic, 73
metabolic changes, 143
metabolism, 21, 66, 72, 74, 100, 106, 111, 126, 155, 168
metal ion(s), 63
metals, 49, 66, 75
metastasis, 23, 118, 124, 132
methodology, 138, 151
methylation, 10
MHC, 121
Miami, 42
mice, 8, 14, 23, 24, 25, 27, 28, 41, 49, 52, 64, 67, 68, 69, 72, 78, 95, 96, 101, 102, 113, 123, 127, 128, 129, 147, 148, 151, 157, 160, 162, 163, 167, 168, 169, 170, 173, 178, 179, 181, 182, 183, 184, 185, 193
microorganisms, 77
microparticles, 143
microRNA, 173
microscopy, 22, 27, 41, 46, 54, 75, 94, 95, 99, 129, 135, 139, 143, 145
miniature, 171
mitosis, 127
models, ix, 9, 13, 24, 25, 26, 66, 71, 85, 89, 99, 109, 123, 127, 159, 160, 162, 164, 168, 169, 170, 171, 172, 173, 195
modifications, 93, 193
molecular biology, 14, 64, 68, 92
molecules, 20, 36, 59, 66, 76, 92, 93, 94, 166
monoclonal antibody, 113, 141, 155, 189, 191
monolayer, 46, 48
Montana, 162
Moon, 77, 131
morbidity, 138
morphology, 52, 137
mortality, 6, 138, 160
mRNA, 65, 91, 102, 119
mucin, 12
mucosa, 4, 12
multicellular organisms, 3, 4
multiple myeloma, 4
multiple sclerosis, 9, 16, 41, 86, 95, 96, 114, 187, 195, 198
multipotent, 3, 4, 5, 6, 7, 11, 120, 153
muscular dystrophy, 72
mutagenesis, 61
mutant, 17, 55
mutation(s), 12, 13, 17, 119, 124
myelin, 24
myocardial infarction, 4, 6, 10, 11, 15, 24, 26, 36, 37, 41, 72, 86, 134, 137, 138, 140, 145, 152, 153, 154, 158, 160, 166, 169, 170, 178, 185, 197
myocardial ischemia, 85
myocardium, 25, 36, 37, 68, 71, 72, 138, 142, 145, 150, 151, 153, 155, 156, 158
myofibroblasts, 132

N

nanomedicine, 54
nanometer, 21
nanometers, 46, 127
nanoparticles, 21, 35, 37, 41, 42, 43, 44, 46, 47, 48, 59, 60, 65, 72, 77, 92, 97, 99, 100, 103, 108, 113, 114, 118, 120, 127, 128, 129, 134, 135, 137, 154, 155, 156, 188, 189, 191, 198
nanotechnology(s), 82, 154
National Academy of Sciences, 102, 113
National Institutes of Health, 11, 45, 137, 159, 177
natural killer cell, 131
neck cancer, 133
necrosis, 63, 111
necrotic core, 166, 167, 172
neoangiogenesis, 166
neovascularization, 83, 166
nephritis, 40
nephropathy, 40
nephrotic syndrome, 40
nerve, 9, 195
nerve fibers, 9
nervous system, 23, 194
neuroblastoma, 66
neurodegenerative disorders, 99
neurogenesis, 107, 194
neurological disability, 195
neurological disease, 89, 96, 97, 195
neuronal stem cells, 127
neurons, ix, 6, 198
neuroprotection, 86
neuroprotective agents, 194
neurosurgery, 97
neurotransmitters, 92
neutral, 107
New Zealand, 134, 169, 170
NK cells, 121, 122, 130
NMR, 39, 40, 41, 43, 44, 53, 54, 55, 64, 73, 74, 75, 76, 78, 79, 101, 114, 155, 156, 157, 173, 184, 196
nodes, 190, 192
nodules, 167
NPC, 78, 92
nuclear magnetic resonance, 95
nuclei, 59, 93, 182

nucleic acid, 92, 93, 94, 154
nucleus, 9, 13, 25, 93
nutrient(s), 13, 83, 139

O

Obama, 8
obstruction, 161
occlusion, 172
oncogenes, 10
one dimension, 140
oocyte, 9
optimization, x, 29, 55, 89, 90, 105
organ(s), ix, xi, 3, 4, 5, 11, 13, 14, 23, 38, 39, 45, 57, 59, 82, 83, 90, 106, 111, 123, 138, 141, 146, 152, 160, 184, 187, 188
organelles, 143
organism, 3, 67, 138, 139
osteoarthritis, ix
ovarian cancer, 13
oxidation, 63
oxidative damage, 77, 78
oxidative stress, 77, 92
oxide nanoparticles, 39, 43, 44, 55, 59, 73, 91, 92, 93, 94, 97, 100, 101, 102, 107, 113, 119, 126, 127, 129, 137, 153, 154, 157, 188, 197
oxygen, 75, 83, 101, 107, 139
oxygen consumption, 75

P

pain, 83
pancreas, 35, 82, 84
pancreas transplant, 84
pancreatic beta-cells, ix
pancreatic cancer, 13
paracrine pathways, x
paradigm shift, 13
paralysis, 4
parenchyma, 24, 111, 127, 195
Parkinson disease, ix, 81, 84, 86
pathogenesis, 159, 173, 184
pathology, xi, 42, 59, 96, 161, 195
pathophysiological, 160, 172
pathophysiology, 26, 160
pathways, x, 21, 62, 93, 168
PCR, 148
peptide(s), 27, 41, 71, 99, 114, 128, 134, 135, 146, 154, 155, 174, 189, 193, 197
perfusion, 72, 82, 162
pericytes, 148
peripheral blood, 4, 5, 6
peripheral nervous system, 102
peripheral vascular disease, 137
permeability, 49, 50, 165
permit, 188
PET, 20, 38, 58, 59, 64, 76, 90, 91, 106, 113, 119, 125, 126, 129, 133, 139, 140, 146, 149, 151, 154, 174, 189
PET scan, 189
pH, 66, 71, 101, 188
phagocytic cells, 23, 35, 92, 107, 126, 189
phagocytosis, 35, 119
pharmaceuticals, 14
pharmacokinetics, 23, 39
phenotype(s), 23, 39, 61, 97, 120, 124, 148, 166, 168
Philadelphia, xv
phosphate, 47, 164
phospholipids, 150
photobleaching, 20
physical characteristics, 82
physical therapy, 51
physicochemical characteristics, 23, 39
physicochemical properties, 137, 140
physiology, 81, 114, 170, 185
pigs, 25, 36, 140, 161, 163, 171, 173, 179
placenta, 8
plants, 4, 63, 77
plaque, 78, 159, 160, 166, 167, 168, 169, 170, 171, 178, 182, 183
plasmid, 64, 69, 154
plasmid DNA, 154
plasticity, 12, 16, 17
platform, 50, 103, 196
polarization, 59
polymer(s), 21, 35, 107, 189, 195
polymorphisms, 15
polysaccharide, 107
polystyrene, 21
population, ix, 10, 17, 122, 124, 125, 132, 153, 169
porosity, 143
portal vein, 28, 82, 84, 111
positron, 58, 63, 64, 90, 91, 106, 119, 125, 139
positron emission tomography, 58, 63, 64, 90, 91, 106, 119, 125, 139
post-transplant, 36, 95, 97, 98, 111, 147, 151
potential benefits, 85
precursor cells, 4, 23, 24, 28, 103, 191
pregnancy, 8
prevention, 118, 123, 159
primary cells, 144
primary tumor, 124, 125
probe, 64, 66, 75, 77, 91, 103, 113
progenitor cells, 5, 7, 23, 27, 41, 52, 54, 84, 92, 93, 99, 100, 127, 128, 129, 132, 134, 135, 138, 143,

149, 151, 153, 154, 160, 164, 165, 173, 178, 179, 181, 182, 183, 184
prognosis, 118, 124, 125, 190
programming, 13, 146
prokaryotes, 77
proliferation, ix, 3, 4, 20, 21, 36, 37, 44, 49, 52, 60, 90, 97, 107, 118, 127, 132, 138, 145, 148, 150, 151, 152, 160, 161, 166, 178, 191, 195, 198
promoter, 61, 91, 94, 119
propagation, 124
prostate cancer, 40, 130, 132, 133
proteins, 13, 60, 61, 66, 71, 91, 94, 119, 120, 123, 160, 166
proteoglycans, 166, 167
proteomics, 82
protons, 27, 30, 31, 32, 34, 46, 47, 66, 109
prototype, 76
public policy, 8
purification, 10, 154

Q

quality of life, 13, 14, 123
quantification, 26, 27, 28, 29, 32, 34, 38, 39, 41, 42, 124, 139, 146, 149, 157
quantum dot(s), 91
quantum yields, 75

R

radiation, 12, 32, 54, 90, 117, 122, 123, 124, 126, 131, 132, 140
radiation therapy, 117, 122
radical formation, 70
radical reactions, 107
radicals, 107, 114
radioactive isotopes, 126
radiopaque, 101
radioresistance, 132
radiotherapy, 118, 123, 124, 133, 196
reactions, 107, 131, 144, 163
reactive oxygen, 21, 166
reagents, 48, 49, 59, 92, 101
receptors, 73, 91, 93, 184
reconstruction, 32, 96
recovery, 24, 41, 43, 72, 84, 86, 99, 103, 146, 154, 156
recurrence, 125, 193
recycling, 93
red blood cells, 166
redistribution, 70, 110
regenerate, 152, 187
regeneration, ix, x, 4, 7, 11, 15, 17, 45, 57, 82, 84, 149, 153, 154
regenerative medicine, ix, xi, 9, 13, 19, 71, 89, 95, 113, 138, 153, 162, 177
regression, 133, 135, 173
regulatory agencies, 14, 144
rejection, 7, 8, 9, 10, 11, 22, 23, 39, 40, 90, 97, 99, 110, 179, 183, 193, 198
relaxation, 21, 26, 28, 29, 34, 46, 47, 65, 68, 75, 78, 93, 105, 109, 140, 141, 148, 188
relaxation rate, 26, 28, 29, 66, 68, 75, 78
relaxation times, 21, 46, 68, 105, 109
remission, 122, 152
repair, x, xi, 4, 6, 11, 12, 38, 45, 84, 112, 113, 122, 123, 152, 160, 162, 163, 164, 177, 178, 184
replication, 7
reporters, 58, 60, 61, 95
reproductive age, 9
reprogramming adult cells, ix
resection, 129
resistance, 124, 132, 133
resolution, x, xi, 20, 22, 27, 28, 29, 30, 41, 42, 46, 59, 72, 90, 95, 96, 106, 125, 126, 127, 129, 134, 139, 140, 142, 146, 151, 175, 188, 190
resources, 14
response, ix, 33, 62, 117, 121, 122, 123, 124, 127, 132, 134, 172, 190, 196
restenosis, 160, 172, 178
restoration, ix, 140, 145, 151, 154
restrictions, 61, 62
retina, 9, 10
retinitis, 4, 10, 11
retinitis pigmentosa, 4, 10, 11
retrovirus, 9, 10
right hemisphere, 52, 96
right ventricle, 25, 98, 145, 163
rings, 181
risk(s), xi, 7, 8, 9, 52, 62, 83, 92, 106, 108, 111, 125, 178
RNA, 92
rodents, 22, 86, 160
root(s), ix, 162, 168, 169, 177, 195
routes, 84, 90, 111

S

safety, 52, 57, 58, 83, 85, 90, 93, 95, 96, 98, 101, 120, 137, 138, 139, 148, 152, 153, 192, 195, 196
salivary gland(s), 123, 131
salts, 107, 114
saturation, 31, 32, 43, 47, 54, 58, 66, 71, 77, 93, 94, 103
scar tissue, ix, 10

sclerosis, 195
secretion, 166
sensing, 42, 71, 101
sensitivity, 20, 26, 27, 29, 30, 34, 38, 44, 46, 47, 66, 78, 92, 93, 95, 97, 106, 109, 125, 126, 127, 132, 140, 188
septum, 145
serine, 91
serum, 132, 193
shear, 165, 168, 171
shock, 49
showing, 9, 24, 25, 48, 51, 76, 97, 98, 117, 122, 147, 168, 179, 180, 181, 192
side effects, 90
signal transduction, 133
signaling pathway, 17
signals, 28, 33, 59, 60, 62, 66, 71, 97, 108, 111, 124, 129, 144, 149, 151, 164, 182, 191, 195
signal-to-noise ratio, 27, 30, 93, 110, 146, 147
silica, 113, 156
silk, 162
Sinai, xiii, xiv, 19
skeletal muscle, 8, 33
skin, 4, 7, 8, 9, 10, 123, 127, 134, 161, 162
smoking, 165
smooth muscle, 157, 160, 161, 162, 163, 164, 165, 166, 171, 178
smooth muscle cells, 157, 160, 161, 162, 163, 164, 165, 166, 171, 178
sodium, 91, 143, 149, 172
solid tumors, 13
solution, 97, 142
somatic cell, 3, 9, 10, 16, 120, 122
specialists, 61, 172
species, 21, 166, 167
spectroscopy, 42, 72, 75
spin, 25, 27, 29, 30, 31, 34, 36, 43, 69, 75, 78, 116
spinal cord, ix, 4, 9, 10, 11, 96, 97, 102, 103, 157, 187, 191, 195, 197
spinal cord injury, ix, 4, 9, 10, 11, 96, 97, 103, 187, 191, 197
spindle, 168
spleen, ix, 14
Sprague-Dawley rats, 150
stability, 102, 152
stabilization, 162, 189
stable complexes, 142
standardization, 14
starvation, 132
state(s), 27, 33, 43, 62, 64, 86, 112, 141, 146, 156, 166
stem cell differentiation, 61, 106
stem cell lines, 8, 14, 16
stem cell therapies, x, 45, 53, 84, 106, 123, 138, 139, 140, 145, 152, 163
stem cell transplants, ix
stenosis, 160
stent, 178, 181
stimulation, 190, 194
storage, 61, 67, 70, 79, 107, 150
stratification, 118
stress, 165, 171
stroke, ix, 37, 41, 54, 84, 86, 90, 95, 96, 101, 102, 103, 160, 166, 178, 184, 188, 195, 196
stroma, 117, 123, 124, 132, 148
stromal cells, 15, 27, 42, 73, 100, 127, 132, 134, 157, 198
structure, 47, 48, 57, 77, 169
style, 162
substrate, 64, 81, 167
subtraction, 181
suicide, 120, 129
sulfate, 20, 23, 48, 54, 73, 75, 108, 127, 128, 142, 148, 155, 189, 197
Sun, xvi, 102, 105, 132, 154, 157, 174, 185
superimposition, 171
superparamagnetic, 21, 32, 36, 39, 40, 41, 42, 43, 44, 46, 53, 55, 59, 62, 66, 73, 75, 79, 91, 92, 100, 102, 107, 114, 119, 126, 127, 129, 131, 134, 135, 137, 139, 141, 154, 155, 156, 157, 158, 164, 178, 188, 196, 197
supplementation, 66, 70, 78
suppression, 8, 43, 69, 78, 146, 156, 195
surface modification, 154
survival, xi, 6, 13, 14, 44, 46, 58, 73, 83, 90, 112, 118, 127, 128, 133, 137, 139, 149, 151, 154, 155, 158, 163, 188, 189
susceptibility, 21, 26, 27, 29, 32, 42, 105, 109, 110, 140, 146, 160, 171, 188
suspensions, 117, 122
symptoms, 84
syndrome, 160, 172
synthesis, 64, 76, 134
systemic lupus erythematosus, 15, 152

T

T cell(s), 6, 35, 121, 122, 130, 134, 189, 190
T lymphocytes, 121
T2 contrast agents, 46
target, ix, 35, 46, 47, 53, 59, 61, 81, 82, 84, 85, 90, 92, 94, 108, 109, 110, 112, 121, 128, 137, 138, 139, 141, 142, 145, 146, 150, 152, 161, 162, 168, 178, 187, 188, 189, 190, 196
target organs, 190
Task Force, 82, 86

technetium, 91
techniques, xi, 22, 26, 27, 28, 29, 30, 31, 32, 36, 38, 43, 45, 46, 53, 58, 59, 61, 64, 66, 82, 83, 92, 95, 100, 106, 108, 112, 118, 125, 127, 129, 137, 139, 141, 144, 146, 152, 159, 160, 162, 172, 177, 178, 180, 184, 187, 196
technology(s), x, xi, 10, 11, 13, 19, 46, 82, 90, 106, 129, 137, 139, 141, 178
territory, 81, 82, 96
testing, 42, 76, 95, 148
therapeutic agents, 81, 85, 154
therapeutic approaches, 139
therapeutic benefits, 111
therapeutic effects, 111
therapeutic use, 129
therapeutics, ix, x, 15, 58, 81, 82, 178, 198
thrombosis, 84, 160, 169, 173, 184
thrombus, 166, 167
tissue, ix, x, 3, 4, 5, 7, 11, 12, 13, 14, 17, 20, 26, 27, 28, 34, 37, 38, 40, 46, 57, 59, 70, 71, 79, 81, 83, 85, 90, 103, 106, 107, 112, 118, 123, 124, 125, 126, 129, 131, 139, 140, 146, 151, 160, 166, 178, 187, 188, 189, 191, 195
tissue homeostasis, 123
tissue perfusion, 59
toxic effect, 70
toxic substances, 63
toxicity, x, 10, 21, 49, 60, 62, 77, 85, 92, 97, 100, 120, 193
trafficking, 35, 42, 53, 82, 83, 85, 95, 96, 129, 135, 178, 185
trajectory, 98
transcatheter, 82
transcription, 3, 9, 61, 119
transcription factors, 9
transducer, 51
transduction, 90, 108, 122
transection, 96
transfection, 10, 23, 39, 41, 48, 49, 53, 55, 59, 60, 61, 62, 73, 76, 90, 91, 92, 100, 102, 108, 128, 134, 137, 141, 142, 143, 144, 148, 154, 155, 156, 189, 190, 196
transferrin, 61, 62, 74, 75, 78, 189
transformation, 61, 62, 146, 166
transgene, 10, 77, 78, 102, 103
translation, xi, 53, 71, 89, 91, 119, 160, 177
translocation, 13
transmission electron microscopy (TEM), 47
transplant, ix, 6, 40, 46, 72, 133, 152, 193, 194
transport, 62, 74, 91, 101, 140, 178
trauma, 97, 172, 191, 195, 197
traumatic brain injury, 97, 187, 191
treatment, 3, 4, 6, 7, 9, 12, 13, 14, 15, 16, 17, 51, 82, 86, 105, 106, 118, 123, 124, 127, 129, 130, 131, 133, 137, 138, 141, 145, 151, 152, 153, 159, 178, 181, 182, 185, 188, 196
trial, 9, 10, 15, 16, 84, 85, 86, 139, 153
tricarboxylic acid cycle, 91
tropism, 123, 127, 131
tumor(s), 10, 12, 13, 16, 23, 27, 32, 35, 42, 62, 63, 64, 66, 68, 74, 76, 77, 78, 82, 85, 95, 113, 117, 118, 119, 120, 121, 123, 124, 125, 126, 127, 128, 129, 130, 131, 132, 133, 134, 135, 138
tumor cells, 66, 68, 76, 117, 120, 121, 124, 125, 129, 132, 133
tumour growth, 17, 132
turnover, 43, 73, 149, 157, 197
type 1 diabetes, 86, 187, 193
tyrosine, 63

U

ultrasound, 50, 51, 52, 53, 55, 58, 91, 125, 126, 134, 139, 140, 144, 162, 163, 181, 185
umbilical cord, 4, 5, 84, 98
unique features, 90
United States (USA), v, x, xiii, xiv, xv, xvi, 14, 39, 41, 44, 54, 57, 72, 74, 102, 137, 159, 161, 162, 197

V

vaccine, 35, 190
valence, 62
validation, 33, 37, 39, 44, 92, 128, 144, 163, 184
valve, 137, 138, 145, 152
variations, 34, 146
vascular biology, x, 184
vascular cell adhesion molecule (VCAM), 166
vascular diseases, 159, 163, 177, 178
vascular endothelial growth factor (VEGF), 123
vasculature, 81, 82, 126, 159, 177, 178
vasospasm, 170
vector, 32, 61, 66, 69, 77, 119, 128, 151, 185
vehicles, 15, 117, 120, 128, 131, 132
vein, 82, 111, 180
ventricle, 98, 145
vessels, 163, 169, 172, 177, 178
victims, 7
viral gene, 60, 61
viral infection, 10
viral vectors, 62, 69, 78, 94, 119, 120
viruses, 120
vision, 4, 82, 86

visualization, 20, 33, 38, 40, 43, 46, 59, 76, 79, 108, 126, 128, 129, 134, 156, 178, 182, 193
vitamin A, 13
VLDL, 168

W

Washington, x, xiii, xiv, xv, xvi, 3, 45, 57, 81, 159, 177, 187
water, 30, 31, 36, 43, 47, 59, 65, 66, 102, 146, 156
water diffusion, 59
white blood cells, 13
white matter, 24, 95
Wisconsin, 8

X

xenografts, 127, 135

Y

yield, 126, 146, 172

Z

zinc, 61, 74